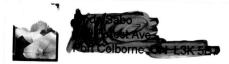
Living a Healthy Life with Chronic Conditions

For Ongoing Physical and Mental Health Conditions

Canadian Third Edition

Kate Lorig, RN. DrPH, Halsted Holman, MD
David Sobel, MD, Diana Laurent, MPH
Virginia González, MPH, and
Marian Minor, RPT, PhD

Canadian content added by
Patrick McGowan, PhD, University of Victoria, Centre on Aging
and Trude LaBossiere Huebner, Cert. T.

Contributor: Peg Harrison, MA, MSW, LCSW

BULL PUBLISHING COMPANY
BOULDER, COLORADO

Copyright © 2007 Bull Publishing Company

Bull Publishing Company
P.O. Box 1377
Boulder, CO 80306
Phone (800) 676-2855 Fax (303) 545-6354

ISBN: 978-1-933503-08-0

Printed in the United States. All rights reserved.
October 2010 Printing

Supported by AHCPR Grant HSO 6680 and California State Tobacco-Related Disease Research Program
Award 1RT 156

Publisher: James Bull
Cover Design: Lightbourne Images
Interior Design and Composition: Shadow Canyon Graphics
Illustrations, Editing, and Proofreading: Publication Services
Index: Emily Plant Sewell
Chapter-opening Illustration: Catherine Mulligan

Note: Information about medications for chronic conditions is provided throughout this text. However, because research about medications is changing rapidly, we suggest that you consult your physician, pharmacist, and/or a recent drug reference book for the latest information.

For additional copies of this book and for copies of the audio relaxation recording
Time for Healing, please call our sales department at 800-676-2855.
Quantity discounts are available for orders of 10 copies or more; call for details.

Bull Publishing Company, P.O. Box 1377, Boulder, CO 80306
800-676-2855 • 303-545-6350 • 303-545-6354 (fax)
www.bullpub.com

To David Bull,
who made this book possible

TABLE OF CONTENTS

ACKNOWLEDGMENTS

The Canadian edition provides contact information to locate resources throughout Canada for the self-management of chronic conditions. Thank you to Helena Bryan for her contributions to Chapter 13: Healthy Eating. Many thanks to Lynne Hussey, for her invaluable research and editing skills throughout the text. Melanie Galloway, Clinical Exercise Instructor, deserves special mention for her dedication to getting people moving, both in water and in the gym. Beth Morrison, Librarian, BC Cancer Agency, helped with the books list. Thanks also to the Heart and Stroke Foundation, Arthritis Society, Canadian Diabetes Association, and Lung Association for sharing your resources with us.

Patrick McGowan, Ph.D.,
Associate Professor, Centre on Aging,
University of Victoria, British Columbia

Trude LaBossiere Huebner, Cert.T.,
Researcher/Writer,
Vancouver, British Columbia

EDITOR'S NOTES

With the publication of the Canadian Diabetes Association 2008 Clinical Practice Guidelines, and the updating of Health Canada's website and the Healthy Eating Guide, a revision of the chapters on Diabetes and Healthy Eating became necessary.

Most clinical and nutrition updates are included to match as closely as possible the handouts from both the Canadian Diabetes Association and Health Canada. You will notice a few omissions; these will be included in the next edition of the textbook. The omissions are for purely technical reasons; we are working on updated charts and tables. Fortunately, they are currently available as handouts from the Canadian Diabetes Association. We appreciate your patience as we strive to be as current as possible, while recognizing printed information is outdated before the ink is dry!

We appreciate the contribution made by Doreen Hatton, RN, BSN, MSN. Doreen is a certified diabetes educator, and bravely took on providing the updated content for both chapters. As a former Clinical Nurse Specialist, Diabetes Program, Children's Hospital (Vancouver, BC) and current Adjunct Professor, School of Nursing, UBC, Doreen has vast clinical experience with diabetes and has contributed to many professional publications. Thank you, Doreen!

This update was initiated by the University of Victoria, Centre on Aging. Please direct all comments to:

Patrick McGowan, Ph.D., Associate Professor
Centre on Aging
University of Victoria, British Columbia
604 940 3574
mcgowan@dccnet.com

Trude LaBossiere Huebner
Vancouver, BC. Canada

OVERVIEW OF SELF-MANAGEMENT

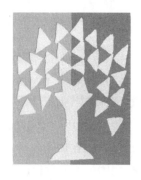

1

NOBODY WANTS TO HAVE A CHRONIC LONG-TERM ILLNESS. Unfortunately, most of us will experience two or more of these conditions during our lives. This book has been written to teach people with chronic illness a healthy way to live with a disease. This may seem like a strange concept. How can one have an illness and live a healthy life at the same time? To answer this, we need to look at the consequences of most chronic diseases. These diseases, be they heart disease, diabetes, liver disease, emphysema, or any one of a host of others, cause most people to lose physical conditioning and experience fatigue. In addition, they may cause emotional distress such as frustration, anger, depression, or a sense of helplessness. Health is soundness of body and mind, and a healthy life is one that seeks that soundness. Therefore, a healthy way to live with a chronic illness is to work at overcoming the physical and emotional problems caused by the disease. The goal is to achieve the greatest possible physical capability and pleasure from life. That is what this book is all about.

You will not find any miracles or cures in these pages. Rather, you will find hundreds of tips and ideas to make your life easier. This advice comes from physicians and other health professionals, and, most important, people like you who have learned to positively manage their illness. Please note that we said "*positively manage*." You see, there is no way you can avoid managing a chronic condition. If you do nothing but suffer, this is a management style. If you only take medication, this is another management style. If you choose to be a positive self-manager and undergo all the best treatments that health care professionals have to offer along with being proactive in your day-to-day management, this will lead you to live a healthy life.

In this chapter, we discuss chronic illness in general as well as point out the most common problems. In addition, we give some guidance on the self-management skills that are unique to particular conditions. You will soon see that the problems and skills have much more in common than you might think. The rest of the book deals with the details you will need in order to master many of the self-management skills.

CHRONIC DISEASE

We think of a health problem as being either "acute" or "chronic." Acute health problems usually begin suddenly; have a single, easily diagnosed cause; are of short duration; and will respond to a specific treatment, such as medication or surgery. For most acute illnesses, a cure with a return to normal health is to be expected. For the patient and the doctor there is relatively little uncertainty; one usually knows what to expect. The illness typically has a cycle of getting worse for a while, being treated, and then getting better. Finally, the care of acute illness depends on a health professional's knowledge and experience in finding and administering the correct treatment.

Appendicitis is an example of an acute illness. It typically begins rapidly, signalled by nausea and pain in the abdomen. The diagnosis of appendicitis, established by physical examination, leads to surgery for removal of the inflamed appendix. There follows a period of recovery and then a return to normal health.

Chronic illnesses are different. They begin slowly and proceed slowly. For example, a person with long-term arteriosclerosis might have a heart attack or a stroke. Arthritis generally starts with brief annoying twinges that gradually increase. Unlike acute disease, chronic illnesses have multiple causes that vary over time and include heredity, lifestyle factors (smoking, lack of exercise, poor diet, stress, etc.), exposure to environmental factors, and physiological factors.

This can be frustrating for those of us who want quick answers. It is difficult for the doctor and the patient when immediate answers aren't available. In some cases, even when diagnosis is rapid, as in the case of a stroke or heart attack, the long-term effects may be hard to predict. The lack of a regular or predictable pattern is a major characteristic of most chronic illnesses.

Unlike acute disease, where full recovery is expected, chronic illness usually leads to more symptoms and loss of physical functioning. Many people assume that the symptoms they are experiencing are due to only one cause: the disease. While the disease can certainly cause pain, shortness of breath, fatigue, etc., it is not the only cause. Each of these symptoms can by itself contribute to the other symptoms, and all can make each one worse. Even more difficult, these symptoms can feed on each other. For example, depression causes fatigue, stress causes tense muscles, and these can lead to more pain or shortness of breath, and so on. The interactions of these symptoms, in turn, make our disease/condition worse. It becomes a *vicious cycle* that only gets worse unless we find a way to break the cycle (see Figure 1.1).

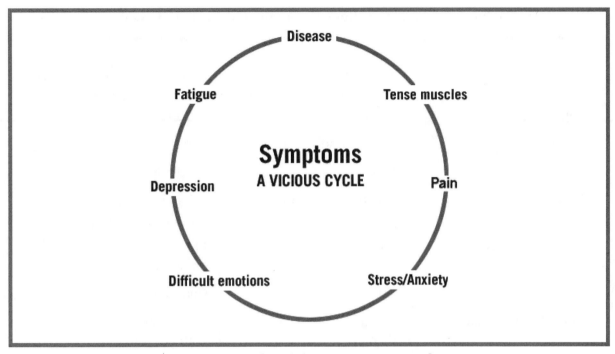

Figure 1.1 **The Vicious Symptom Cycle**

Throughout this book we examine ways of breaking the cycle and getting away from the problems of physical and emotional helplessness which can result from chronic illness.

WHAT CAUSES A CHRONIC DISEASE?

To answer this question, we need to understand how the body operates. As you know, cells are the building blocks of tissues and organs: the heart, lungs, brain, blood, blood vessels, bones, muscles—in fact, everything in the body. For a cell to remain alive and function normally, three things must happen: It must be nourished, receive oxygen, and get rid of waste products. If anything goes wrong with any of these three functions, the cell becomes diseased. If cells are diseased, the organ or tissue suffers, which you may experience as limitations in your ability to be active in daily life. The difference in chronic diseases depends on which cells and organs are affected and the processes by which the effect occurs. For example, in a stroke, a blood vessel in the brain becomes blocked or breaks. Oxygen and nutrition are cut off from part of the brain, and, as a result, the part of your body controlled by the damaged brain cells, such as an arm or a leg or a portion of the face, loses function.

Table 1.1 **Differences Between Acute and Chronic Disease**

	Acute Disease	Chronic Disease (long-term)
Beginning	Rapid	Gradual
Cause	Usually one	Many
Duration	Short	Indefinite
Diagnosis	Commonly accurate	Often uncertain, especially early on
Diagnostic Tests	Often decisive	Often of limited value
Treatment	Cure common	Cure rare
Role of Professional	Select and conduct therapy	Teacher and partner
Role of Patient	Follow orders	Partner of health professionals, responsible for daily management

If you have heart disease, several things might happen. For instance, heart attacks occur when the vessels supplying blood to the heart muscle become blocked. This is called a coronary thrombosis. When this happens, oxygen is cut off, the heart muscle is injured, and pain results. After the injury the heart may be less effective in supplying the rest of your body with oxygen-carrying blood. Because the heart is pumping blood less efficiently through the body, fluid accumulates in tissues, and one experiences shortness of breath.

With bronchitis, asthma, and emphysema, there is either a problem getting oxygen to the lungs, as with bronchitis or asthma, or the lungs cannot effectively transfer oxygen to the blood, as with emphysema. In both cases the body is deprived of oxygen. In diabetes, the pancreas does not produce enough insulin or produces insulin that cannot be used efficiently by the body. Without this insulin the body's cells are not able to use the glucose (sugar) in the blood for energy. In liver and kidney disease, the cells of these organs do not work properly, making it difficult for the body to get rid of waste products.

The basic consequences of these diseases are similar: loss of function due to a reduction in oxygen, accumulation of waste products, or inability of the body to utilize glucose for energy. Loss of function also occurs in arthritis, but for other reasons. In osteoarthritis, cartilage (the tough material found on the ends of bones and as the "disks" between the vertebrae of the back) becomes worn, frayed, or displaced, causing pain. We do not know exactly why the cartilage cells begin to weaken or die. But the results are pain and disability.

So far, you can see that all chronic illness starts at a cellular level. But an illness is more than cellular malfunction. It also involves the problems of everyday life, which may include not doing the things you want to do and needing to change your social activities. However, until you observe symptoms (shortness of breath, fatigue, pain, etc.) you won't know you have a disease.

Although the biological causes of chronic diseases differ, the problems they cause for people are similar. For example, most people with chronic disease suffer fatigue and loss of energy. Sleeping problems are not uncommon. In one case there is pain, while in another case there is trouble breathing. Disability, to some extent, is a part of chronic disease. It may be the inability to use your hands well because of arthritis or stroke, or difficulty in walking due to shortness of breath, stroke, arthritis, or diabetes. Sometimes disability is caused by a lack of energy or extreme fatigue.

Another common problem with chronic illness is depression, or just "feeling blue." It is hard to have a cheerful disposition when your condition causes problems that probably won't go away. Along with the depression come fear and concern for the future. Will I be able to remain independent? If I can't care for myself, who will care for me? What will happen to my family? Will I get worse? Disability and depression bring loss of self-esteem.

One of the most important things to learn is that there are similarities among chronic illnesses. Thus, the central management tasks and skills one must learn in order to live with different chronic illnesses are also similar. Besides overcoming physical and emotional problems, you must learn problem-solving skills and how to respond to the trends in your disease. These tasks and skills include developing and maintaining exercise and nutrition programs, managing symptoms, making decisions about when to seek medical help, working effectively with your doctor, using medications and minimizing side effects, finding and using community resources, talking about your illness with family and friends, and, if necessary, changing social activities. Maybe the most important skill of all is learning to respond to your illness on an ongoing basis to solve day-to-day problems as they arise. After all, you live with your condition 24 hours a day. Your health care provider sees you only a small portion of this time. Thus you must manage your condition. Chart 1.1 illustrates some of the self-management problems for common chronic conditions.

Chart 1.1 **Self-Management Problems for Common Chronic Conditions**

Chronic Condition	POSSIBLE PROBLEMS CAUSED BY CHRONIC CONDITIONS				
	Pain	Fatigue	Shortness of Breath	Physical Function	Emotions
Arthritis	X	X		X	X
Asthma and Lung Disease		X	X	X	X
Cancer	X	X	sometimes	X	X
Chronic Heartburn and Acid Reflux	X				X
Chronic Pain	X	X		X	X
Congestive Heart Failure		X	X		X
Diabetes	X	X		X	X
Heart Disease	X	X	X	X	X
Hepatitis	X	X			X
High Blood Pressure					X
HIV Disease (AIDS)	X	X	X	X	X
Inflammatory Bowel Disease	X				X
Irritable Bowel Syndrome	X				X
Kidney Stones	X				
Multiple Sclerosis		X		X	X
Parkinson's Disease	X	X		X	X
Peptic Ulcer Disease	X				X
Renal Failure		X			X
Stroke		X		X	X

From this brief introduction, you can see that chronic illnesses have more in common than first meets the eye. In this book, we talk about managing these illnesses. For most of the book, however, we will talk more about the management tasks common across many illnesses. If you have more than one health problem, you need not be confused about how to start. The approaches that work for heart disease will also help with lung disease, arthritis, or a stroke. Start with the problem or condition that bothers you most. Chart 1.2 (pages 9–11) outlines some of the management skills that may be needed to deal with disease-specific problems. Some of these skills are also discussed later in the book in the chapters dealing with specific diseases.

Before we discuss management techniques, however, let us talk more about what we mean by self-management.

THE CHRONIC ILLNESS PATH

The first responsibility of any chronic disease self-manager is to understand the disease. This means more than learning about what causes the disease and what you can do. It also means observing how the disease and its treatment affect you. A disease is different for each person, and with experience you and your family will become experts at determining the effects of the disease and its treatment. In fact, you are the only person who lives with your disease every day. Therefore, observing your disease and making accurate reports to your health care providers are essential parts of being a good manager. As we mentioned before, most chronic illnesses go up and down in intensity. They do not have a steady path.

The visits on the graph in Figure 1.2 represent Pat's regular follow-up appointments with the doctor or other health professional. Even though the intensity of Pat's symptoms are at the same level for all three visits, what has happened in the time between appointments can mean entirely different things when the health care team is evaluating whether to maintain or change treatment. In the case of the first visit, the symptoms are getting better, so keeping the treatment stable or even lessening it may be in order. In the case of the second visit, things seem to be getting worse, so additional treatment may be the choice. In the case of the third visit, things have been stable for a while, so maintaining treatment may be the best treatment option.

Your experience and understanding, communicated clearly to the physician, are often the best indicators of the path's course, and skilled clinicians commonly depend on them. In fact, if the clinician encourages and facilitates learning by the patient, and the patient

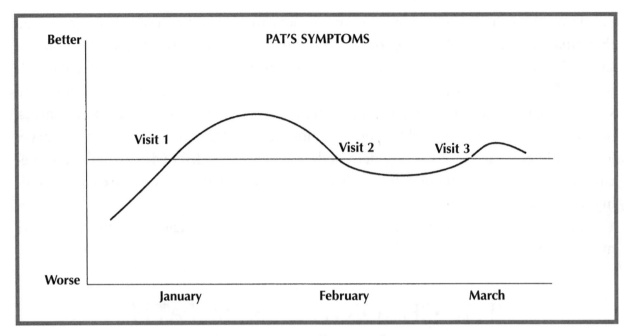

Figure 1.2 **Illness Path**

responds by participating in decisions, a partnership is born. To be most effective, self-management of chronic illness requires such a partnership.

When you develop a chronic illness, you become more aware of your body. Minor symptoms that were formerly ignored may now cause concerns. For example, is this chest pain a signal of a heart attack? Is this pain in my knee a sign that the arthritis has spread? There are no simple reassuring answers to apply to all patients. Nor is there a fail-safe way of sorting out serious signals from minor temporary symptoms that can be ignored.

It is helpful to understand the natural rhythms of your chronic illness. In general, symptoms should be checked out with your doctor if they are unusual, severe, or persistent, or if they occur after starting a new medication.

Throughout this book, we give some specific examples of what actions to take if you experience certain symptoms. But this is where your partnership with your health care provider becomes critical. He or she can guide you in responding to specific problems or symptoms. Self-management does not mean going it alone. Get help or advice when you are concerned or uncertain.

From what has just been said, self-management may seem like a simple enough concept. Both at home and in the business world, managers direct the show. They don't do

Chart1.2 Management Skills for Dealing with Chronic Conditions

MANAGEMENT SKILLS

Chronic Condition	Pain Management	Fatigue Management	Breathing Techniques	Relaxation and Managing Emotions	Nutrition	Exercise	Medications	Other Management Tools
Arthritis	X	X		X	X	X	X	• Use of assistive devices • Appropriate use of joints • Use of cold/heat • Pacing of activities
Asthma & Lung Disease		X	X	X		X	X	• Use of inhalers and peak ow meters • Avoid triggers
Cancer	X	X		X	X	X	X	• Varies with site of the cancer • Managing effects of surgery, radiation, and chemotherapy
Chronic Pain	X	X		X		X	X	• Pacing of activities • Specific exercises • Use of pain management techniques
Congestive Heart Failure		X	X	X	X	X	X	• Monitoring of daily weight • Sodium/salt restriction
Diabetes	X	X		X	X	X	X	• Home blood glucose monitoring • Insulin injection • Foot care • Regular eye (retinal) exams

Chart 1.2 Management Skills for Dealing with Chronic Conditions (continued)

MANAGEMENT SKILLS

Chronic Condition	Pain Management	Fatigue Management	Breathing Techniques	Relaxation and Managing Emotions	Nutrition	Exercise	Medications	Other Management Tools
Heartburn and Acid Reflux					X	X		• Avoid stomach irritants (e.g., coffee, alcohol, aspirin, nonsteroidal anti-inflammatory medications) • Elevation of bed
Heart Disease	X	X	X	X	X	X	X	• Know and watch for warning signs of heart attack
Hepatitis	X	X		X	X		X	• Avoid use of alcohol, IV drugs, medications toxic to liver • Preventing spread of infection (e.g., for hepatitis B and C, safer sex practices, hygiene)
High Blood Pressure				X	X	X	X	• Home blood pressure monitoring • Sodium/salt restriction
HIV Disease (AIDS)	X	X	X	X	X	X	X	• Preventing spread of infection (e.g., safer sex practices, hygiene) • Watch for signs of early infection • Avoid IV drugs

Chart 1.2 **Management Skills for Dealing with Chronic Conditions** (continued)

MANAGEMENT SKILLS

Chronic Condition	Pain Management	Fatigue Management	Breathing Techniques	Relaxation and Managing Emotions	Nutrition	Exercise	Medications	Other Management Tools
Inflammatory Bowel Disease	X			X	X		X	
Irritable Bowel Syndrome	X			X	X		X	
Kidney Stones	X				X		X	• Maintain fluid intake • Avoid calcium or oxalates, depending on type of stone
Multiple Sclerosis								• Management of incontinence • Management of mobility
Parkinson's Disease		X		X		X	X	• Mobility
Peptic Ulcer Disease	X			X	X		X	• Avoid stomach irritants (e.g., coffee, alcohol, aspirin, nonsteroidal anti-inflammatory medications) and early infection
Renal Failure		X		X		X		• Dialysis
Stroke		X		X		X	X	• Use of assistive devices

everything themselves; they work with others, including consultants, to get the job done. What makes them managers is that they are responsible for making the decisions and making sure these decisions are carried out.

As a manager of your illness, your job is much the same. You gather information and hire a consultant, or a team of consultants consisting of your physician and other health professionals. Once they have given you their best advice, it is up to you to follow through. All chronic illness needs day-to-day management. We have all noticed that some people with severe physical problems get on well while others with lesser problems seem to give up on life. The difference often lies in management style.

Managing a chronic illness, like managing a family or a business, is a complex undertaking. There are many twists, turns, and midcourse corrections. By learning self-management skills, you can ease the problems of living with your condition.

The key to success in any undertaking is, first, deciding what you want to do, second, deciding how you are going to do it, and, finally, learning a set of skills and practising them until they have been mastered. These tasks are all based on learning skills and mastering them. Success in chronic disease self-management is the same. In fact, mastering such skills is one of the most important tasks of later life.

We will describe hundreds of skills and strategies to help relieve the problems caused by chronic illness. We do not expect you to practise all of them. Pick and choose. Experiment. Set your own goals. What you do may not be as important as the sense of confidence and control that comes from successfully doing something you want to do. However, we have learned that knowing the skills is not enough. We need a way of incorporating these skills into our daily lives. Whenever we try a new skill, the first attempts are clumsy and slow and show few results. It is easier to return to old ways than to continue trying to master new and sometimes difficult tasks. The best way to master new skills is through practice and evaluation of the results.

SELF-MANAGEMENT SKILLS

What you do about something is largely determined by how you think about it. For example, if you think that having a chronic illness is like falling into a deep pit, you may have a hard time motivating yourself to crawl out, or you may even think the task is impossible. The thoughts you have can greatly determine what happens to you and how you handle your health problems.

Some of the most successful self-managers are people who think of their illness as a path. This path, like any path, goes up and down. Sometimes it is flat and smooth. At other times the way is rough. To negotiate this path one has to use many strategies. Sometimes you can go fast; other times you must slow down. There are obstacles to negotiate.

Good self-managers are people who have learned the skills to negotiate this path. These skills fall into three main categories:

- **Skills needed to deal with the illness**

  Any illness requires that you do new things. These may include taking medicine, using an inhaler, or using oxygen. It means more frequent interactions with your doctor and the health care system. Sometimes there are new exercises or a new diet. Even diseases like cancer require self-management. Chemotherapy, radiation, and surgery can all be made easier by good day-to-day self-management. All of these constitute the work you must do just to manage your illness.

- **Skills needed to continue your normal life**

  Just because you have a chronic illness does not mean that life does not go on. There are still chores to do, friendships to maintain, jobs to perform, and a multitude of family relationships to continue. Things that you once took for granted can become much more complicated in the face of chronic illness. You may need to learn new skills in order to maintain your daily activities and to enjoy life.

- **Skills needed to deal with emotions**

  When you are diagnosed as having a chronic illness, your future changes, and with this comes changes in plans and changes in emotions. Many of these emotions are negative. They may include anger ("Why me? It's not fair"), depression ("I can't do anything any more, what's the use"), frustration ("No matter what I do it doesn't make any difference. I can't do what I want to do"), or isolation ("No one understands, no one wants to be around someone who is sick"). Negotiating the path of chronic illness, then, also means learning skills to work with these negative emotions.

With this as background, you can think of self-management as the use of skills to

1. manage the work of dealing with your illness,

2. manage the work of continuing your daily activities, and

3. manage the changing emotions brought about by chronic illness.

Self-Management Tasks

1. **To take care of your illness** (such as taking medicine, exercising, going to the doctor, communicating your symptoms accurately, changing diet).

2. **To carry out your normal activities** (such as chores, employment, social life, etc.).

3. **To manage your emotional changes** (changes brought about by your illness, such as anger, uncertainty about the future, changed expectations and goals, and sometimes depression, and also including changes in your relationship with family and friends).

Throughout this book you will find information to help you learn and practise self-management skills. This is not a textbook. You do not need to read every word in every chapter. Instead, read the first two chapters and then use the table of contents to find the information you need. Feel free to skip around. In this way you will learn the skills you need to negotiate your individual path.

Suggested Further Reading

Cousins, Norman. *Anatomy of an Illness as Perceived by the Patient: Reflections on Healing and Regeneration*. New York: W.W. Norton and Co., 1979.

Hister, Art. *Dr. Art Hister's Guide to Living a Long and Healthy Life*. Vancouver: Greystone Books, 2003.

Maté, Gabor. *When The Body Says No: The Cost of Hidden Stress*. Toronto: A.A. Knopf Canada, 2003.

Peck, Scott M. *The Road Less Traveled: A New Psychology of Love, Traditional Values and Spiritual Growth.* New York: Simon & Schuster, 1998.

Pulos, Lee. *The Biology of Empowerment.* Audio CD, www.drpulos.com, 2005.

Register, Cheri. *Living With Chronic Illness.* Center City, Minn.: Hazelden, 1999.

Selak, Joy H., and Overman, Steven M. *You Don't Look Sick: Living Well With Invisible Chronic Illness.* Binghamton, N.Y.: Illness. Haworth Medical Press, 2005.

Sobel, David., and Robert Ornstein. *The Healthy Mind, Healthy Body Handbook.* Los Altos, Calif.: DRX, 1996.

Sobel, David, and Robert Ornstein. *Healthy Pleasures,* 2nd ed. Reading, Mass.: Addison-Wesley, 1997.

Sobel, David., and Robert Ornstein. *Mind & Body Health Handbook: How to Use Your Mind & Body to Relieve Stress, Overcome Illness, and Enjoy Healthy Pleasures,* 2nd ed. Los Altos, Calif.: DRX, 1998.

Weil, Andrew. *Healthy Aging: A Lifelong Guide to Your Physical and Spiritual Well-Being,* 1st Knopf ed. New York: Alfred A. Knopf, 2005.

Other Useful Resources

Balance: Television for Living Well. CTV weekday program hosted by Toronto physician Maria Shapiro.

Namaste. A-Channel (available in parts of southern Ontario and Ottawa, as well as Vancouver and Victoria). Hatha yoga instruction on Sundays and Mondays at 6 a.m.

BECOMING AN
ACTIVE SELF-MANAGER

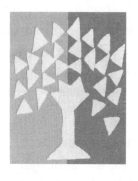

2

IT IS IMPOSSIBLE TO HAVE A CHRONIC CONDITION WITHOUT BEING A SELF-MANAGER. Some people manage by withdrawing from life. They stay in bed or socialize less. The disease becomes the centre of their existence. Other people with the same condition and symptoms somehow manage to get on with life. They may have to change some of the things they do or the way that things get done. Nevertheless, life continues to be full and active. The difference between these two extremes is not the disease but rather how the person with a chronic condition decides to manage the disease. Please note the word "decide." Self-management is always a decision, a decision to be active or a decision to do nothing, a decision to seek help or a decision to suffer in silence. This book will help you with these decisions.

Like any skill, active self-management must be learned and practised. This chapter will start you on your way. Remember: **You are the manager.** Like the manager of an organization or a household, you must

1. decide what you want to accomplish,

2. look for alternative ways to accomplish this goal,

3. start making short-term plans by making an action plan or agreement with yourself,

4. carry out your action plan,

5. check the results,

6. make changes as needed, and

7. remember to reward yourself.

Problems sometimes start with a general uneasiness. Let's say you are unhappy but not sure why. Upon closer examination, you find you miss contact with some relatives who live far away. With the problem identified, you decide to take a trip to visit these relatives. You know what you want to accomplish.

In the past you have always driven, but you now find it tiring, so you seek alternative ways of travel. Among other things, you consider leaving at noon instead of early in the morning and making the trip in two days instead of one. You consider asking a friend along to share the driving. There is also a train that goes within 20 kilometres of your destination, or you might fly (although the airport is not very convenient). You decide to take the train.

The trip still seems overwhelming, as there is so much to do to prepare. You decide to write down all the steps necessary to make the trip a reality. These include finding a good time to go, buying a ticket, figuring out how to handle luggage, seeing if you can make it up and down the stairs to get on the train, wondering if you can walk on a moving train to get food or go to the bathroom, and figuring out how you will get to the station.

You start by making an action plan that this week you will call and find out just how much the railroad can help. You also decide to start taking a short walk each day and walking up and down a few steps so that you can be steadier on your feet. Having done this, you carry out your action plan by calling the railroad and starting your walking program.

A week later you check the results. Looking back at all the steps to be accomplished, you find that a single call answered many questions. The railroad is used to people who have mobility problems and has dealt with many of your concerns. However, you are still worried about walking. Even though you are walking better, you are still unsteady. You make a change in your plan by asking a physical therapist about this, and he suggests using a cane. Although you hate it, you find that a cane gives you that extra security needed on a moving train.

Now you are ready to make a new action plan for accomplishing some of the other tasks necessary to make the trip possible. What once seemed like a dream is becoming a reality.

Let's go through these seven problem-solving steps in detail. They are the backbone of any self-management program.

DECIDING WHAT YOU WANT TO ACCOMPLISH

Deciding what you want to accomplish may be the most difficult part. You must be realistic and very specific.

Think of all the things you would like to do. One of our self-managers wanted to climb 20 steps to her daughter's home so that she could join her family for a holiday meal. Another wanted to lose weight to help his cardiac condition. Still another wanted to be more socially active but felt limited by the need to take her oxygen tank everywhere. In each case, the goal was one that would take several weeks or even months to accomplish.

In fact, one of the problems with goals is that they often seem like dreams. They are so far off that we don't even try to accomplish them. We'll tackle this problem next. For now, take a moment and write your goals here.

Goals:

1. _____

2. _____

3. _____

Put a star (★) next to the goal you would like to work on first.

LOOKING FOR ALTERNATIVE WAYS OF ACCOMPLISHING THE GOAL

Sometimes what keeps us from reaching our goal is a failure to see alternatives, or we reject alternatives without knowing much about them. In the earlier example, our traveller was able to make a list of alternative travel arrangements, and then chose the train.

There are many ways to reach any specific goal. For example, our self-manager who wanted to climb 20 steps could start off with a slow walking program, could start to climb a few steps each day, or could look into having the family gathering at a different place. The man who wanted to lose weight could decide not to eat between meals, to give up desserts, or to start an exercise program. The self-manager who wanted more social contact could find out about community recreation programs, or could call or write friends.

As you can see, there are many options for reaching each goal. The job here is to list the options and then choose one or two on which you would like to work.

Sometimes it is hard to think of all the options yourself. If you are having problems, it is time to use a consultant. Share your goal with family, friends, and health professionals. You can call community organizations such as the Heart and Stroke Foundation or the Arthritis Society. You can use the Internet. Don't ask what you should do. Rather, ask for suggestions. It is always good to have a list of options.

Now a note of caution. Many options are never seriously considered because you assume they don't exist or are unworkable. Never make this assumption until you have thoroughly investigated the option. One woman we know had lived in the same town all her life and felt that she knew all about the community resources. When she was worried about living alone, a friend from another city suggested she subscribe to a community-based 24-hour emergency assistance system. However, the woman dismissed this suggestion because she knew that this service did not exist in her town. It was only when, months later, the friend came to visit and called the local hospital, that the woman learned the service was offered through some community hospitals. In short, never assume anything. Assumptions are major self-management enemies.

Write the list of options for your main goal here. Then put a star (★) next to the two or three options on which you would like to work.

Options:

1. _____

2. _____

3. _____

4. _____

5. _____

6. _____

Making Short-Term Plans—Action Planning

The next step is to turn your options into short-term plans. These we call action plans. An action plan calls for a specific action or set of actions that you can realistically expect to accomplish within, say, the next week. The action plan should be about something **you** want to do or accomplish. This is a tool to help you do what **you** wish. You do not make action plans to please your friends, family, or doctor.

Action plans are probably your most important self-management tool. Most of us can do things to make us healthier, but fail to do them. For example, most people with chronic illness can walk—some just across the room, others for a half block. Most can walk several blocks, and some can walk a kilometre or more. However, few people have a systematic exercise program.

An action plan helps us to do the things we know we should do. Let us go through all the steps for making a realistic action plan. This is an important skill that may well determine the success of your self-management program.

First, decide what you will do this week. For a step climber, this might be climbing three steps on four consecutive days. The man trying to lose weight may decide not to eat between meals for three days and to walk around the block before dinner on the following four days. This action must be something you want to do that you feel is realistic, a step on the way to your long-term goal.

Make sure that your plans are "behaviour specific"; that is, rather than just deciding "to relax," you will "listen to the progressive muscle relaxation tapes."

Next, make a specific plan. This is the most difficult and important part of making an action plan. Deciding what you want to do is worthless without a plan to do it. The plan should contain all of the following steps:

1. Exactly **what** are you going to do? How far will you walk, how will you eat less, what breathing technique will you practise?

2. **How much** will you do? Will you walk around the block, walk for 15 minutes, not eat between meals for three days, practice breathing exercises for 15 minutes?

3. **When** will you do this? Again, this must be specific, such as before lunch, in the shower, or when I come home from work. Connecting a new activity with an old habit is a good way to make sure it gets done. Another trick is to do your new activity before an old favourite activity such as reading the paper or watching a favorite TV program.

4. **How often** will you do the activity? This is a bit tricky. We would all like to do things every day, but it is not always possible. It is usually best to decide to do something three or four times a week. If you do more, so much the better. However, if you are like most of us, you will feel less pressure if you can do your activity three or four times and still be successful at your action plan. (Please note! Taking medications is an exception. This must be done exactly as directed by your doctor.)

There are a couple of guidelines for writing your action plan that may help you achieve success. First, start where you are or start slowly. If you can walk only for one minute, start your walking program with walking one minute once every hour or two, not by walking a kilometre. If you have never done any exercise, start with a few minutes of warm-up. A total of five or ten minutes is enough. If you want to lose weight, set a goal based on your existing eating behaviours, such as not eating after dinner. "Losing a pound this week" is not an action plan. There is no behaviour.

Also, give yourself some time off. All people have days when they don't feel like doing anything. That is a good reason for saying that you will do something three times a week instead of every day. In this way, if you don't feel like walking one day, you can still achieve your action plan.

Once you've made your action plan, ask yourself the following question: "On a scale of 0 to 10, with 0 being totally unsure and 10 being totally certain, how certain am I that I can complete this plan?"

If your answer is 7 or above, this is probably a realistic action plan. Congratulate yourself; you have done the hard work. If your answer is below 7, then you should look again at your action plan. Ask yourself why you're not confident. What problems do you foresee? Then see if you can either solve the problems or change your plan to make yourself more confident of success.

Once you have made a plan you are happy with, write it down and post it where you will see it every day. Keep track of how you are doing and the problems you encounter. (Page 27 is a completed example of an action plan. Pages 28–30 are blanks; make copies of them to use weekly.)

Carrying Out Your Action Plan

If the action plan is well written and realistic, fulfilling it is generally pretty easy. Ask family or friends to check with you on how you are doing. Having to report your progress is good motivation. Keep track of your daily activities while carrying out your plan. All good managers have lists of what they want to accomplish. Check things off as they are completed. This will give you guidance on how realistic your planning was and will also be useful in making future plans. Make daily notes, even of the things you don't understand at the time. Later these notes may be useful in establishing a pattern to use for problem solving.

For example, our stair-climbing friend never did her climbing. Each day she had a different problem: not enough time, being tired, the weather being too cold, and so on. When she looked back at her notes, she began to realize that the real problem was her fear of falling with no one around to help her. She then decided to use a cane while climbing stairs and to do it when a friend or neighbour was around.

Basics of a Successful Action Plan

1. Something YOU want to do

2. Reasonable (something you can expect to be able to accomplish that week)

3. Behaviour-specific (losing weight is *not* a behaviour; not eating after dinner is)

4. Answers the questions:

    What?

    How much? (think about your day/week—which days, times, etc.)

    When?

    How often?

5. Confidence (certainty) level of 7 or more (that you will fulfill the entire contract)

Checking the Results

At the end of each week, see if you completed your action plan and if you are any nearer to accomplishing your goal. Are you able to walk farther? Have you lost weight? Are you less fatigued? Taking stock is important. You may not see progress day by day, but you should see a little progress each week. At the end of each week, check on how well you have fulfilled your action plan. If you are having problems, this is the time to problem-solve.

MAKING MIDCOURSE CHANGES (PROBLEM SOLVING)

When you are trying to overcome obstacles, the first plan is not always the most workable plan. If something doesn't work, don't give up. Try something else; modify your short-term plans so that your steps are easier, give yourself more time to accomplish difficult tasks, choose new steps toward your goal, or check with your consultants for advice and assistance.

The first and most important step in problem solving is to identify the problem. This is usually the most difficult step as well. You may know, for example, that stairs are a problem for you, but it will take a little more effort to determine that the real problem is fear of falling.

Once you have identified the problem, the next step is to list ideas for solving the problem. You may be able to come up with a good list yourself, but often calling in help from consultants is helpful. Consultants can be friends, family, members of your health care team, or community resources. One note about using consultants: These folks cannot help you if you do not describe the problem well. For example, there is a big difference between saying that you can't walk because your feet hurt and saying that your feet hurt because you cannot find proper-fitting walking shoes.

When you have a list of ideas, pick one to try. As you try something new, remember that new activities are usually difficult. Be sure to give your potential solution a fair chance before deciding it won't work.

Assess the results after you've given your idea a fair trial. If all goes well, your problem will be solved.

If you still have the problem, substitute another idea from your list and try again.

If you still do not have a solution, utilize other resources (your consultants) for more ideas. If all of the above does not work, then you may have to accept that your problem may not be solvable right now. This is sometimes hard to do. Just because a problem is not immediately solvable doesn't mean that it won't be solvable later or that other problems can't be solved in the same way. Even if your path is blocked, there are probably alternative paths. Don't give up. Keep going.

✳ Summary of Problem-Solving Steps

1. Identify the problem (this is the most difficult and most important step).

2. List ideas to solve the problem.

3. Select one method to try.

4. Assess the results.

5. Substitute another idea if the first didn't work.

6. Utilize other resources (ask friends, family, or professionals for ideas if your solutions didn't work).

7. Accept that the problem may not be solvable now.

REWARDING YOURSELF

The best part of being a good self-manager is the reward that comes from accomplishing your goals and living a fuller and more comfortable life. However, don't wait until your goal is reached; rather, reward yourself frequently. For example, decide that you won't read the paper until after your exercise. Thus, reading the paper becomes your reward. One self-manager buys only one or two pieces of fruit at a time and walks the four blocks to the supermarket every day or two to get more fruit. Another self-manager who stopped smoking used the money he would have spent on cigarettes to have his house professionally cleaned, and there was even enough left over to go to a baseball game with a friend. Rewards don't have to be fancy, expensive, or fattening. There are many healthy pleasures that can add enjoyment to your life.

In review, a successful self-manager

1. sets goals,

2. makes a list of alternatives for reaching the goal,

3. makes short-term action plans toward that goal,

4. carries out the plan,

5. checks on progress weekly,

6. makes midcourse changes as necessary, and

7. uses rewards for a job well done.

One last note: Not all goals are achievable. Chronic illness may mean having to give up some options. If this is true for you, don't dwell too much on what you can't do. Rather, start working on another goal you would like to accomplish. One self-manager we know who uses a wheelchair talks about the 90% of the things he can do. He spends his life developing this 90% to the fullest.

Now that you understand the meaning of self-management, you are ready to begin using the tools that will make you a self-manager. Even if your particular illness or condition is not covered by a specific chapter, this book is still for you. The chart on pages 9–11 may contain information pointing you toward the specific self-management skills you'll need. Remember: Most self-management skills are similar for all diseases. Chapters 15 to 18 contain information on some of the more common chronic illnesses. In Chapter 14 we talk about medications and their uses. The rest of the book is devoted to tools of the trade. These include exercise, nutrition, symptom management, communication, making decisions about the future, finding resources and information about representation agreements and durable power of attorney for health care, and, of course, sex and intimacy.

ACTION PLAN FORM

In writing your action plan, be sure it includes

    1. what you are going to do,
    2. how much you are going to do,
    3. when you are going to do it, and
    4. how many days a week you are going to do it.

For example: This week, I will walk (*what*) around the block (*how much*) before lunch (*when*) three times (*how many*).

This week I will _____ *walk around the block* _____ (what)

_____ *3 times* _____ (how much)

_____ *before lunch* _____ (when)

_____ *3 days this week* _____ (how many)

How confident are you? (0 = not at all confident; 10 = totally confident) ___*9*___

	Check Off	Comments
Monday	—	*raining*
Tuesday	✓	*walked slowly & noticed everything around me*
Wednesday	✓	*it was cool out, but the walk felt good*
Thursday	—	*raining again*
Friday	✓	*only walked around the block 2 times*
Saturday	✓	*took a friend along—we had a nice chat*
Sunday	—	*felt tired*

ACTION PLAN FORM

In writing your action plan, be sure it includes

    1. what you are going to do,
    2. how much you are going to do,
    3. when you are going to do it, and
    4. how many days a week you are going to do it.

For example: This week, I will walk (*what*) around the block (*how much*) before lunch (*when*) three times (*how many*).

This week I will _____(what)

_____(how much)

_____(when)

_____(how many)

How confident are you? (0 = not at all confident; 10 = totally confident) _____
[*Just a note: You may want to make copies of this form.*]

	Check Off	Comments
Monday		
Tuesday		
Wednesday		
Thursday		
Friday		
Saturday		
Sunday		

ACTION PLAN FORM

In writing your action plan, be sure it includes

1. what you are going to do,
2. how much you are going to do,
3. when you are going to do it, and
4. how many days a week you are going to do it.

For example: This week, I will walk (*what*) around the block (*how much*) before lunch (*when*) three times (*how many*).

This week I will _____(what)

_____(how much)

_____(when)

_____(how many)

How confident are you? (0 = not at all confident; 10 = totally confident) _____
[*Just a note: You may want to make copies of this form.*]

	Check Off	Comments
Monday		
Tuesday		
Wednesday		
Thursday		
Friday		
Saturday		
Sunday		

ACTION PLAN FORM

In writing your action plan, be sure it includes

1. what you are going to do,
2. how much you are going to do,
3. when you are going to do it, and
4. how many days a week you are going to do it.

For example: This week, I will walk (*what*) around the block (*how much*) before lunch (*when*) three times (*how many*).

This week I will _____(what)

_____(how much)

_____(when)

_____(how many)

How confident are you? (0 = not at all confident; 10 = totally confident) _____
[*Just a note: You may want to make copies of this form.*]

	Check Off	Comments
Monday		
Tuesday		
Wednesday		
Thursday		
Friday		
Saturday		
Sunday		

FINDING RESOURCES

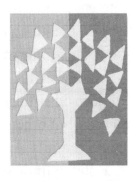

3

A MAJOR PART OF BECOMING A SELF-MANAGER OF YOUR CHRONIC ILLNESS IS KNOWING WHEN YOU NEED HELP AND HOW TO FIND HELP. Seeking help to perform daily tasks, to assist with chores, or to help with other areas of your life does not mean that you have fallen victim to your illness. Knowing where to go for help in specific areas of your life takes initiative and requires you to evaluate your condition and your own capabilities. By becoming more aware of the symptoms you experience throughout the day, you can better predict the amount of energy and patience you will have later to accomplish tasks. If you find that you come up short on energy, time, patience, or capability for some tasks, you can evaluate where help from other resources will spare you for those things most important to you.

The first resource we probably go to for help is family, followed by close friends. Some find it difficult, however, to ask for help from people they know. Finding the right words to ask for help is discussed in Chapter 10. Unfortunately, some people either do not have family or close friends to call on, or cannot bring themselves to ask. If this is the case, you must look for other resources in your community.

Finding resources in your community can be a little like a "treasure hunt." Just as in a treasure hunt, creative thinking wins the game. Finding what you need may be as simple as looking in the telephone book and making a couple of phone calls. Other times, it may take detective talents to find it. The community resource detective must find clues and follow them, including starting over when a clue leads to a dead end.

Finding and recognizing clues are the detective's most important tasks. For example, suppose you find it difficult to prepare meals because prolonged standing is too tiring or painful. However, after some thought, you decide that you want to continue cooking for yourself rather than have someone else cook your meals. So you must explore getting your kitchen altered to enable you to prepare meals from a seated position.

Where can you find an architect or contractor who has knowledge and experience in kitchen alterations for people with physical limitations? You need a starting point for your treasure hunt. Looking in the yellow pages and the classified section of the newspaper reveals pages of ads and listings for architects and contractors; some advertisers say they specialize in kitchens, but others don't mention any specialty. None mention anything about designing for physical limitations. A couple of phone calls to those listing kitchens as a specialty are unsuccessful in finding anyone experienced in kitchens for the physically limited.

Now what? Well, you have a couple of choices in your hunt for clues. First, you can call everyone listed until you find what you need. Not only would this be time-consuming, but you may not feel comfortable about the person you find until you talk to someone who knows his or her work.

Who else do you know who might have information of this kind? Maybe someone who works with people with disabilities would know, such as an occupational or physical therapist, a medical supplies store, a pharmacist, the local college accessibility office or Paraplegic Associaton, or service clubs such as Rotary, Kiwanis, or Lions Clubs. The Canadian Red Cross and your local health information line (like the BC NurseLine or Tele-care NET) are other resources for you.

You may talk to someone who doesn't have the answer but says, "Gosh, Jack so-and-so just had his kitchen remodelled to accommodate his wheelchair. Maybe he can help you find someone." Jack's name is probably a great clue. He may be able to give you not only the name of someone who does the work, but also some ideas about the cost and hassle before you go any further in the process. He's probably done much of the detective work already.

Suppose, however, that your search still isn't successful. There are people in every community who are natural resources. These "Naturals" seem to know everyone and where everything is in their community. They tend to be folks who have lived a long time in the community and have been closely involved in it. They are natural problem solvers.

You may already know such a person. The "Natural" is the one people always seek out for advice, and this person always seems to be helpful. You probably count him or her among your friends or acquaintances. If you were to call this person, he or she would probably know the answer or set you on the right path to get the answer. Sometimes the "Natural" will taste the thrill of the hunt and, like a modern-day Sherlock Holmes, will announce that "the game is afoot!" and promptly join you in your search.

The "Natural" could be a friend, a business associate, the letter carrier, your physician, your pet's veterinarian, the clerk at the corner grocery store, the pharmacist, the bus or taxi driver, your kid's school secretary, a real estate agent, or the librarian. All you need do is think of this person as an information resource.

Watch out, though! Once you get good at thinking about community resources creatively, you will become a "Natural" in your community!

RESOURCES FOR RESOURCES

When we need to find goods or services, there are certain resources we can call on in order to find more resources. The "Natural" is one of those resources, but our community resource "detective's kit" needs a variety of other tools to be fully useful.

Probably the most frequently used tool we pull from our community resource detective's kit is the telephone book. Particularly if you can hire someone to do something for you, the phone book is full of people and organizations ready to help. For most searches, this is where to start.

While you have your telephone book out, another tool to look up is your local community services numbers and local information and referral services. There are several types of agencies, depending on your community, offering helpful services. In B.C.'s lower Mainland, you can contact Information and Referral Services. This agency maintains a large database of health and social service agencies, government ministries, and information on drug and alcohol abuse, gambling and VictimLink (if you've been a victim of crime). A community directory, 211, provides information about social services, health, and related government services in Edmonton, Calgary, and Toronto. For seniors, a federal government resource called Seniors' Health is a source for issues such as home safety and choosing assistive devices. Most communities have an information and referral service; just check in the blue pages of your telephone book. Once you have an information and referral telephone number, your searches will become much easier. These services maintain a huge file of referral addresses and telephone numbers for just about any help you might need. Even if they don't have the answer to your need, they will almost always be able to refer you to another agency that can speed you along in your search.

One of the most important resources you can find for either information or help is the voluntary agencies dedicated to your disease. In Canada, these include the Heart and Stroke Foundation, the Canadian Lung Association, the Canadian Diabetes Association, and the Arthritis Society. These agencies have provincial bureaus and often local offices in many cities and towns. Funded by contributions from individuals and corporate sponsors, they provide up-to-date information about your disease. They also conduct research in the hope it will help people live better with their disease and someday lead to a cure. Ask about being put on the newsletter mailing list, and if membership or a donation is required. You do not, however, have to be a member to qualify for their services. They are here to serve you. Many of these organizations have great websites. In this era of information sharing with the Internet, you can live in rural Yukon and get help from all corners of the globe.

There are other organizations in your community offering information and direct services. These include seniors' centres, community centres, and religious service agencies. These organizations offer information, classes, recreational opportunities, nutrition programs, legal and tax help, and social programs. There is probably a senior centre or community centre close to you. Your city government office or local librarian will know where they are, and the calendar section of your local or community newspaper (sometimes referred to as a shopper) will usually have information about programs these organizations offer.

Most religious groups offer information and social services to those who need it, either directly through the local church or synagogue or through the Council of Churches, Catholic Diocese, or Jewish social service groups. To get help from religious organizations, start with the local church or synagogue, and they will help you or refer you to someone who can help you. You ned not be a member of the religion or of its local organization to receive help.

Your hospital or regional health care authority may also offer services. Call your local hospital, clinic, or regional health authority or health board, for more in-depth information and the services available. Your doctor will also be aware of the available services in the various health authority regions.

The next resource to call upon in your search is the library. Particularly when you are looking for information about your disease, this is a valuable resource. The library, and the reference librarian in particular, can provide an information and referral service as well. Often the reference section of the library will have a little gem of a book or pamphlet that gives listings of the resources you are looking for. If you're a good detective, you will find this gem on your own. The reference librarian, on the other hand, can probably take you right to it (and maybe show you some others, too). Even if you think you are an excellent library detective, it's a good idea to ask the reference librarian to make sure you haven't overlooked something. These people see volumes of material cross their desks constantly, and are knowledgeable about the community (and probably "Naturals" as well).

In addition to the city or county library we are most familiar with, there are other, more specialized libraries available to us. Ask your information and referral service if there is a "health library" in your community. These libraries specialize in health-related resources, usually having a computerized database search service available along with the usual print, audiotape, and videotape materials. These libraries are usually offered through nonprofit organizations and hospitals, and will sometimes charge a small fee for use.

Universities and colleges also have libraries open to the public. The "government documents" section of universities and community colleges provide access to publications at no charge. However, some provincial governments increasingly insist that end-users download and print documents themselves. Government publications exist on just about any subject, and the health-related publications are particularly extensive. You can find information on everything from organic gardening to detailed nutritional recipes. The librarians are usually very helpful, and these publications represent "your tax dollars at work."

If you are fortunate enough to have a medical school in your community, you may be able to use its medical library. This, however, is a place to go for information, rather than a place to look for help with tasks. Naturally, you can expect to find a great deal of information about disease and treatment at a medical library. Unless you have special knowledge about medicine, however, the information you find in a medical library can be intimidating, confusing, and possibly frightening. Use medical libraries with care.

Many books related to your disease will have reading lists and resource lists at the backs. Sometimes we miss these lists because they are found near the index. "Backs of books" are helpful for either finding information or finding agencies or other organizations.

Your local newspaper is also an excellent resource, and the health editor, science editor, or "calendar of events" editor may be very knowledgeable about resources in the community. The two sections of the newspaper that can be most helpful in your search for resources are the "calendar of events" and the classified section. Organizations advertise classes, lectures, and other events in these sections. Even if you are not interested in the particular event advertised, the contact telephone number given may be an important clue in your search for something else. Look in other logical places for news stories that might be of interest also, such as the pages around the calendar section or the sports and fitness section (if you are looking for an exercise program for people with your health problem, for example).

Sometimes you can find clues in the classified section. Look under "announcements," "health," or any other heading that seems promising. Review the index of classified headings, which is usually printed at the front of the section near the rate information, to see which headings your newspaper uses.

INFORMATION OVERLOAD—THE INTERNET

The fastest-growing resource in our society today is the Internet. Information is being added to this worldwide network at a dizzying rate every day, every second. The Internet (all electronic information transfer, including e-mail and graphical web pages) and the World Wide Web (the graphical interface to the Internet that we are most familiar with) offer not only a nearly endless supply of information about health and anything else you can imagine, but also opportunities to interact with people all over the world. Someone who has a rare health condition might find it difficult to find others with the same disease where she or he lives. With the Internet, though, there might be a whole group of such people to talk to—it doesn't matter whether they are across the street or on the other side of the world.

The good thing about the Internet is that anyone can have a website. The bad thing about the Internet is that anyone can have a website. The Internet has virtually no controls over who is posting information or whether the information is correct, or even safe. This can mean that there is a lot of information out there that might be very useful, because individuals can share information quickly. It can also mean that someone might post incorrect, outdated, or dangerous information. You should never assume that information found on the Internet is true. Approach the information with skepticism and caution: Is the author/sponsor of the website clearly identified? Is the author reputable? Is the information contrary to what everyone else seems to be saying about the subject? Does common sense support the information? What is the purpose of the website? Is it trying to sell you something? Is it linked to a website selling books or products for healing chronic or acute conditions? Key words and phrases to look out for are: "secrets doctors won't tell you;" "what the government doesn't want you to know;" the cure for cancer is here." If the site is selling a product, be especially careful. When we are trying to cope with a chronic condition, we can be at our most vulnerable.

You may have heard about "evidence-based medicine," which uses the best available current research, rather than relying only on observation, experience, or authority such as a textbook. While this may be beyond most people's ability, you can still take an "evidence-based approach" to medical research you read about online by making sure that it comes from a well-known medical website (like the Canadian Institute of Health Research) or a book by an author from a well-known institution, like a university. For example, the author of *Take Control of Your Health*, a book that explains evidence-based medicine, is Dr. William Feldman, professor emeritus at the University of Toronto.

One way to start analyzing the purpose of the Web site is to look at the URL (the address, starting with http://). The URL usually will look something like this:

http://www.hc-sc.gc.ca

"http://" begins every Web URL. It stands for "hypertext transfer protocol." "www" means that the server (computer) that Health Canada's main website lives on is dedicated to the World Wide Web. "gc" identifies the server as belonging to the federal government, and "ca" indicates that a website is Canadian.

Looking at the last part of the main website's URL, you will most often see .edu, .org, .gov, .com, or .ca. This gives you a clue about the nature of the organization that owns the website. A college or university will have .edu, a non-profit organization will have .org, and a government site will have .gov. As a general rule of thumb, these will be trustworthy sites, although non-profit organizations can be formed to promote just about anything. The endings .com and .ca (Canadian designation) represent a wide variety of companies, organizations, and associations that offer information, products, and services. With millions of different websites out there, below are some of our favourites that can get you started. Often these websites will have posted links to other resourceful web pages.

Health Canada
    http://www.hc-sc.gc.ca
Canadian Red Cross
    http://www.redcross.ca/
Insidermedicine:
    http://www.insidermedicine.ca
Canadian Institutes of Health Research
    http://www.cihr-irsc.gc.ca/
College of Family Physicians of Canada
    http://www.cfpc.ca/

Dieticians of Canada
  http://www.dieticians.ca/
World Health News (Harvard)
  http://www.worldhealthnews.harvard.edu/
Mayo Clinic
  http://www.mayoclinic.com/
Bandolier
  http://www.jr2.ox.ac.uk/Bandolier/
Centers for Disease Control and Prevention
  http://cdc.gov/nccdphp
Snopes
  http://www.snopes.com
Seniors' Health
  http://www.phac-aspc.gc.ca/sh-sa_e.html

CANADIAN DIRECTORY

BC Centre for Disease Control
  Telephone: 604-660-0584
Quebec: Infectious Diseases Research Centre at Laval University
  Telephone: 418-656-7888
Canadian Physiotherapy Association
  Telephone: 1-888-474-9746

24/7 Telephone Health Information

Alberta: Health Link Alberta
  Toll Free: 1-866-408-5465
British Columbia: BC NurseLine
  Toll Free: 1-866-215-4700
Manitoba: Health Links-Info Santé
  Toll Free: 1-888-315-9257

New Brunswick: Tele-Care
   Toll Free: 1-800-244-8353
Newfoundland and Labrador: HealthLine
   Toll Free: 1-888-709-2929
Northwest Territories: Tele-Care NWT
   Toll Free: 1-888-255-1010
Ontario: Telehealth Ontario
   Toll Free: 1-866-797-0000
Quebec: Info Santé
   Telephone: (514) 934-0354
Saskatchewan: HealthLine
   Toll Free: 1-877-800-0002

Nunavut has 26 Health Centres, each with its own telephone number, such as Cambridge Bay Health Centre at 867-983-2531.

1.	Arctic Bay Health Centre	(867) 439-8816
2.	Arviat Health Centre	(867) 857-3100
3.	Baker Lake Health Centre	(867) 793-2816
4.	Broughton Island Health Centre	(867) 927-8916
5.	Cambridge Bay Health Centre	(867) 983-2531
6.	Cape Dorset Health Centre	(867) 897-8820
7.	Chesterfield Inlet Health Centre	(867) 898-9968
8.	Clyde River Health Centre	(867) 924-6377
9.	Coral Harbour Health Centre	(867) 925-9916
10.	Gjoa Haven - Haputtit Health Centre	(867) 360-7441
11.	Grise Fiord Health Centre	(867) 980-9923
12.	Hall Beach Health Centre	(867) 928-8827
13.	Igloolik Health Centre	(867) 934-8837
14.	Iqaluit Public Health Clinic	(867) 979-5306
15.	Kimmirut Health Centre	(867) 939-2217
16.	Kugluktuk Health Centre	(867) 982-4531
17.	Nanisivik Health Centre	(867) 436-7482
18.	Pangnirtung Health Centre	(867) 473-8977
19.	Pelly Bay - St. Theresa Health Centre	(867) 769-6441

20. Pond Inlet Health Centre   (867) 899-8840
21. Rankin Inlet Health Centre   (867) 645-2816
22. Repulse Bay Health Centre   (867) 462-9916
23. Resolute Health Centre   (867) 252-3844
24. Sanikiluaq Health Centre   (867) 266-8965
25. Taloyoak - Judy Hill Memorial Health Centre   (867) 561-5111
26. Whale Cove Health Centre   (867) 896-9916

Health Canada

Alberta: 780-495-2651

British Columbia: 604-666-2083

Manitoba: 204-983-2508

Ontario: Toll free: 1-866-999-7612

Quebec: 1-800-561-3350

Nova Scotia, New Brunswick, Prince Edward Island, Newfoundland and Labrador:
    902-426-2038

Yukon, Nunavut, and the Northwest Territories: 613-946-8081

Becoming an effective community resource detective is one of the jobs of a good self-manager. Hopefully, this chapter has given you some ideas about the process of finding resources in your community. Knowing how to search for resources will serve you better than being handed a list of resource agencies.

UNDERSTANDING AND MANAGING COMMON SYMPTOMS

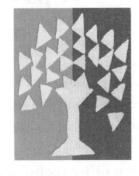

4

CHRONIC ILLNESSES COME WITH SYMPTOMS. These symptoms are signals from the body that something unusual is happening. They cannot be seen by others, are often difficult to describe to others, and are usually unpredictable. While some symptoms are common, the times when they occur, and the way in which they affect us, are very personal. These symptoms, which include fatigue, stress, shortness of breath, pain, itching, anger, depression, and sleep problems, can interact with each other; this in turn can worsen existing symptoms and/or lead to new symptoms or problems.

Regardless of the causes of these symptoms, the ways in which we can manage them are similar. These are our self-management tools. This chapter discusses some of the symptoms most common among different conditions, as well as some of their causes. In addition, some ways to deal with the symptoms (tools you can use to self-manage) are discussed. In Chapter 5, cognitive techniques are discussed; these are the ways you can use your mind to help deal with these symptoms.

DEALING WITH COMMON SYMPTOMS

Learning to manage symptoms is very similar to the process of problem solving that was discussed in Chapter 2 (page 24). Before you can manage a symptom, it is important to identify which symptom you are experiencing. Next, it is necessary to try to determine the cause of the symptom at this particular time. While this may sound like a simple process, it

Tips for Practising Different Symptom Management Techniques

- **Choose a technique to try first.** Be sure to give this method a fair trial. We recommend that you practise it twice a day for at least two weeks before deciding whether or not the technique is going to be helpful to you.

- **Try some other techniques, giving each the same trial period.** It is important to try more than one technique because some may be more useful for certain symptoms, or you may find that you simply prefer some techniques over others.

- **Think about how and when you will use each technique you have chosen.** For example, some of these methods may require more substantial lifestyle changes. As you practise the different techniques, you may find that some work best for specific symptoms and not so well for others. The best symptom managers learn to use a variety of techniques according to their needs and situation on a daily basis.

- **Place some cues in your environment to remind you to practise these techniques, as both practice and consistency are important for the mastery of new skills.** For example, place stickers or notes where you'll see them, such as on your mirror, near the phone, in your office, or on the car's dashboard. Also, change the notes periodically so that you'll continue to notice them.

- **Try linking the practice of each technique with some other established behaviour or activity in your daily routine.** For example, practise relaxation as part of your cool-down from exercise. Also, ask a friend or family member to remind you to practise each day; he or she may even wish to participate.

is not always easy because symptoms and the problems caused by chronic disease can be numerous, complex, and often interrelated.

The person with a chronic condition can experience many different symptoms, and each symptom can have various causes. The way in which these symptoms affect one's life is also different. All of these factors can become very tangled, like the loose threads of a cloth. To be able to successfully manage these symptoms, we must figure out how to untangle the threads. One way to untangle the threads is to keep a daily diary or journal. This can be as simple as writing your symptoms and what you are doing on a calendar. After a week or two, you will probably see a pattern. For example, you go out to dinner on Saturday evening and wake up in the night with stomach pain. You realize that when you go out you overeat, and then adjust what you order. Every time you go dancing your feet hurt, but this does not occur when you walk. Maybe the different shoes you wear make the difference. Seeing patterns is for many the first step in symptom self-management. See page 44 for an example of a sample calendar journal.

Looking at the sample calendar, we can see that the following patterns may occur:

1. Something happens when the person is baby-sitting that causes pain—maybe it is lifting, chasing after small children, or leaning over to change diapers.

2. When this person has pain she tends to be tired the next day.

3. Water exercise makes her feel better, although she may be a little stiff the next day.

4. Eating dinner out seems to result in poor sleep and being tired the next day. Maybe she eats too much, or maybe this is the only time she drinks alcohol. Even a little alcohol at night can interfere with good-quality sleep.

As you read through this chapter, you will note that many symptoms have the same causes. Also, one symptom may actually cause other symptoms. By gaining a better understanding of the possible causes of your symptoms, you will be better able to identify more effective ways to deal with these symptoms and their causes. As you learn more about the causes, you may also find ways to prevent certain symptoms from recurring.

Now let's look at some of the more common symptoms experienced by people with different chronic conditions.

SAMPLE CALENDAR JOURNAL

Mon	Tue	Wed	Thur	Fri	Sat	Sun
Grocery shop	Baby-sit grand kids Pain PM	Tired	Water exercise Feel great	Little stiff Clean house	Dinner out Poor sleep	Tired

Mon	Tue	Wed	Thur	Fri	Sat	Sun
Grocery shop	Baby-sit grandkids Pain PM	Tired	Water exercise Feel great	Clean house	Feel Great	Feel Great Dinner out Poor sleep

FATIGUE

Having a chronic condition can drain your energy. Therefore, fatigue is a very real problem for many people. It is not, as some might say, "all in the mind." Fatigue can keep you from doing things you'd like to do. Often, it is misunderstood by those who do not have a chronic illness. After all, others cannot usually see your fatigue. Unfortunately, spouses, family members, and friends sometimes do not understand the unpredictable way in which the fatigue associated with your condition can affect you. They may think that you are just not interested in certain activities or that you want to be alone. Sometimes you may not even know why you feel this way.

To be able to manage fatigue, it is important to understand that your fatigue may be related to several factors, such as:

- **The disease itself.** No matter what disease or diseases you have, whatever you do demands more energy. When a chronic illness is present, the body is less efficient in its use of the energy reserved for everyday activities. This is because some of your energy is used to help the body heal itself.

- **Inactivity.** Muscles that are not used become deconditioned and less efficient in doing what they are supposed to do. The heart, which is made of muscular tissue, can also become deconditioned. When this happens, the ability of the heart to pump blood, necessary nutrients, and oxygen to other parts of the body is decreased. When muscles do not receive these necessary nutrients and oxygen, they cannot function properly. Deconditioned muscles tire more easily than muscles in good condition—those that receive an adequate supply of blood, oxygen, and nutrients.

- **Poor nutrition.** Food is our basic source of energy. If the fuel we take in is not good quality and/or consumed in the proper quantities, fatigue can result. For some people, obesity results in fatigue. Extra weight causes an increase in the amount of energy needed to perform daily activities. For others, being underweight can cause problems associated with fatigue. This is especially true for those with chronic obstructive pulmonary disease (COPD). Many people with COPD experience sudden weight loss because of a change in their eating habits and therefore have increased fatigue.

- **Insufficient rest.** For a variety of reasons, there are times when we do not get enough sleep or have poor-quality sleep. This can also result in fatigue. Later in this chapter, sleep problems will be discussed in more detail.

- **Emotions.** Stress, anxiety, fear, and depression can also cause significant fatigue. Most people are aware of the connection between stress and feeling tired, but fewer are aware of the fact that fatigue is a major symptom of depression.

- **Medications.** Some medications can cause fatigue. If you think your fatigue is medication-related, talk to your doctor. Sometimes medications or the dose can be changed.

If fatigue is a problem, your first job is to determine the cause. Again, a journal may be helpful. Are you eating healthy foods? Are you exercising? Are you getting enough good-quality sleep? If you answer "no" to any of these questions, you may be well on your way to determining one or more of the reasons for your fatigue.

The important thing to remember about your fatigue is that it may be caused by things other than your illness. Therefore, in order to combat and prevent fatigue, you must address the different causes of your fatigue. This may mean trying a variety of self-management tools.

If your fatigue is caused by not eating well, such as eating too many "empty calories" in the form of "junk food" or alcohol, then the solution is to eat better-quality foods in the proper quantities. For others, the problem may be a decreased interest in food, leading to a lack of calories and subsequent weight loss. Chapter 13 discusses, in greater detail, some of the problems associated with eating, as well as tips for improving your eating habits.

People often say they can't exercise because they feel fatigued. Believing this creates a vicious cycle: People are fatigued because of a lack of exercise, and yet they don't exercise because of the fatigue. Believe it or not, if this is your problem, then motivating yourself to do a little exercise the next time you are fatigued might be the answer. You don't have to run a marathon. The important thing is to get outdoors and take a short walk. If this is not possible, then walk around your house. See Chapter 6 for more information on getting started on an exercise program.

If emotions are causing your fatigue, rest will probably not help. In fact, it may make you feel worse, especially if your fatigue is a sign of depression. We will talk about how to deal with depression a little later in this chapter. If you feel that your fatigue may be related to stress, then read the next section for some tips on managing stress.

STRESS

Stress is a common problem for everyone. But what is stress? In the 1950s, physiologist Hans Selye described stress as "the nonspecific response of the body to any demand made upon it." Others have expanded this definition to explain that the body adapts to demands, whether pleasant or unpleasant. For example, sitting in the sun on a warm spring day may cause you to relax. Your blood pressure and pulse will go down. Being caught in a cold, driving rain will cause your body to speed up. Your BP and pulse will go up. In short, you are stressed.

How Does Your Body Respond to Stress?

Your body is used to functioning at a certain level. When there is a need to change this level, your body must adjust to meet the demand. Your body reacts by preparing itself to take some action: Your heart rate increases, your blood pressure rises, your neck and shoulder muscles tense, your breathing becomes more rapid, your digestion slows, your mouth becomes dry, and you may begin sweating. These are signals of "stress."

- Why does this happen? To take an action, your muscles need to be supplied with oxygen and energy. Your rate of breathing increases in an effort to inhale as much oxygen as possible and to get rid of as much carbon dioxide as possible. Your heart rate increases to deliver the oxygen and nutrients to the muscles. Furthermore, physiological processes that are not immediately necessary, such as the digestion of food and the body's natural immune responses, are slowed down. Strangely enough, these things happen even when you do not need more oxygen, such as when you are afraid or anxious.

- How long will these responses last? In general, these responses are present only until the stressful event passes. Then your body returns to its normal level of functioning. Sometimes, though, your body does not return to its former comfortable level. If the stress is present for any length of time, your body begins adapting to this stress. This adaptation can contribute to other problems, such as hypertension, shortness of breath, or muscle and joint pain.

Common Types of Stressors

Regardless of the type of stressor, the changes in the body are the same. Stressors, however, are not completely independent of one another. In fact, one stressor can often lead to other types of stressors or even magnify the effects of existing stressors. Several stressors can also occur simultaneously. This is much the same as the "vicious cycle" described in Chapter 1. Let us look now at some of the more common sources and types of stress.

- **Physical stressors.** The physical stressors can range from something as pleasant as picking up your grandchild for the first time, to grocery shopping, to the physical symptoms of your chronic illness. The one thing these three stressors have in common is that they all increase your body's demand for energy. If your body is not prepared to deal with this demand, the results may range from sore muscles to fatigue to a worsening of some disease symptoms.

- **Mental and emotional stressors.** The mental and emotional stressors can range from pleasant to uncomfortable. The joys you experience from seeing a child get married or meeting new friends induce the same stress response in the body as feeling frustrated or worried because of your illness. While it seems strange that this is true, the difference comes in the way the stress is perceived by your brain.

- **Environmental stressors.** The environmental stressors can also be both good and bad. These stressors may be as varied as a sunny day, uneven sidewalks that make it difficult to walk, loud noises, bad weather, a snoring spouse, or secondhand smoke.

Isn't "Good Stress" a Contradiction?

As we mentioned earlier, some types of stress can be good, such as a job promotion, a wedding, a vacation, a new friendship, or a new baby. These stressors make you feel good, but still cause the physiological changes in your body that were discussed above. Another example of a "good stressor" is exercise.

When you exercise, or do any type of physical activity, there is a demand placed on the body. The heart has to work harder to deliver blood to the muscles; the lungs are working harder, and you breathe more rapidly to keep up with your muscles' demand for oxygen. Meanwhile, your muscles are working hard to keep up with the signals from your brain, which are telling them to keep moving.

As you maintain an exercise program for several weeks, you will begin to notice a change: What once seemed virtually impossible is now relatively simple. Your body has adapted to this stress. In addition, there is less strain on your heart, lungs, and other muscles to do this extra work. They've become more efficient, and you have become more fit.

Recognizing When You Feel Stressed

Everyone has a certain need for stress. It helps your life run more efficiently. As long as you do not go past the "breaking point," stress is helpful. On some days you can tolerate more stress than on others. But sometimes, if you are not aware of the different types of stress, you can go beyond this breaking point and feel like your life is completely out of control. Often it is difficult to recognize when you are under too much stress. Some warning signs include

- Biting your nails, pulling your hair, tapping your foot, or other repetitive habits;

- Grinding your teeth or clenching your jaw;

- Tension in your head, neck, or shoulders;

- Feelings of anxiousness, nervousness, helplessness, or irritability; and

- Frequent accidents or forgetting things you usually don't forget.

Sometimes, you can catch yourself when you are behaving or feeling these ways. If you do, take a few minutes to think about what it is that is making you feel tense. Take a few deep breaths and try to relax. (Some relaxation methods are presented in Chapter 5.)

Let us now examine some tools for dealing with stress.

Dealing with Stress

USE PROBLEM SOLVING

There are some situations that you recognize as stressful, such as being stuck in traffic, going on a trip, or preparing a meal. First, look as objectively as possible at what it is about the particular situation that is stressful. Is it that you hate to be late? Are trips stressful because of the uncertainty involved with your destination? Does meal preparation involve too many steps and demand too much energy?

Once you have decided on the problem, begin looking for possible ways to reduce the stress. Can you leave earlier? Can you let someone else drive? Can you call someone at your destination site and ask about wheelchair access, local mass transit, and so on? Can you prepare food in the morning? Can you take a short nap in the early afternoon?

After you have identified some possible solutions, select one to try the next time you are in this situation. Don't forget to evaluate the results. (This is the problem-solving approach that was discussed in Chapter 2.)

MANAGING THE STRESS

While you can successfully manage some types of stress by modifying the situation, other types of stress seem to sneak up on you when you don't expect them. The approach to dealing with this type of stress also involves problem solving.

If you know that certain situations will be stressful, develop ways to deal with them before they happen. Try to rehearse, in your mind, what you will do when the situation arises so that you will be ready. Inherent in this approach is the ability to listen to and recognize your body's signals that the tension and stress are building. The better you become at listening and understanding your body signals, the better you'll become at managing your stress and stressful situations.

Certain chemicals you may consume can also increase stress. These chemicals include nicotine, alcohol, and caffeine. Although some people tend to smoke a cigarette, drink a glass of wine, eat chocolate, or drink a cup of coffee to soothe their tension, this, in fact, actually increases the body's stress response. Eliminating or cutting down on these stressors can leave you feeling calmer.

There are also techniques where you use your mind to deal with stress. These are discussed in the next chapter. They include self-talk, progressive muscle relaxation, guided imagery, and visualization. We will discuss these in the next chapter.

Some additional ways to deal with stress include getting enough sleep, exercising, and eating well. These are also discussed in other chapters of this book. Sometimes stress is so overwhelming that these tools are not enough. This is the time good self-managers use consultants such as counselors, social workers, psychologists, or psychiatrists.

In summary, stress, like every other symptom, has many causes and therefore can be managed in many different ways. It is up to you to examine the problem and try those solutions that meet your needs and lifestyle.

SHORTNESS OF BREATH

Shortness of breath, like fatigue and stress, can be related to several factors. In all cases, your body is not getting the oxygen it needs. The difference comes in the types of physiological changes that take place as the result of a chronic illness. These changes can lead to an increased sensitivity to different stimuli, such as walking uphill or secondhand smoke. (Before reading further about shortness of breath, you may wish to turn to Chapter 15, which discusses normal lung functioning, as well as changes that take place in the lungs with chronic lung disease.) Some of the most common changes that can take place are discussed below.

Damage to the air sacs in the lungs, as occurs with emphysema, causes the lungs to be less efficient at getting oxygen into the blood and carbon dioxide out. While the body can adjust to this change to some extent, when there is a sudden change in the "normal" breathing pattern, the lungs cannot always keep up.

Narrowing of the airways to the air sacs and excess mucus production are associated with chronic bronchitis. Because the airways become narrowed, there is less room for air to flow through them to get to the lungs. Therefore, your body receives less oxygen.

People with asthma have problems similar to those of chronic bronchitis. One difference between these two diseases is that with asthma, the narrowing of the airways, coupled with an increase in mucus production, is in response to some sort of stimulus.

People with heart disease can also experience problems with shortness of breath, but for different reasons. With heart disease, the heart becomes less efficient at pumping blood throughout the body. If there is a sudden change in the demand for oxygen by the body, the heart has to work harder to deliver this oxygen. Because the heart cannot work hard enough to meet the oxygen needs of the body, a person can feel short of breath, as the breathing rate speeds up to try to meet these needs. This increase in the breathing rate can make a person feel even more short of breath.

People who are overweight can experience shortness of breath because the added weight increases the amount of energy, and therefore oxygen, required by the body to do even simple tasks. This also increases the workload for the heart. If obesity is coupled with chronic lung disease or heart disease, there is added difficulty in supplying the body with the oxygen it needs.

Deconditioning of muscles can also lead to shortness of breath. This deconditioning process can affect the breathing muscles or any of the other muscles in your body. When muscles become deconditioned, they are less efficient in doing what they are supposed to do, so they require more energy (and oxygen) to perform activities than do well-conditioned muscles. In the case of the breathing muscles, the problem is complicated by muscle deconditioning because clearing the lungs becomes less efficient. This leaves less space for fresh air to be inhaled.

Just as there are many causes of shortness of breath, there are many things you can do to manage this problem.

When you feel short of breath, don't stop what you are doing or hurry up to finish, but slow down. If shortness of breath continues, then stop for a few minutes. If you are still short of breath, take your medication, if it has been prescribed by your doctor. Often, shortness of breath is frightening, and this fear can cause two additional problems. First, the hormones that fear itself can release may cause more shortness of breath. Second, fear may cause you to stop your activity and thus never build up the endurance necessary to help your breathing. The basic rule is to take things slowly and in steps.

Increase your activity level gradually, generally not by more than 25% each week. Thus, if you are now able to garden comfortably for 20 minutes, next week increase it by a maximum of 5 minutes. Once you can garden comfortably for 25 minutes, you can again add a few more minutes.

Don't smoke, and equally important, avoid smokers. This may sometimes be difficult, because smoking friends may not realize how difficult they are making your life. Your job is to tell them. Explain that their smoke is causing breathing problems for you and that you would appreciate it if they would not smoke when you are around. Also, make your house and especially your car "No Smoking" zones. Ask people to smoke outside.

Use your medications and oxygen as prescribed by your doctor. We are constantly being bombarded by messages that drugs are bad and not to be used. In many cases, this is correct. However, when you have a chronic disease, drugs can be, and often are, life savers.

Don't try to skimp, cut down, or go without. Likewise, more is not better, so don't take more than the prescribed amount of medication(s). Drugs, taken as prescribed, can make all the difference. This may mean using medications even when you are not having symptoms. This also means resisting the temptation to take more of the medication if the prescribed amount does not seem to be working. If you have questions about your medications or feel they are not working for you, discuss these concerns with your doctor before you stop taking the medication or take more than has been prescribed. Preventing problems before they start is much better than having to manage the problems.

Drink plenty of fluids if mucus and secretions are a problem, unless your doctor has advised you to restrict your fluid intake. This will help to thin the mucus and, therefore, make it easier to cough up. The use of a humidifier may also be helpful.

Breathing Control

Diaphragmatic breathing is also called breathing control and belly breathing. As mentioned earlier, one of the problems that causes shortness of breath, especially for people with emphysema, chronic bronchitis, or asthma, is deconditioning of the diaphragm and breathing muscles. When this deconditioning occurs, the lungs are not able to function properly. That is, they do not fill well, nor do they get rid of old air.

Diaphragmatic breathing or controlled breathing requires a little practice to master. Diaphragmatic breathing strengthens the breathing muscles. Strengthening these muscles makes them more efficient, so less effort is needed to breathe. The following are the steps for diaphragmatic breathing:

1. Lie on your back with pillows under your head and knees.

2. Place one hand on your stomach (at the base of your breastbone) and the other hand on your upper chest.

3. Inhale slowly through your nose, allowing your stomach to expand outward. Imagine that your lungs are filling with fresh air. The hand on your stomach should move upward, and the hand on your chest should not move or should move only slightly.

4. Breathe out slowly, through pursed lips. At the same time, use your hand to gently push inward and upward on your abdomen.

5. Practise this technique for 10 to 15 minutes, three or four times a day, until it becomes automatic. If you begin to feel a little dizzy, rest.

Once you feel comfortable doing this, you may wish to place a light weight on your abdomen. This will help to further strengthen the muscles used to inhale. Start with a weight of about one pound, like a book or a bag of rice or beans. Gradually increase the weight as your muscle strength improves. You can also practise diaphragmatic breathing while sitting in a chair:

- Relax your shoulders, arms, hands, and chest. Do not grip the arms of the chair or your knees.

- Put one hand on your abdomen and the other on your chest.

- Breathe in through your nose—filling the area around your waist with air. Your chest hand should remain still and the hand on your abdomen should move.

- Breathe out without force or effort.

Once you are comfortable with this technique, you can practise it almost anytime, while laying down, sitting, standing, or walking. Diaphragmatic breathing can help strengthen and improve the coordination and efficiency of the breathing muscles, as well as decrease the amount of energy needed to breathe. In addition, it can be used with any of the relaxation techniques that use the power of your mind to manage your symptoms (described in Chapter 5).

A second technique, pursed-lip breathing, usually happens naturally for people who have problems emptying their lungs. It can also be used if you are short of breath or breathless.

- Purse your lips as if blowing across a flute or into a whistle.

- Use diaphragmatic breathing (breathing control). Breathe out through pursed lips without any force.

- Remember to relax the upper chest, shoulders, arms, and hand while breathing out. Check for tension.

- Breathing out should take longer than breathing in.

By mastering this technique while doing other activities, you will be better able to manage your shortness of breath.

Here are two techniques that may be helpful for removing secretions (mucus, phlegm).

HUFF

This technique combines one or two forced huffs with diaphragmatic breathing (breathing control). It is useful for removing secretions from small airways.

- Take in a breath as you would do for diaphragmatic breathing.

- Hold your breath for a moment.

- Huff—keep your mouth open while squeezing your chest and abdominal muscles to force out the air (this is a little like panting).

- If possible, do another huff before taking in another breath.

- Take two or three diaphragmatic breaths.

- Huff once or twice.

CONTROLLED COUGH

This helps to remove secretions (phlegm) from larger airways.

- Take in a full, slow breath (diaphragmatic breath).

- Keep shoulders and hand relaxed.

- Hold the breath for a moment.

- Cough (tighten the abdominal muscles and force the air out).

Positions That Will Help If You Are Breathless or Short of Breath

Lying

Forward lean sitting

Standing

Forward lean standing

Note: If you you have a bout of uncontrolled coughing, this may help:

- Avoid very dry air or steam.

- Swallow as soon as the bout starts.

- Sip water.

- Suck lozenges or hard candy.

- Try diaphragmatic breathing, being sure to breathe in through your nose.

PAIN/PHYSICAL DISCOMFORT

Pain or physical discomfort is a problem shared by many people with chronic illness. In fact, for many people, this is their number one concern. As with most symptoms of chronic illness, this pain or discomfort can have many causes. The five most common causes are

- **The disease itself.** Pain can come from inflammation, damage in or around joints and tissues, insufficient blood supply to the heart, or trapped nerves, to name just a few sources.

- **Tense muscles.** When something hurts, the muscles in that area become tense. This is your body's natural reaction to pain—to try to protect the damaged area. When muscles are tensed for a period of time, lactic acid builds up in the muscles, which can also cause soreness or pain.

- **Muscle deconditioning.** With chronic disease, it is common to become less active, leading to a weakening of the muscles, or muscle deconditioning. When a muscle is weak, it tends to complain any time it is used. This is why even the slightest activity can sometimes lead to pain and stiffness.

- **Lack of sleep or poor-quality sleep.** Pain often interferes with the ability to get either enough sleep or good-quality sleep. This, in turn, can make pain worse, as well as lessen your ability to cope with it.

- **Stress, anxiety, and emotions such as depression, anger, fear, and frustration.** These are all normal responses to living with a chronic condition, and they can affect your perception of the pain or discomfort. When we are stressed, angry, afraid, or depressed, everything, including the pain, seems worse.

- **Medications.** The medicine you are taking can sometimes cause pain or discomfort. If you suspect this, talk with your doctor.

Because the pain comes from many sources, the methods we use to manage or reduce this pain must be aimed at all of those that apply. The use of medications can help with some of the disease pain. For example, medications can help open blood vessels and bronchial tubes. Other medications may reduce pain caused by inflammation.

With chronic disease, painkillers, such as narcotics, are generally not useful. Furthermore, narcotics can be dangerous for people with impaired respiratory function, because these drugs slow down the breathing rate, making existing breathing problems worse. Painkillers also tend to be less effective over time and are usually addictive. Since chronic disease is long-term and the associated pain can also be long-term, the potential for addiction to high doses of painkillers is greatly increased.

Two of the best ways to deal with pain are the use of exercise and symptom management techniques that use your mind, such as relaxation and visualization. The benefits of exercise as well as tips for starting an exercise program are discussed in Chapters 6 through 9. Using your mind to manage symptoms is discussed in Chapter 5.

In addition to exercise and techniques that use your mind, there are several other methods that are sometimes useful for localized pain. These include the use of heat, cold, and massage. These three applications work by stimulating the skin and other tissues surrounding the painful area, which in turn increases the blood flow to these areas.

Stimulation with heat can be done by applying a heating pad or by taking a warm bath or shower (with the water flow directed at the painful area). You can make a heating "pad" by placing rice or dry beans in a sock, knotting the top of the sock, and placing it in a microwave oven for 3 to 4 minutes. Before use, be sure to test the heat so as not to burn yourself. Do not use popcorn. Some people, however, prefer cold for soothing pain, especially if there is inflammation. A bag of frozen peas or corn makes an inexpensive, reusable cold pack. Whether using heat or cold, limit the application to 15 or 20 minutes at a time.

Massage is one of the oldest forms of pain management. Hippocrates (c. 460–380 B.C.) said, "Physicians must be experienced in many things, but assuredly also in the rubbing that can bind a joint that is loose and loosen a joint that is too hard." Self-massage is a simple procedure that can be performed with little practice or preparation. It stimulates the skin, underlying tissues, and muscles with applied pressure. Some people like to use a mentholated cream with self-massage because it also gives a cooling effect.

Massage, while relatively simple, is not appropriate for all cases of pain. Do not use self-massage for a "hot joint" (one that is red, swollen, and hot to the touch) or an infected area or if you are suffering from phlebitis, thrombophlebitis, or skin eruptions.

If pain continues to have a major influence on your life, you might ask for a referral to a pain management clinic.

ITCHING

Of all the symptoms one may have, itching is one of the most difficult to understand and is even harder to define. Basically, itching is any sensation that causes an urge to scratch. Itching, like other symptoms, can have many different causes. Some of these we understand, such as the itching caused by the release of histamines that irritate nerve endings. This happens when you get an insect bite or come in contact with a substance such as poison ivy or poison oak. People with liver diseases may also experience itching that is caused by the deposit of bile products in the skin when the liver is damaged and cannot function properly to remove them. There is, however, no association between the amount of bile products deposited and the amount of itching that one may experience. In kidney disease, itching may be severe, but the exact cause is not clear. There are also other conditions, such as psoriasis, where the causes of itching are not easily explained. We do know that other factors such as warmth, wool clothing, and stress can make itching worse. The following are some ways that may help you relieve your itching. Before trying any remedies, however, it is important to ask a doctor about your itching, to be certain you know what is causing it.

Moisture

Dry skin tends to be itchy; therefore, it is important to keep the skin moisturized by applying moisturizing creams several times a day. When you choose a moisturizer, be careful. Just because a product is advertised as a moisturizer does not necessarily mean it is. Be sure to read the list of ingredients when buying a cream or lotion. Avoid products that contain alcohol or any other ingredient that ends in "ol," which is usually some variation of alcohol. These types of ingredients actually tend to dry the skin, rather than moisturize it. In general, the greasier the product, the better it works as a moisturizer. Creams are better moisturizers than lotions, and products such as Vaseline, olive oil, or vegetable shortening are also very effective.

When taking a bath or shower, use warm water and soak for not less than 10 or more than 20 minutes. You also may want to add bath oil, baking soda, or "Sulzberger's household bath oil" to the water. This household bath oil is made from 2 teaspoons of olive oil and a large glass of milk, which is added to the bath. When you get out of the water, pat yourself dry immediately and apply your cream.

If your itching is caused by the release of histamines during an allergic reaction or from having had contact with an irritating substance, it is important to wash off the oils or offending agent, apply cold compresses, and take an antihistamine.

During cold weather it can be especially difficult to deal with the itching because indoor heating tends to dry the skin. If this is a problem for you, the use of a humidifier might help. Also, try to keep your home and office as cool as you can without being uncomfortable.

Clothing

The type of clothing you wear can also add to the itching sensations; therefore, it is important to select the appropriate clothing. Obviously, the best rule of thumb is to wear what is comfortable. This is usually clothing made from material that is not scratchy. Most people find that natural fibres such as cotton allow the skin to "breathe" better and are the least irritating to the skin.

Medications

Antihistamines will help if your itching is caused by the release of histamines. You can buy many of these products over the counter. They include diphenhydramine and triprolidine.

You can also buy creams that help to soothe the nerve endings by cooling or numbing the skin, which contain menthol, camphor, benzyl alcohol, or pramoxine. However, be careful, because some people can have allergic reactions to these creams. Capsaicin creams can also help itching, although they will cause a burning sensation. Steroid creams can also help control some types of itching. These are creams that contain cortisone or other steroids.

If you are confused about what over-the-counter products to buy, ask your doctor or pharmacist.

With the exception of moisturizing creams, no cream should be used on a long-term basis without talking to your doctor. If your itching continues with use of these over-the-counter products, you may want to talk to your doctor about trying the stronger prescription versions of these medications.

Stress

Anything that you can do to reduce the stress in your life will also help reduce the itching. We have already discussed some of the ways to deal with stress earlier in this chapter, and there are some other techniques described in Chapter 5 (Using Your Mind to Manage Symptoms).

Scratching

While our natural tendency is to scratch what itches, this really does not help, especially for chronic itching. Rather, it leads to a vicious cycle whereby the more you scratch, the more you tend to itch. Unfortunately, it is hard to resist scratching. However, you might try rubbing, pressing, or patting the skin when you feel the need to scratch. If you are not able to break this cycle yourself, consult a dermatologist, who may be able to help you find alternative ways to control the itching.

Itching is a common and, undoubtedly, a very frustrating symptom for both patients and physicians to manage. When the self-management tips described here do not seem to help, it may be time to utilize the help of a physician. Often he or she can offer some prescription medications that can help with some specific types of itching. Also, if you are interested in learning more about itching, we recommend the book written for physicians titled *Itch Mechanisms and Management of Pruritus* by Jeffrey D. Bernard (McGraw-Hill, 1994). You might also recommend this book to your doctor.

ANGER—"WHY ME?"

Anger is one of the most common responses to chronic illness. The uncertainty and unpredictability of living with a chronic disease threatens what you have fought all your life to achieve—independence and control. The loss of control over your body and loss of independence in life create feelings of frustration, helplessness, and hopelessness, all of which fuel the anger. In fact, at various times during the course of your illness, you may find yourself asking, "Why me?" You may wonder what you did to deserve this or why God is punishing you. All of these are normal anger responses to chronic disease.

You may be angry with yourself, family, friends, health care providers, God, or the world in general—all for a variety of reasons. For example, you may be angry at yourself for not taking better care of yourself when you were younger. You may be angry at your family and friends because they don't do things the way you would like them done. Or you might be angry at your doctor because he or she cannot "fix" your problems. Sometimes your anger may be misplaced, as when you find yourself yelling at the cat or dog. Misplaced anger is quite common, especially if you are not even aware that you are angry or why.

Sometimes, the anger is not just a response to having a chronic illness, but is actually the result of the disease process itself. For example, if someone has suffered a stroke that affected a certain part of the brain, that person's ability to express or suppress emotions may be affected. Thus, some people who have had strokes may appear to cry inappropriately or have flares in temper.

Recognizing (or admitting) that you are angry and identifying why, or with whom, are important steps to learning how to manage your anger effectively. This task also involves finding constructive ways to express your anger. If not expressed, the anger becomes unhealthy. It can build up until it becomes explosive and offends others, or is turned inward, thereby intensifying the experience of other disease symptoms like depression.

There are several things that you can do to help manage your anger. One important way is to learn how to communicate your anger verbally, preferably without blaming or offending others. This can be done by learning to use "I" (rather than "you") messages to express your feelings. (Refer to Chapter 10 for a discussion of "I" messages.) However, if you choose to express your anger verbally, know that many people will not be able to help you. Most of us are not very good at, or comfortable with, dealing with angry people, even if the anger is justified. Therefore, you may also find it useful to seek counselling or join a support group. Community organizations such as the Canadian Mental Health Association, Family Services, or Ministry/Department of Health clinics, or your Employee Assistance Plan may be useful for you in this area.

Another way to deal with anger is to modify your expectations. You have done this throughout your life. For example, as a child you thought you could become anything—a fireman, a ballet dancer, a doctor, etc. As you grew older, however, you reevaluated these expectations, along with your capabilities, talents, and interests. Based on this reevaluation, you modified your plans.

This same process can be used to deal with the effects of chronic illness on your life. For example, it may be unrealistic to expect that you will get "all better." However, it is realistic to expect that you can still do many pleasurable things. You have the ability to affect the progress of your illness, by slowing its decline or preventing it from becoming worse.

Changing your expectations can help you to change your perspective. Instead of dwelling on the 10% of things you can no longer do, think about the 90% of things you still can do. You may even be able to find new activities or hobbies to replace those old ones. Developing a more positive attitude and positive self-talk can also help to change your perspective; this is discussed more in the next chapter.

Anger can also be channelled through new activities, such as exercise, writing, music, or painting. Some people find these to be extremely therapeutic outlets for this emotion.

In short, anger is a normal response to having a chronic condition. Part of learning to manage the condition involves acknowledging this anger and finding constructive ways to deal with it.

DEPRESSION

Depression can be a scary word. Some people prefer saying that they are "sad," "blue," or "feeling down." Whatever you call it, depression is a normal reaction to chronic illness.

Sometimes it is not easy to recognize when you are depressed. Even more difficult is recognizing when you may be becoming depressed and then catching yourself before you fall into a deep depression. Just as there are many degrees of pain, there are different degrees of depression. If your disease is a significant problem in your life, you almost certainly have or have had some problems with depression. Depression is felt by everyone at some time. It is how you handle it that makes the difference.

While there are many signs of depression, which will be discussed later in this section, there are also several emotions that can lead to depression. These include the following:

- **Fear, anxiety, and/or uncertainty about the future.** Whether these feelings result from worries about finances, the disease process, treatment, or your family, these issues can lead to depression if they are not addressed by you and those involved. Chapter 19 deals with some decisions all of us will have to make at some time in our lives. By confronting these issues early on, both you and your family will have less time to worry about them and more time to enjoy life.

- **Frustration can have any number of causes.** You may find yourself thinking, "I just can't do what I want," "I feel so helpless," "I used to be able to do this myself," or "Why doesn't anyone understand me?" Feelings like these can leave you feeling more alone and isolated the longer you hold on to them.

- **Loss of control over your life.** Whether it comes from having to rely on medications to ease symptoms, having to see a doctor on a regular basis, or having to count on others to help you perform daily activities such as bathing, dressing, and preparing meals, this feeling of losing control can make you lose faith in yourself and your abilities. Instead of being an individual sport, your life has suddenly become a team sport. You need help to play, but you can still be the coach.

While these feelings have been described separately, they are often experienced in combination, making it more difficult to determine what is really at the root of the depression. Also, we often do not recognize when we are depressed, or we do not wish to admit to ourselves that we are actually depressed.

The following are 13 common signs of depression. Learning to recognize the signs of depression is the first step in learning how to manage it.

1. **Loss of interest in friends or activities.** Not wanting to talk to anyone or to answer the phone or doorbell—in short, isolation—is an important symptom of depression.

2. **Difficulty sleeping, changed sleeping patterns, interrupted sleep, or sleeping more than usual.** Often, going to sleep easily but awakening and being unable to return to sleep becomes a problem.

3. **Change in eating habits.** This change may range from a loss of interest in food to unusually erratic or excessive eating.

4. **Unintentional weight change.** Either a gain or loss of more than 5 kilograms in a short period of time. (This can also be a sign of physical illness and should be checked out by your doctor.)

5. **Loss of interest in personal care and grooming.**

6. **A general feeling of unhappiness lasting longer than six weeks.**

7. **Loss of interest in being held or in sex.** Sometimes these problems can be due to medication side effects, so it is important that you talk them over with your doctor.

8. **Suicidal thoughts.** If your unhappiness has caused you to think about killing yourself, get some help from your doctor, good friends, a member of the clergy, a psychologist, or a social worker. These feelings will pass and you will feel better, so get help and don't let a tragedy happen to you and your loved ones.

9. **Frequent accidents.** Watch for a pattern of increased carelessness, accidents while walking or driving, dropping things, and so forth. Of course, you must take into account the physical problems caused by your disease, such as unsteady balance or slowed reaction times, which could also account for some accidents.

10. **Low self-image.** A feeling of worthlessness, a negative image of your body, and wondering if it is all worth it.

11. **Frequent arguments or increased irritability.** A tendency to blow up easily over minor matters, over things that never bothered you before.

12. **Loss of energy.** Fatigue; feeling tired all the time.

13. **Inability to make decisions.** Feeling confused and unable to concentrate.

Here is a quick test for depression. Ask yourself what you do to have fun. If you do not have a quick answer, suspect that you may have some type of depression.

Not all depression behaviour is negative. Sometimes unrealistic "cheeriness" will mask what the person is really feeling, and the wise observer will recognize the brittleness or "phoniness" of the mood. Refusal to accept offers of help, even in the face of obvious need for it, is a frequent symptom of unrecognized depression.

Depression behaviour tends to be excessive in one direction or another from what would be considered normal for that individual.

The paradox of depression-related behaviour is that the more you engage in the behaviour, the more likely it is that you will ultimately drive away the people who are most able to provide the comfort and support that the depressed person needs. Most of our friends and family want to help us feel better, but often they don't really know what to do to help. As their efforts to comfort and reassure us are frustrated, they may at some point throw up their hands and quit trying. Then the depressed person winds up saying "See, nobody cares," thus reinforcing the feelings of loss and loneliness.

Some of these signs of depression may seem familiar to you. Whether you've experienced these feelings in the past or are currently experiencing one or more of them, depression is a very real and common symptom associated with chronic illness.

Having a chronic illness while living alone can be very depressing. Although this is not a matter of dictating how you should or should not feel, being depressed is not pleasant, and depression is something that can be managed. In fact, there are at least a dozen things you can do to change the situation. But if you are depressed, you may not feel like making the effort to do so. Force yourself or get someone to help you into action. Find someone to talk with.

Here are 14 things you can do:

1. If you feel like hurting yourself or someone else, call your mental health centre, doctor, suicide prevention centre, friend, spiritual counsellor, or senior centre. Do not delay. Do it now. Often, just talking with an understanding person or health professional will be enough to help you through this mood.

2. Are you taking tranquillizers such as meprobamate, diazepam, and chlordiazepoxide, or narcotic painkillers such as codeine, morphine, sleeping medications, or other "downers"? These drugs intensify depression, and the sooner you can stop taking them, the better off you will be. Your depression may be a drug side effect. If you are not sure what you are taking or are uncertain if what you're experiencing could be a side effect, check with a doctor or pharmacist. Before discontinuing a prescription medication, always check, at least by phone, with the prescribing physician, as there may be important reasons for continuing its use or there may be withdrawal reactions. Please note that there are drugs that help depression and are taken over months or years. Talk to your doctor about these.

3. Are you drinking alcohol in order to feel better? Alcohol is also a downer. There is virtually no way to escape depression unless you unload these negative influences from your brain. For most people, one or two drinks in the evening is not a problem, but if your mind is not free of alcohol during most of the day, you are having trouble with this drug. Talk this over with your doctor or call Alcoholics Anonymous.

4. Continue your daily activities. Get dressed every day, make your bed, get out of the house, go shopping, walk your dog. Plan and cook meals. Force yourself to do these things even if you don't feel like it.

5. Visit with friends, call them on the phone, plan to go to the movies or on other outings. Do it!

6. Join a group. Get involved in a church group, a discussion group at a senior center, a community college class, a self-help class, or a senior nutrition program. If you can't get out, consider a group on the Internet. If you do this, be sure the Internet group is moderated, that is, someone is in charge to enforce the rules of the group.

7. Volunteer. People who help other people are seldom depressed.

8. Make plans and carry them out. Look to the future. Plant some young trees. Look forward to your grandchildren's graduation from college even if your own kids are in high school.

If you know that one time of the year is especially difficult, such as Christmas or a birthday, make specific plans for that period. Don't wait to see what happens. Be prepared.

9. Don't move to a new setting without first visiting for a few weeks and learning about the resources available to you in this new community. Moving can be a sign of withdrawal, and depression often intensifies when you are in a location away from friends and acquaintances. Besides, many types of troubles usually move with you, whereas the support you may need to deal with them effectively does not.

10. Take a vacation with relatives or friends. A vacation can be as simple as a few days in a nearby city or a resort just a few miles down the road. Rather than go alone, look into trips sponsored by colleges, city recreation departments, the "Y," senior centers, or church groups. Many people have found that Elder Hostel programs offer a vacation, as well as opportunities to expand your knowledge of an interesting topic and to make new friends.

11. Do 20 to 30 minutes of physical activity or exercise every day.

12. Make a list of self-rewards. Take care of yourself. You can reward yourself by reading at a set time, seeing a special play, or doing anything else, big or small, that you can look forward to during the day.

13. Use positive self-talk. This cognitive technique is a very powerful weapon against depression. See Chapter 5 for more information on self-talk.

14. Seek professional help. Often some "talk therapy" and/or the proper medications can go a long way toward relieving depression. Seeking professional help and/or taking medications are not signs of weakness. They are signs of strength.

Depression feeds on depression, so break the cycle. The success of your self-management program depends on it. Depression is not permanent, and you can hasten its disappearance. Focus on your pride, your friends, your future goals, and your positive surroundings. How you respond to depression can be a self-fulfilling prophecy. When you believe that things will get better, they will.

SLEEP PROBLEMS

Sleep is a time during which the body can concentrate on healing. Minimal amounts of energy are required to maintain body functioning when we sleep. When we do not get enough sleep, we can experience a variety of other symptoms, such as fatigue and a lack of concentration. But this does not mean that fatigue or lack of concentration are always caused by a lack of sleep. Remember, the symptoms associated with chronic disease can have many causes. If you have noticed a change in your sleep patterns, then the fatigue you are experiencing may be, at least in part, related to your problems with sleep. Some tricks to help you get a good night's sleep follow.

Before you even get into bed:

- **Get a comfortable bed** that allows for ease of movement and good body support. This usually means a good-quality, firm mattress that supports the spine and does not allow the body to stay in the middle of the bed. A bed board, made of half-inch to three-quarter-inch (1 or 2 cm) plywood, can be placed between the mattress and the box spring to increase the firmness.

- **Heated waterbeds or airbeds** are helpful for some people with arthritis, because they support weight evenly by conforming to the body's shape. Other people can find them very uncomfortable. If you are interested, try one out at a friend's home or a hotel for a few nights to decide if it is right for you. An electric blanket or mattress pad, set on low heat, or a wool mattress pad are other effective ways of providing heat while sleeping, especially on cool or damp nights. If you decide to use electric bedding, be sure to follow the instructions carefully.

- **Find a comfortable sleeping position.** The best position depends on you and your condition. Sometimes the use of small pillows placed in the right places can relieve pain and discomfort. Experiment with different positions and the use of pillows. Also, check with your health care provider for specific recommendations given your condition.

- **Elevate the head of the bed** on wooden blocks a total of four to six inches to make breathing easier. This same effect can be accomplished by the use of pillows that elevate the chest, shoulders, and head. This is especially helpful if you have heartburn or gastric reflux.

- **Keep the room at a comfortable, warm temperature.**

- **Use a vaporizer if you live where the air is dry.** Warm, moist air often makes breathing easier, leaving you with one less thing to worry about when trying to fall asleep.

- **Make your bedroom a place in which you feel safe and comfortable.** Keep a lamp and telephone by your bed, within easy reach.

- **If you are nearsighted and wear glasses or contact lenses, keep a pair of glasses by the bed when you go to sleep.** This way, in case you need to get up in the middle of the night, you can easily put on your glasses and see where you are going!

Things to avoid before bedtime:

- **Avoid eating.** While you may feel sleepy after eating a big meal, this is no way to help you fall asleep and get a good night's sleep. Sleep is supposed to allow your body time to rest and recover, and when you eat, this takes valuable time away from this healing process. Since going to sleep feeling hungry may also keep you awake, try drinking a glass of warm milk at bedtime.

- **Avoid alcohol.** Contrary to the popular belief that alcohol helps you to sleep better because it makes you feel more relaxed, alcohol actually disrupts your sleep cycle. Alcohol before bedtime can lead to shallow and fragmented sleep, as well as frequent awakenings throughout the night.

- **Avoid caffeine late in the day.** Caffeine is a stimulant, and it can keep you awake. This includes coffee, some types of teas, colas and other sodas, and chocolate.

- **Avoid eating foods with MSG (monosodium glutamate) late in the day.** Although Chinese food often has been singled out as containing MSG (in fact, it usually does not), many other types of food, especially pre-packaged foods, may contain this food additive. Before purchasing a pre-packaged meal, be sure to read the ingredient label to make sure it does not contain monosodium glutamate. In Asian restaurants ask if they use MSG.

- **Avoid smoking to help you sleep.** Aside from the fact that smoking itself can cause complications and a worsening of your chronic disease, falling asleep with a lit cigarette can be a fire hazard. Additionally, the nicotine contained in cigarettes is a stimulant.

- **Avoid diet pills.** Diet pills often contain stimulants, which may interfere with falling asleep as well as staying asleep.

- **Avoid sleeping pills.** While the name "sleeping pills" sounds like the perfect solution for sleep problems, they tend to become less effective over time. Also, many sleeping pills have a rebound effect—that is, if you stop taking them, it is more difficult to get to sleep. Thus, as they become less effective, you can have even more problems than you had when you first started taking the sleeping pills. All in all, it is best to avoid using sleeping pills if at all possible.

- **Avoid diuretics (water pills) before bedtime.** You may want to take them in the morning so that your sleep is not interrupted so often by the need to go to the bathroom. Unless your doctor has recommended otherwise, don't reduce the overall amount of fluids you drink, as these are important for your health. However, you may want to limit your fluid intake right before you go to bed.

Develop a routine:

- **Set up and maintain a regular rest and sleep schedule.** That is, go to bed at the same time every night and get up at the same time every morning. If you wish to take a nap, take one in the afternoon, but do not take a nap after dinner. Stay awake until you are ready to go to bed.

- **If your sleep schedule is way off the norm (for example, you go to bed at 4 a.m. and sleep until noon), reset your sleep clock.** To do so, try going to bed one hour earlier or later each day until you reach the hour you want to go to sleep. This may sound strange, but it seems to be the best way to reset your sleep clock.

- **Exercise at regular times each day.** Not only will the exercise help you obtain better-quality sleep, it will also help to set a regular pattern during your day. However, avoid exercising immediately before bedtime, as well as other activities that excite you.

- **Get out in the sun every afternoon,** even if it is only for 15 or 20 minutes.

- **Get used to doing the same things every night before going to bed.** This can be anything from watching the news, to reading a chapter of a book, to taking a warm bath. By developing and sticking to a "time to get ready for bed" routine, you will be telling your body that it's time to start winding down and relax.

- **Use your bed and your bedroom only for sleeping.** If you find that you get into bed and you can't fall asleep, get out of bed and go into another room until you begin to feel sleepy again.

"But I can't fall (back) asleep":

- Many people can get to sleep without a problem but then wake up and have the "early morning worries," where they can't turn off their minds. Then they get more worried because they cannot go back to sleep once they have awakened. Keeping your mind fully occupied will ward off the worries and help you get back to sleep. For example, try a distraction technique such as quieting your mind by counting backward from 100 by 3's or by naming a flower for every letter of the alphabet. The relaxation techniques described in the next chapter may also be helpful.

- Don't worry about not getting enough sleep. If your body needs sleep, you will sleep. Also, remember that people tend to need less sleep as they get older.

Do You Sleep "Like a Baby"?

If you fall asleep "as soon as your head hits the pillow" or fall asleep regularly in front of the TV, and are tired when you wake up in the morning, even after a full night's sleep, you may have a sleep disorder. People who have the most common sleep disorder, obstructive sleep apnea, often do not know it. When they are asked about their sleep, they respond "I sleep just fine." Sleep specialists believe that obstructive sleep apnea is very common and alarmingly underdiagnosed.

With sleep apnea, the soft tissue in the throat or nose relaxes during sleep and blocks the airway, requiring extreme effort to breathe. The person struggles against the blockage for up to a minute, then wakes just long enough to gasp air, and falls back to sleep to start the cycle all over again. The person is never aware that he or she has awakened dozens of times during the night and does not get the deep sleep needed to restore the body's energy and help with the healing process. This, in turn, leads to more symptoms such as fatigue and pain.

Sleep apnea is a serious medical problem and can be life-threatening. It has been linked to heart disease and stroke and is believed to be the cause of death for many who die in their sleep from a heart attack. Sleep experts suggest that people who are tired all the time in spite of a full night's sleep, or who find they need more sleep now than when they were younger, should be evaluated for sleep apnea or other sleep disorders, especially if they (or their spouses) report snoring.

In this chapter, we have discussed common causes for some of the more common symptoms experienced by people with different chronic conditions. In addition, we have described some actions that you can take to cope with your symptoms. Taking action to physically deal with your symptoms is necessary in coping with your illness on a day-to-day basis. But sometimes, this just doesn't seem to be enough. There are times when you may wish to escape from your surroundings and just have "your time"—a time that allows you to clear your mind, to gain a fresh perspective. The following chapter presents different ways to complement your physical-symptom management with cognitive techniques, or using the power of your mind, to help reduce and even prevent some of the symptoms you may experience.

Suggested Further Reading

Bernard, Jeffrey D. *Itch Mechanisms and Management of Pruritus.* New York: McGraw-Hill, 1994.

Carter, Les. *The Anger Trap: Free Yourself from the Frustrations That Sabotage Your Life,* 1st ed. San Francisco: Jossey-Bass, 2003.

Coren, Stanley. *Sleep Thieves.* New York: Simon & Schuster, 1997.

Caudill, Margaret. *Managing Pain Before It Manages You,* rev. ed. New York: Guilford Press, 2002.

DePaulo, J. Raymond, and Leslie Alan Horvitz. *Understanding Depression: What We Know and What You Can Do About It.* New York: Wiley, 2002.

Donoghue, Paul J., and Mary E. Siegel. *Sick and Tired of Feeling Sick and Tired: Living with Invisible Chronic Illness,* new ed. New York: Norton, 2000.

Hall, Hamilton. *A Consultation with the Back Doctor.* Toronto: McClelland & Stewart, 2003.

Hoffstein, Victor and Linde, Shirley. *No More Snoring: A Proven Program for Conquering Snoring and Sleep Apnea.* New York, Toronto: John Wiley & Sons, Inc., 1999.

Kabat-Zinn, Jon. *Coming to Our Senses: Healing Ourselves and the World Through Mindfulness,* 1st ed. New York: Hyperion, 2005.

Kabat-Zinn, Jon. *Full Catastrophe Living: Using the Wisdom of Your Body and Mind to Face Stress, Pain, and Illness.* New York: Delta Trade Paperbacks, 2005.

Klein, Donald F., and Paul H. Wender. *Understanding Depression: A Complete Guide to Its Diagnosis and Treatment*, 2nd ed. New York: Oxford University Press, 2005.

Posen, David. *The Little Book of Stress Relief.* Toronto: Key Porter Books, 2003.

Schafer, Walter E. *Stress Management for Wellness*, 4th ed. Fort Worth, TX: Harcourt College Publishers, 2000.

Worthen, Mary. *Journey Not Chosen . . . Destination Not Known: Living with Bipolar Disorder,* 2nd ed. Dallas, TX: Brown Books, 2004.

USING YOUR MIND TO MANAGE SYMPTOMS

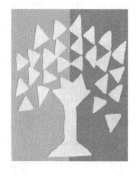

5

THERE IS GROWING SCIENTIFIC EVIDENCE THAT SHOWS A STRONG LINK BETWEEN OUR THOUGHTS, ATTITUDES, AND EMOTIONS AND OUR MENTAL AND PHYSICAL HEALTH. One of our self-managers said, "It's not always mind over matter, but mind matters." While thoughts and emotions do not directly cause our chronic conditions, they can influence the symptoms we experience. Research has shown that thoughts and emotions trigger certain hormones or other chemicals that send messages throughout the body. These messages affect how our body functions; for example, thoughts and emotions can change our heart rate, blood pressure, breathing, blood sugar levels, muscle responses, concentration, the ability to get pregnant, and even our ability to fight off other illnesses (that is, our immune response).

All of us, at one time or another, have experienced the power of the mind and its effects on the body. Both pleasant and unpleasant thoughts or emotions can cause the body to react in different ways. Our heart rate and breathing can increase or slow down; we may experience sensations such as sweating (warm or cold), blushing, tears, and so on. Sometimes just a memory or an image can create these physiological responses. For example, take a moment now and try this simple exercise. Imagine that you are holding a big, bright yellow lemon. You hold it close to your nose and smell its strong citrus aroma. Now, you bite into the lemon. It's juicy! The juice fills your mouth and dribbles down your chin. Now you begin to suck on the lemon and its tart juice. What happens? The body responds. Your mouth puckers and starts to water. You may even smell the scent of the lemon. All of these reactions are triggered by the mind and its memory of your experience with a real lemon.

These examples demonstrate the power that the mind has over the body and why we should work to develop our mental abilities to help us manage the different symptoms people with chronic conditions experience. With training and practice, we can learn to use the mind to relax the body, to reduce stress and anxiety, and to reduce the discomfort or unpleasantness caused by our physical and emotional symptoms. The mind can also greatly help to relieve the pain and shortness of breath associated with different diseases, and may even help a person depend less on the medications used to relieve some symptoms.

In this chapter we describe several ways in which you can begin to use your mind to manage symptoms. These are usually referred to as cognitive techniques because they involve the use of our thinking abilities to make changes in the body.

RELAXATION TECHNIQUES

Many of us have heard and read about relaxation, yet some of us are still confused as to what relaxation is, its benefits, and how to do it. Relaxation is not a cure-all, but it can be an effective part of a treatment plan.

There are different types of relaxation techniques, each having specific guidelines and uses. Some techniques are used only to achieve muscle relaxation, while others are aimed at reducing anxiety and emotional stress, or diverting attention, all of which aid in symptom management.

The term "relaxation" means different things to different people. We can all identify ways we relax. For example, we may walk, watch TV, listen to music, knit, or garden. These methods, however, are different from the techniques discussed in this chapter because they include some form of physical activity or require a stimulus such as music that is outside of the mind. Relaxation techniques are also different from taking a nap because we are using the mind actively to help the body achieve a relaxed state.

The goal of relaxation is to turn off the outside world so the mind and body are at rest. This allows you to reduce the tension that can increase the intensity or severity of symptoms.

Below are some guidelines to help you practise the relaxation techniques described in this chapter.

- **Pick a quiet place and time during the day** when you will not be disturbed for at least 15–20 minutes. (If this seems too long, start with 5 minutes. By the way, in some homes the only quiet place is the bathroom. This is just fine.)

- **Try to practise the technique twice daily** and not less than four times a week.

- **Don't expect miracles.** Some of these techniques take time in order for you to acquire the skill. Sometimes it takes 3–4 weeks of consistent practice before you really start to notice benefits.

- **Relaxation should be helpful.** At worst, you may find it boring, but if it is an unpleasant experience or makes you more nervous or anxious, then you might try one of the other symptom management techniques described in this chapter.

Muscle Relaxation

Muscle relaxation is one of the most commonly used cognitive techniques for symptom management. It is popular because it makes sense to us. If we are told that physical stress or muscular tension intensifies our pain, shortness of breath, or emotional distress, we will be motivated to learn how to recognize this tension and release it.

In addition, muscle relaxation is easy to learn and remember for practice in different situations. It is also one technique from which we can recognize some immediate results, such as the positive sensations of reduced pain, stress, or muscle tension and calm, normal breathing. Muscle relaxation is not likely to fail because of distractions caused by symptoms or thoughts. It is a useful strategy to reduce pain, muscular tension, and stress, while helping to control shortness of breath and to promote more restful sleep.

Following are three examples of muscle relaxation techniques. Try each technique and choose the one that works best for you. Then you might want to tape-record the script for that routine. Although this is not necessary, it is sometimes helpful if you find it hard to concentrate. Also, you won't be distracted by having to refer to the book when you are trying to relax.

You might even want to buy your own relaxation tape or CD to use regularly. Nowadays there are many different ones available in stores and on the Internet. There are some listed in the references at the end of this chapter. Be sure to ask if you can try it out first to make sure you find it pleasant before buying it. If this is not possible, ask about the return policy in case you find the tape or CD unpleasant after trying it at home.

Jacobson's Progressive Relaxation

Many years ago, a physiologist named Edmund Jacobson discovered that in order to relax, one must first know how it feels to be tense. He believed that if one learned to recognize body tension, then one could learn to let it go and relax. He designed a simple exercise to assist with this learning process.

To relax muscles, you need to know how to scan your body, recognize where you are holding tension, and release that tension. The first step is to become familiar with the difference between the feeling of tension and the feeling of relaxation. This brief exercise will allow you to compare those feelings and, with practice, spot and release tension anywhere in your body. Pause for about 10 seconds whenever there is a series of dots (. . .).

PROGRESSIVE MUSCLE RELAXATION

Give yourself permission to take the next few minutes for yourself. For just a little while, let go of all outside concerns. Make yourself as comfortable as possible. Loosen any clothing that feels tight. Uncross your legs, ankles, arms. . . . Allow your body to feel completely supported by the surface beneath you.

You may want to close your eyes as a way of shutting out any unnecessary distractions. Begin by taking a deep breath—in through your nose, filling your chest, and breathing all the way down to the abdomen. Hold . . . and when you're ready, breathe out through pursed lips slowly and completely. As you breathe out, let as much tension as possible flow out with your breath. Let all your muscles feel heavy. And let your whole body just sink into the surface beneath you. . . . Good.

This exercise will guide you through the major muscle groups from your feet to your head, asking you to first tense and then relax those muscles. If you have pain in any part of your body today, don't tense that area. Instead, just notice any tension that may already be there and let go of that tension.

Become aware of the muscles of your feet and calves. . . . Pull your toes back up towards your knees. Hold your feet in this position . . . noticing the sensations. Now relax your feet and release the tension. Observe any changes in sensations as you let go of the tension. . . . Good.

Now tighten the large muscles of your thighs and buttocks. Hold these muscles tense and, as you do, be aware of the sensations. . . . Now relax these muscles, allowing them to feel soft as if they're melting into the surface beneath you. . . . That's it.

Now turn your attention to your abdomen and chest. Tense these muscles by holding in your abdomen and tightening the muscles of your chest wall. . . . Notice a tendency to hold your breath as you tense these muscles. Now relax and release the tension. . . . Notice that you may feel a natural desire to take a deep breath to release even more of the tension. Take a deep breath now. Breathe in deeply through your nose, and when you breathe out, allow your abdomen and chest to soften. . . . Good.

Now, stretching your fingers out straight, tighten the muscles of your hands and arms. . . . Hold. Now release and feel the tension flowing out and the circulation returning. . . .

Next, press your shoulder blades together, tightening the muscles in your upper back, shoulders, and neck. . . . This is a place many people carry tension. Now relax. You may notice that your muscles feel a little warmer and more alive.

Finally, tighten all the muscles of your face and head. . . . Notice the tension around your eyes and in your jaw. Now, release the tension, allowing the muscles around your eyes to soften and your mouth to remain slightly open as your jaw relaxes. Notice the difference. . . .

Now take another deep breath . . . and when you're ready to breathe out, allow any remaining tension to flow out with your breath. And your whole body to be even more deeply relaxed. . . .

And now, just enjoy this feeling of relaxation for a little while. . . . Remember this pleasant feeling. You can quiet your mind and body in this way any time you do this exercise. With practice, you'll be able to create this feeling just by taking a deep breath. As you prepare to end this exercise, picture yourself bringing this feeling of quiet and calm to whatever you are going to do next. Take one more deep breath . . . and when you're ready, open your eyes.

As Jacobson emphasizes, the purpose of voluntarily tensing the muscles is to learn to recognize and locate tension in your body. You will then become aware of tension and use this same procedure for letting it go. Once you learn the technique, it will no longer be necessary to tense voluntarily; just locate the existing tension and let it go.

For some people with a lot of pain, especially pain in the joints, the Jacobson technique may not be appropriate. If it causes any pain, this may distract from the relaxation. If this happens, try a different technique or don't tense those areas, but just try to locate and release the tension.

Body Scan

This is another relaxation technique, similar to Jacobson's progressive muscle relaxation exercise, but it does not require the tensing or movement of muscle groups. Like Jacobson, it is best done lying down on your back, but any comfortable position can be used. First, you must focus on your breathing. Spend a few minutes concentrating on each breath as it enters and leaves your body. Try directing your breath past your chest all the way down to your abdomen. (This is diaphragmatic or belly breathing, which is described in Chapter 4 and is an important part of all relaxation exercises.)

After three or four minutes of concentrating on your breathing, move your attention to your toes. Don't move these, just think about how they feel. . . . Don't worry if you don't feel anything at all. If you find any tension there, let it go on the out breaths. . . .

After a few moments of concentrating on your toes, move your attention to the bottoms of your feet. Again, don't move, just concentrate on any sensations you have. . . . Let go of any tension you may find on the out breaths. Next concentrate on the tops of your feet and your ankles. . . . Release any tension on the out breaths. . . . After a few more moments, bring your attention to your lower legs.

Continue this process, shifting your attention every few moments to another part of your body, working slowly upward to your head. If you find tension, let it go as you breathe out. If your mind starts to wander, just bring your attention back to the feelings in your body and your breathing.

This technique can also be used to help you get to sleep because it helps to clear your mind of any worries or distracting thoughts. The key is to give your full attention to scanning your body for tension and releasing it.

The Relaxation Response

In the early 1970s, Dr. Herbert Benson studied extensively what he calls the "relaxation response." According to Dr. Benson, our bodies have several natural states. One example is the "fight or flight" response experienced by people when faced with a great danger. The body becomes quite tense, which is followed by the body's natural tendency to relax; this is the relaxation response. As our lives become more and more hectic, our bodies tend to stay in an extended or constant state of tension, and we lose our ability to relax. In order to help our bodies relieve this tension and elicit the relaxation response, we may consciously need to practise the following exercise, which consists of four basic elements:

1. Finding a quiet environment where there are few or no distractions.

2. Finding a comfortable position. You should be comfortable enough to remain in the same position for 20 minutes.

3. Choosing a word, object, or pleasant feeling to dwell upon. For example, repeat a word or sound (like the word "one"), gaze at a symbol (like a flower), or concentrate on a feeling (such as peace).

4. Adopting a passive attitude. This is the most essential element. Empty all thoughts and distractions from your mind. You may become aware of thoughts, images, and feelings, but don't concentrate on them. Just allow them to pass on.

To elicit the relaxation response:

1. Sit quietly in a comfortable position.

2. Close your eyes.

3. Relax all your muscles, beginning at your feet and progressing up to your face. Keep them relaxed.

4. Breathe in through your nose. Become aware of your breathing. As you breathe out through your mouth, say the word you chose silently to yourself. Try to empty all thoughts from your mind; concentrate on your word.

5. Continue this for 10–20 minutes. You may open your eyes to check the time, but do not use an alarm. When you finish, sit quietly for several minutes, at first with your eyes closed. Do not stand up for a few minutes.

6. Maintain a passive attitude and let relaxation occur at its own pace. When distracting thoughts occur, ignore them by not dwelling upon them, and return to repeating the word you chose. Do not worry about whether you are successful in achieving a deep level of relaxation.

7. Practise this once or twice daily, but ideally not within two hours after any meal. Digestive processes can interfere with relaxation responses.

This exercise is very much like meditation, which provides the principles on which the relaxation response is based. Meditation is discussed later in this chapter.

While relaxation is the most common method for relieving muscle tension, other techniques can also be used to provide additional emotional and mental health benefits. These benefits include a reduction in fear and anxiety and a refocusing of attention away from the discomfort or unpleasantness of symptoms. These techniques include guided imagery and visualization.

Imagery

Guided Imagery

The guided-imagery relaxation technique is like a guided daydream. It allows you to divert your attention, refocusing your mind away from your symptoms and transporting you to another time and place. It has the added benefit of helping you to achieve deep relaxation by picturing yourself in a peaceful environment.

The guided-imagery script presented here can help take you on this mental stroll. Again, consider each of the following ways to use imagery:

1. Read the script over several times to familiarize yourself with it. Then sit or lie down in a quiet place and try to reconstruct the scene in your mind. The script should take 15–20 minutes to complete.

2. Have a family member or friend read you the script slowly, pausing for about 10 seconds wherever there is a series of dots (. . .).

3. Make a tape of the script and play it to yourself whenever convenient.

Guided-Imagery Script:

A Walk in the Country

You're giving yourself some time to quiet your mind and body. Allow yourself to settle comfortably wherever you are right now. If you wish, you can close your eyes. Breathe in deeply through your nose, expanding your abdomen and filling your lungs. And, pursing your lips, exhale through your mouth slowly and completely, allowing your body to sink heavily into the surface beneath you. Letting go of tension, . . . letting go of anything that's on your mind right now, . . . and just allowing yourself to be present in this moment. . . .

Imagine yourself walking along a peaceful old country road. . . . The sun is warm on your back. The birds are singing. The air is calm and fragrant. . . . As you walk along, your mind naturally wanders to the concerns and worries of the day. Then you come upon a box by the side of the road, and it occurs to you that this box is a perfect place to leave your cares behind, while you enjoy this time in the country.

So you open the box and put into it any concerns, worries, or pressures that you're carrying with you. You close the box and fasten it securely, knowing that you can come back and deal with those concerns whenever you're ready. . . .

You feel lighter as you progress down the road. . . . Soon, you come across an old gate. The gate creaks as you open it and go through. You find yourself in an overgrown garden. Flowers are growing where they've seeded themselves. Vines are climbing over a fallen tree. Soft, green wild grasses. Shade trees. Breathe deeply, smelling the flowers. . . . Listen to the birds and insects. . . . Feel the gentle breeze, warm against your skin. . . . All of your senses are alive and responding to the pleasure of this peaceful time and place. . . .

Guided-Imagery Script:

A Walk in the Country

(continued)

When you're ready to move on, you leisurely follow a path behind you to the garden, eventually coming to a more wooded area. The air feels mild and a little cooler. You become aware of the sound and fragrance of a nearby stream. You pause, breathing deeply of the cool and fragrant air several times. . . . Continuing along the path for a while, you come to the stream. It's clear and clean as it flows and tumbles over the rocks and some fallen logs. . . .

You follow the path along the creek for a way, and after a while, you come out into a sunlit clearing, where you discover a small waterfall emptying into a quiet pool of water. . . . You find a comfortable place to sit for a while. A perfect niche where you can feel completely relaxed. You feel good as you allow yourself to just enjoy the warmth and solitude of this peaceful place. . . .

After a while, you become aware that it's time to return. . . . You walk back down the path through the cool and fragrant trees, out into the sun-drenched overgrown garden, one last smell of the flowers, and out the creaky gate. . . .

You leave this retreat for now and return down the road, noticing that you feel calm and rested. You know that you can visit this special place whenever you wish to take some time to refresh yourself and renew your energy.

When you are ready to return, take a deep breath and open your eyes.

Alternative Guided-Imagery Script:

A Walk on the Beach

You're giving yourself some time to quiet your mind and body. Allow yourself to settle comfortably wherever you are right now. If you wish, you can close your eyes. Breathe in deeply through your nose, expanding your abdomen and filling your lungs. And, pursing your lips, exhale through your mouth slowly and completely, allowing your body to sink heavily into the surface beneath you. Letting go of tension, . . . letting go of anything that's on your mind right now, . . . and just allowing yourself to be present in this moment. . . .

Imagine yourself walking along a peaceful white sand beach. . . . The waves are gently lapping on the sand. The birds are singing. The air is calm and fragrant. As you walk along, your mind naturally wanders to the concerns and worries of the day. Then, you come upon a box in the sand, and it occurs to you that this box is a perfect place to leave your cares behind while you enjoy this time at the beach.

So you open the box and put into it any concerns, worries, or pressures that you're carrying with you. You close the box and fasten it securely, knowing that you can come back and deal with those concerns whenever you're ready. . . .

You feel lighter as you progress along the beach. . . . Soon you come across a wooded area. You enter through an opening in the trees. You find yourself in a lovely fern grotto. Wildflowers growing where they've seeded themselves. Vines climbing over a fallen tree. Soft, green wild grasses. Shade trees. . . . Breathe deeply, smelling the fragrance of the ocean and the forest. . . . Listen to the birds and insects. . . . Feel the gentle breeze, warm against your skin. . . . All of your senses are alive and responding to the pleasure of this peaceful time and place.

Alternative Guided-Imagery Script:

A Walk on the Beach

(continued)

When you're ready to move on, you leisurely follow a path, . . . eventually coming to a more wooded area. The air feels mild and a little cooler. . . . You become aware of the sound and fragrance of a nearby stream. You pause, breathing deeply of the cool and fragrant air several times. . . . Continuing along the path for a while, you come to the stream. It's clear and clean as it flows and tumbles over the rocks and some fallen logs. . . .

You follow the path along the creek for a way, and after a while you come out into a sunlit clearing, where you discover a small waterfall emptying into a quiet pool of water. . . . You find a comfortable place to sit for a while. A perfect niche where you can feel completely relaxed. . . . You feel good as you allow yourself to just enjoy the warmth and solitude of this peaceful place. . . .

After a while, you become aware that it's time to return. . . . You walk back down the path through the cool and fragrant trees, out into the fern grotto. . . . One last smell of the forest and out to the beach. . . .

You leave this retreat for now and return down the beach, noticing that you feel calm and rested. You know that you can visit this special place whenever you wish to take some time to refresh yourself and renew your energy. . . .

When you are ready to return, take a deep breath and open your eyes.

Visualization

This technique, also referred to as vivid imagery, is similar to guided imagery. It is another way of using your imagination to create a picture of yourself in any way you want, doing the things you want to do. All of us use a form of visualization every day, without realizing it—when we dream, worry, read a book, or listen to a story. In all these activities the mind creates images for us to see. We also use visualization intentionally when making plans for the day, considering the possible outcomes of a decision we have to make, or rehearsing for an event or activity. Visualization can be done in different ways and can be used for longer periods of time, or while you are engaged in other activities.

One effective way to use visualization to manage symptoms is to remember pleasant scenes from your past or create new scenes in your mind. Visualization allows you to create your own images, which is different from guided imagery, where the images are suggested to you. To practise visualization, try to remember every detail of a special holiday or party that made you happy. Who was there? What happened? What did you do or talk about? You can also try this by remembering a vacation or other important and pleasant event.

Visualization can be used to plan the details of some future event or to fill in the details of a fantasy. For example, how would you spend a million dollars? What would be your ideal romantic encounter? What would your ideal home or garden look like? Where would you go and what would you do on your dream vacation?

Another form of visualization involves using your mind to think of symbols that represent the discomfort or pain felt in different parts of your body. For example, a painful joint might be red or a tight chest might have a constricting band around it. After forming these images, you then try to change them. The red colour might fade until there is no more colour, or the constricting band will stretch and stretch until it falls off; these new images then cause your perception of the pain or discomfort to change.

Visualization helps build confidence and skill and therefore is a useful technique to help you set and accomplish your personal goals (see Chapter 2). After you write your weekly action plan, take a few minutes to imagine yourself taking a walk, doing your exercises, or taking your medications. Here you are mentally rehearsing the steps you need to take in order to achieve your goal successfully.

Numerous scientific studies have shown that this technique can help people cope better with stressful situations, master skills, and accomplish personal goals. In fact, the people who have become skilled at visualization find they can actually reduce some of the discomfort and distress associated with symptoms.

All the relaxation techniques mentioned above can be used in conjunction with diaphragmatic breathing. This breathing technique is described in detail in Chapter 4, page 52; it can help you achieve a more relaxed state and keep your mind off any potential for shortness of breath.

OTHER COGNITIVE STRATEGIES

While learning to relax is an important part of symptom management, other cognitive strategies can also be useful. These techniques, however, may require more practice than relaxation before you notice the benefits; they include distraction, positive thinking or self-talk, meditation, and prayer.

Distraction

Our minds have trouble focusing on more than one thing at a time; therefore, we can lessen the intensity of symptoms by training our minds to focus attention on something other than our bodies and their sensations. This technique, called distraction or attention refocusing, is particularly helpful for those people who feel their symptoms are overwhelming, or worry that every bodily sensation might indicate a new or worsening symptom or health problem. (It is important to mention that with distraction you are not ignoring the symptoms, but choosing not to dwell on them.)

Distraction works best for short activities or episodes in which symptoms may be anticipated. For example, if you know climbing stairs will be painful or cause discomfort, or that falling asleep at night is difficult, you might try one of the following distraction techniques:

1. Make plans for exactly what you will do after the unpleasant activity passes. For example, if climbing stairs is uncomfortable or painful, think about what you need to do once you get to the top. If you have trouble falling asleep, try making plans for some future event, being as detailed as possible.

2. Think of a person's name, a bird, a flower, or whatever, for every letter of the alphabet. If you get stuck on one letter, go on to the next. (These are good distractions for pain as well as for sleep problems.)

3.   Count backward from 1,000 or 100 by threes (e.g., 100, 97, 94, . . .).

4.   To get through unpleasant daily chores (such as sweeping, mopping, or vacuuming), imagine your floor as a map of a country or continent. Try naming all the states, provinces, or countries, moving east to west or north to south. If geography does not appeal to you, imagine your favorite store and where each department is located.

5.   Try to remember words to favourite songs or the events in an old story.

There are, of course, a million variations to these examples, all of which help you to refocus attention away from your problem.

So far we have discussed short-term refocusing strategies that involve using only the mind for distraction. Distraction also works well for long-term projects or symptoms that tend to last longer, such as depression and some forms of chronic pain.

In these cases, the mind is focused not internally, but rather externally, on some type of activity. If you are somewhat depressed or have continuous unpleasant symptoms, find an activity that interests you and distract yourself from the problem. The activity can be almost anything, from gardening to cooking to reading or going to a movie, even doing volunteer work. One of the marks of a successful self-manager is that he or she has a variety of interests and always seems to be doing something.

Developing Positive and Healthy Thinking or Self-Talk—"I Know I Can"

All of us talk to ourselves all the time. For example, when waking up in the morning, we think, "I really don't want to get out of bed. I'm tired and don't want to go to work today." Or at the end of an enjoyable evening, we think, "Gee, that was fun. I should get out more often." What we think or say to ourselves is called our "self-talk." The way we talk to ourselves tends to come from how and what we think about ourselves. Our thoughts can be positive or negative, and so is our self-talk. Therefore, self-talk can be an important self-management tool when it's positive, or a weapon that hurts or defeats us when it's negative.

All of our self-talk is learned from others and becomes a part of us as we grow up. It comes in many forms, unfortunately mostly negative. Negative self-statements are usually in the form of phrases that begin with something like: "I just can't do . . .," "If only I could/didn't . . .," "I just don't have the energy . . .," "How could I be so stupid?" This type of self-talk represents the doubts and fears we have about ourselves in general, and about our abilities to deal with our condition and its symptoms in particular. It damages our self-esteem, attitude, and mood. Negative self-talk makes us feel bad and our symptoms worsen.

What we say to ourselves plays a major role in determining our success or failure in becoming good self-managers. Negative self-talk tends to limit our abilities and actions. If we tell ourselves, "I'm not very smart" or "I can't" all the time, then we probably won't try to learn new skills because this just doesn't fit with what we think about ourselves. Soon we become prisoners of our own negative beliefs. Fortunately, self-talk is not something fixed in our biological makeup, and therefore it is not completely out of our control. We can learn new, healthier ways to think about ourselves so that our self-talk can work for us instead of against us. By changing the negative, self-defeating statements to positive ones, we can manage symptoms more effectively. This change, as with any habit, requires practice and includes the following steps:

1. **Listen carefully to what you say to or about yourself, both out loud and silently.** Then write down all the negative self-talk statements. Pay special attention to the things you say during times that are particularly difficult for you. For example, what do you say to yourself when getting up in the morning with pain, while doing those exercises you don't really like, or at those times when you are feeling blue? Challenge these negative thoughts by asking yourself questions to identify (1) why you believe this, and (2) what about the statement is really true or not true. For example, are you exaggerating the situation, generalizing, worrying too much, or assuming the worst? Maybe you are making an unrealistic or unfair comparison, assuming too much responsibility, taking something too personally, or expecting perfection. Look at the evidence so that you are better able to change these negative thoughts and statements.

2. **Next, work on changing each negative statement you identified to a positive one, or find some positive statement to replace the negative one.** These positive statements are called affirmations. Write these down. Positive statements should reflect the better you and your decision to be in control. For example, negative statements such as "I don't want to get up," "I'm too tired and I hurt," "I can't do the things I like anymore so why bother," or "I'm good for nothing" become positive messages such as "I'm feeling pretty good today, and I'm going to do something I enjoy," "I may not be able to do everything I used to, but there are still a lot of things I can do," "People like me, and I feel good about myself," or "Other people need and depend on me; I'm worthwhile."

3. **Read and rehearse these positive statements, mentally or with another person.** It is this conscious repetition or memorization of the positive self-talk that will help you replace those old, habitual negative statements.

4. **Practise these new statements in real situations.** This practice, along with time and patience, will help the new patterns of thinking become automatic.

Once established, positive thinking can be one of the most powerful tools that you add to your self-management program; it will help you to manage symptoms as well as master the other skills discussed in this book.

As with exercise and other acquired skills, using your mind to manage your health condition requires both practice and time before you begin to notice the benefits. Thus, if you feel you are not accomplishing anything, don't give up. Be patient and keep on trying.

Prayer and Meditation

For many people, religious and spiritual beliefs are a vital part of how they think about their lives and how they cope. Our beliefs bring a sense of meaning and purpose to life, and help us put things into perspective and set priorities. Our beliefs may help us to find comfort during difficult times and can motivate us to make those difficult but necessary changes, as well as to get support in doing so.

Recent medical and scientific research suggests that maintaining religious or spiritual beliefs may improve health. People who belong to a religious or spiritual community and/or regularly pray or meditate have better health and live longer than those who do not. One possible explanation is that prayer and meditation help increase people's confidence and emotional well-being by fighting feelings of helplessness and restoring a sense of control over their lives, which have positive effects on the body. Other explanations are that religious or spiritual beliefs encourage a healthy lifestyle, and the social support people receive from a group or community positively affects their health.

We do know that people experience the relaxation response when they pray or meditate; their blood pressure, heart rate, and levels of stress hormones drop. At the same time, the brain waves associated with relaxation increase. These physiological changes reduce anxiety and increase blood protein levels in the body, indicating a healthy immune system. In addition to promoting relaxation, prayer and meditation also work as a form of distraction for people with long-term health conditions. They are able to refocus their attention away from their symptoms, thereby reducing the intensity of the discomfort caused by those symptoms.

Regardless of the rationale, prayer and meditation remain the oldest of the self-management tools and are practised in all parts of the world. While these cannot be "prescribed" for you, we encourage you to explore your own beliefs. If you are religious, try practising prayer and meditation more consistently. If you are not religious, consider adopting some form of meditation or reflection to practise regularly. Below are some specific types of prayer and meditation you may want to use.

Centering Prayer

All the major religions of the world use some form of prayer. Basically, prayer is talking with your God, a way to spend time with your God and express or share your feelings. If you are not religious, then prayer may simply involve statements of your feelings, wants, and needs. Prayer can be done publicly with others or privately at home alone. You might pray to give thanks and praise, to ask for help for yourself or others, or to ask for forgiveness. There are many kinds of prayer, but there is one form, in particular that produces positive effects in your daily life. This is called the centering prayer and is very similar to some types of meditation. It requires you to first choose a sacred or special word. The word might be something like *Lord, Father, Mother, Abba, Omm, love, peace, shalom*, etc., or any other word that inspires you and expresses your intention for the prayer. To begin the centering prayer, you'll need to set aside at least 20 minutes of quiet time, maybe right after you wake up in the morning or in the late afternoon or early evening, but not right after eating. A full stomach can interfere with the body's ability to relax and can make you drowsy during your prayer time. Next, find a quiet, comfortable place to sit, keeping your back straight and closing your eyes. You close your eyes to let go of whatever is going on around and within you. Once you are comfortable, you will gently introduce and focus on your sacred word. When you become aware of other thoughts, sensations, feelings, images, memories, etc., do not try to analyze them, but return gently to your sacred word. At the end of the prayer period, remain in silence with your eyes closed for a couple of minutes. During your prayer, you may notice physical sensations, like slight pains, itches, or twitches in parts of your body. These may occur as your body releases both its physical and emotional tension. As you become more relaxed and spiritually attentive, you may also notice either a heaviness or lightness in your arms and legs. When this happens, just allow yourself to notice the sensations briefly, but then return to your sacred word.

It is recommended that you practice the centering prayer two times a day, once in the morning and once in the afternoon or early evening. If this is not possible, start with just once a day. Over time, you will begin to experience the positive results in your life.

Mindfulness Meditation

There are many types of meditation. The purpose of meditation is to quiet the mind. It may also help the individual to quiet the body. For this reason, meditation is often a useful technique for managing stress and other symptoms such as pain, fatigue, or shortness of breath. Mindfulness meditation is one type of meditation that can be practiced by anyone. All that you need to begin is a quiet place and five or more minutes. Start by sitting in a chair with your feet flat on the floor and your hands in your lap or on your knees. If you wish and are able to do so, you can sit on the floor with crossed legs or in a more traditional yoga position. How you sit, however, does not matter.

The essence of mindfulness meditation is to concentrate fully on your breathing. It is best if you can do diaphragmatic or belly breathing, but you do not have to take deep breaths. It is important to keep your full attention on your breathing. Breathe in slowly; hold the breath for a moment, then breathe out slowly. At all times concentrate on your breathing.

While this seems fairly simple, you will soon find that your mind easily wanders. This is called "having a monkey mind." As soon as you notice that your mind is wandering, bring your attention back to your breathing. At first you may not be able to attend to your breathing for more than a minute or two. You will improve, however, with practice.

When you are doing this type of meditation, you may become very aware of your body. For example, your eye may itch or you may become uncomfortable in your sitting position. When this happens, first do nothing but pay attention to your breathing. In many cases you will find that the discomfort goes away. If it continues, however, scratch the itch or change your position. As you do this, pay full attention to what you are doing. With mindfulness meditation it is important to be fully aware of what you are doing at that moment!

Like all other self-management techniques, mindfulness meditation requires practice. You will not get results immediately; however, if you practice this for 15 to 30 minutes a day, four or five times a week, you will find that over time this can be a great symptom management tool.

As we mentioned earlier, symptoms, their causes, and the ways they interact to affect your daily life can become a vicious cycle. Therefore, to successfully manage symptoms, it is important to identify them and their causes, in order to use our different self-management tools to break this cycle.

Following are several key principles to remember from this and the previous chapter:

1. **Symptoms have many causes.** Thus, there are many ways to manage most symptoms. An understanding of the nature and varied causes of your symptoms and how these interact will help you to better manage them.

2. **Not all management techniques will work for everyone.** It is up to you to experiment and find out what works best for you. Be flexible. This includes trying different techniques and monitoring the results to determine which technique is most helpful for which symptom(s) and under what circumstances.

3. **When trying to determine which techniques work best for you, remember that learning a new skill and gaining control of the situation take time.** Therefore, give yourself several weeks to practice a new technique before you decide if it is working for you.

4. **As with exercise and other acquired skills, using your mind to manage your health condition requires both practice and time before you notice the benefits.** Thus, if you feel you are not accomplishing anything, don't give up. Be patient and keep on trying!

5. **These techniques should not have negative effects.** If you become frightened, angry, or depressed when using one of these techniques, please do not continue to use it. Try another technique instead.

Suggested Further Reading

Benson, H., and M.Z. Kiper. *The Relaxation Response.* San Francisco: HarperCollins, 2000.

Berger, Janice with Hall, Harry. *Emotional Fitness: Discovering Our National Healing Power.* Toronto: Penguin Canada, 2005.

Borysenko, Joan. *Inner Peace for Busy People: 52 Simple Strategies for Transforming Your Life.* Carlsbad, Calif.: Hay House, 2001.

Burns, David D. *The Feeling Good Handbook*, rev. ed. New York: Plume, 1999.

Chopra, Deepak. *Journey to the Boundless: Exploring the Intimate Connection Between Your Mind, Body and Spirit.* Niles, Il: Nightingale-Conant Corporation, 1966.

Cousins, Norman. *Head First: The Biology of Hope and the Healing Power of the Human Spirit.* New York: E.P. Dutton, 1990.

Craze, Richard. *Teach Yourself Relaxation.* Chicago: Contemporary Publishing, 1998.

Davis, Martha, et al. *The Relaxation and Stress Reduction Workbook.* Oakland, Calif.: New Harbinger, 2000.

Dossey, Larry. *Prayer Is Good Medicine.* San Francisco: HarperCollins, 1996.

Funk, Mary Marget. *Tools Matter for Practicing the Spiritual Life.* New York: Continuum, 2001.

Kabat-Zinn, Jon. *Coming to Our Senses: Healing Ourselves and the World Through Mindfulness,* 1st ed. New York: Hyperion, 2005.

Kabat-Zinn, Jon. *Full Catastrophe Living: Using the Wisdom of Your Body and Mind to Face Stress, Pain, and Illness.* New York: Delta Trade Paperbacks, 2005.

Keating, Thomas. *Open Mind, Open Heart: The Contemplative Dimension of the Gospel.* New York: Amity House, 1986.

Keating, Thomas, and Gustave Reininger (eds). *Centering Prayer in Daily Life and Ministry.* New York: Continuum, 1998.

McKay, Matthew. *The Anger Control Workbook.* Oakland, CA: New Harbinger, 2000.

McKay, Matthew, and Patrick Fanning. *The Daily Relaxer.* Oakland, Calif.: New Harbinger, 1997.

McKay, Matthew, Patrick Fanning, Carole Honeychurch, and Catherine Sutker. *The Self-Esteem Companion: Simple Exercises to Help Challenge Your Inner Critic and Celebrate Your Personal Strengths.* Oakland, Calif.: New Harbinger, 1999.

Peale, Norman V. *Positive Imaging: The Powerful Way to Change Your Life.* New York: Ballantine Books, 1996.

Regan, Catherine. *Time for Healing: Relaxation for Mind and Body.* Audio CD. Boulder, Colo.: Bull Publishing Co., 1996.

Remen, Rachel Naomi. *Kitchen Table Wisdom: Stories That Heal.* New York: Riverhead Books, 1996.

Rosenberg, Marshall B. *Getting Past the Pain Between Us: Healing and Reconciliation Without Compromise.* Encinitas, Ca: Puddle Dancer Press, 2003.

Siegel, Bernie S. *Help Me to Heal: A Practical Guidebook for Patients, Visitors, and Caregivers.* Carlsbad, Calif.: Hay House, 2003.

Sobel, David S. *The Healthy Mind, Healthy Body Handbook.* Los Altos, CA: DRX, 1996.

EXERCISING FOR FUN AND FITNESS

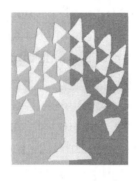

6

*"The weakest and oldest among us can become some sort of athlete,
but only the strongest can survive as spectators. Only the hardiest can withstand
the perils of inertia, inactivity, and immobility."*

J. H. Bland and S.M. Cooper,
Semin Arthritis Rheum (1984)

REGULAR EXERCISE AND PHYSICAL ACTIVITY ARE VITAL TO YOUR PHYSICAL AND EMO-
TIONAL HEALTH AND CAN BRING YOU FUN AND FITNESS AT THE SAME TIME. Having a
chronic illness and growing older can make an active lifestyle seem far away.
Some people have never been very active, and others have given up leisure activities
because of illness.

Unfortunately, long periods of inactivity in anyone can lead to weakness, stiffness,
fatigue, poor appetite, high blood pressure, obesity, osteoporosis, constipation, and
increased sensitivity to pain, anxiety, and depression. These problems arise from chronic illnesses as well. So it can be difficult to tell whether it is the illness, inactivity, or a combination of the two that is responsible for these problems. Although we do not have cures for
many of these illnesses yet, we know the cure for inactivity—exercise!

Most people have a sense that exercising and being active is healthier and more satisfying than being inactive, but often have a hard time finding information and support to
get started on a more active way of life.

Thanks to the knowledge gained from many people with chronic illnesses who have worked with health professionals in exercise research, we can now advise exercise for fun and fitness, as well as exercise for helping manage your illness and for making everyday activities less stressful. This applies to all ages. Some of our self-managers are in their nineties.

In this chapter, you will learn how to improve your health and fitness and make wise exercise choices. This advice is not intended to take the place of therapeutic recommendations from your health care providers. If you've had an exercise plan prescribed for you that differs from the suggestions here, take this book to your doctor or therapist and ask what she or he thinks about this program. Later in this book, we will provide additional information and helpful exercise ideas for people with specific chronic illnesses.

Regular exercise benefits everyone, especially people with chronic health problems. Regular exercise improves levels of strength, energy, and self-confidence, and lessens anxiety and depression. Exercise can help maintain a good weight, which takes stress off weight-bearing joints and improves blood pressure, blood sugar, and blood fat levels. There is evidence that regular exercise can help to "thin" the blood, or prevent blood clots, which is one of the reasons exercise can be of particular benefit to people with heart disease, cerebrovascular disease, and peripheral vascular disease.

In addition, strong muscles can help people with arthritis to protect their joints by improving stability and absorbing shock. Regular exercise also helps nourish joints and keeps cartilage and bone healthy. Regular exercise has been shown to help people with chronic lung disease improve endurance and reduce shortness of breath (and trips to the emergency room!). Many people with claudication (leg pain from severe atherosclerotic blockages in the arteries of the lower extremities) can walk farther without leg pain after undertaking a regular exercise program. Studies of people with heart disease who exercise in cardiac rehabilitation programs suggest that exercise may even increase life expectancy. Regular exercise is an important part of controlling blood sugar levels, losing weight, and reducing the risks of cardiovascular complications for people with diabetes.

The good news is that it doesn't take hours of painful, sweat-soaked exercise to achieve most of these health benefits. Even short periods of gentle physical activity can significantly improve health and fitness, reduce disease risks, and boost your mood.

Exercise reconditions your body, helping to restore function previously lost to disuse and illness. This will help you improve your health, feel better, and manage your chronic illness more effectively. Feeling more in control and less at the mercy of your chronic illness is one of the biggest and best benefits of becoming an exercise self-manager.

DEVELOPING AN ACTIVE LIFESTYLE

OK, so you want to be more physically active. One way is to set aside a special time for a formal exercise program, involving such planned activities as walking, jogging, swimming, tennis, aerobic dance, chair exercises, exercising to an exercise video or CD, and so on. But don't underestimate the value and importance of just being more physically active throughout the day as you carry out your usual activities. Both can be helpful.

The formal programs are usually more visible and get more attention. But being more physical in everyday life can also pay off. Consider taking the stairs a floor or two instead of waiting impatiently for a slow elevator. Park and walk several blocks to work or to the store instead of circling the parking lot looking for the perfect, up-close parking space. Mow the lawn, work in the garden, or just get up once in a while and walk around the house.

These types of daily activities, often not viewed as "exercise," can add up to significant health benefits. Recent studies show that even small amounts of daily activity can raise fitness levels, decrease heart disease risk, and boost mood—and the activities can be pleasurable, enjoyable ones! Playing with the children, dancing, gardening, bowling, golf—all these enjoyable activities can make a big difference. One person commented that she never exercised. When asked why she went square-dancing several times a week she replied, "Oh, that's not exercise, that's fun." The average day is filled with excellent opportunities to be more physical.

DEVELOPING AN EXERCISE PROGRAM

For many people, a more formal exercise program can be helpful. This usually involves setting aside a period of time, at least several times a week, to deliberately focus on increasing fitness. A complete, balanced exercise program should help you improve these three aspects of fitness:

1. **Flexibility.** This refers to the ability of the joints and muscles to move comfortably through a full, normal range of motion. Limited flexibility can cause pain, increase risk of injury, and make muscles less efficient. Flexibility tends to diminish with inactivity, age, and certain diseases, but you can increase or maximize your flexibility by doing gentle stretching exercises like those described later in Chapter 7.

2. **Strength.** Muscles need to be exercised to maintain their strength. With inactivity, muscles tend to weaken and shrink (atrophy). The weaker the muscles get, the less we feel like using them and the more inactive we tend to become, creating a vicious circle. Much of the disability and lack of mobility for people with chronic illness is due to muscle weakness. This weakness can be reversed with a program of gradually increasing exercise.

3. **Endurance.** Our ability to sustain activity depends on the function of our heart and lungs. The heart and lungs must work efficiently to distribute oxygen-rich blood to the muscles. The muscles must be conditioned to use the oxygen.

Aerobic (meaning "with oxygen") exercise improves this cardiovascular and muscular conditioning. This type of exercise uses the large muscles of your body in a rhythmical, continuous activity. The most effective activities involve your whole body: walking, swimming, dancing, mowing the lawn, and so on. Aerobic exercise improves cardiovascular fitness, lessens heart attack risk, and helps control weight. Aerobic exercise also promotes a sense of well-being, easing depression and anxiety, promoting restful sleep, and improving mood and energy levels.

YOUR FITNESS PROGRAM

A complete fitness program combines exercises to improve each of the three aspects of fitness: flexibility, strength, and endurance. Chapter 7 explains and illustrates a number of flexibility and strengthening exercises. Chapter 8 contains information about endurance or aerobic exercise. If you haven't exercised regularly in some time, or have pain, stiffness, shortness of breath, or weakness that interferes with your daily activities, it is a good idea to discuss your ideas about increasing your amount of exercise with your health care providers. Begin your fitness program by choosing a number of flexibility and strengthening exercises that you are willing to do every day or every other day. Once you are able to comfortably exercise for at least 10 minutes at a time, you are ready to start adding some endurance or aerobic activities.

Many people wonder how to choose the right exercises and how to know what's best for them. The truth is that the best exercises for you are the ones that will help you do what you want to do. Often, the most important decision to start a successful fitness program is to choose a goal (something you want to do) that exercise can help you reach. Once you have a goal in mind, it is much easier to choose exercises that make sense to you. There is no doubt that we all are more successful exercisers if we know where we want exercise to take us. If you don't see how exercise can be helpful to you, it is hard to get excited about adding yet another task to your day.

Choose Your Goal and Make a Plan

1. **Choose something that you want to do but don't or can't do now because of some physical reason.** For example, you might want to enjoy a shopping or fishing trip with your friends, mow the lawn, or take a family vacation.

2. **Think about why you can't or don't do it or don't enjoy doing it now.** It might be that you get tired before everybody else, that it's too hard to get up from a low chair or bench, that climbing steps is painful or makes your legs tired, or that your shoulders are too weak or stiff to cast your fishing line or stow a carry-on bag.

3. **Decide what it is about your abilities that makes it difficult to do what you want.** For example, if getting up from a low seat is difficult, you may realize that your hips or knees are stiff and that your leg muscles are weak. In this case, look for flexibility and strengthening exercises for hips and knees. If you decide that a major problem is that your shoulders are stiff and your arms too weak to handle a carry-on bag for a plane trip, choose flexibility and strengthening exercises for your shoulders and arms.

4. **Design your exercise plan.** Choose no more than 10 to 12 exercises at first. Start by doing 3 to 5 repetitions of each and review the information in Chapter 7. As you get comfortable, you can increase repetitions and kinds of exercise. If you want to improve your endurance, read Chapter 8 about aerobic exercise. Start off with short periods and build up gradually. Health and fitness take time to build, but every day you exercise you are healthier and on your way to fitness. That's why it's so important to make sure you keep it up.

WHAT ARE YOUR EXERCISE BARRIERS?

Health and fitness make sense. Yet, when faced with actually being more physically active, most people can come up with scores of excuses, concerns, and worries. These barriers can prevent us from even taking the first step. Here are some common barriers and possible solutions:

"I don't have enough time."

Everyone has the same amount of time. We just choose to use it differently. It's a matter of priorities. Some find a lot of time for television, but nothing to spare for fitness. It doesn't really take a lot of time. Even five minutes a day is a good start, and it's much better than no physical activity. You may be able to combine activities, like watching television while pedalling a stationary bicycle, or arranging "walking meetings" to discuss business or family matters.

"I'm too tired."

When you're out of shape, you feel listless and tend to tire easily. Then you don't exercise because you're tired, and this becomes yet another vicious cycle. You have to break out of the "too tired" cycle. Regular physical activity increases your stamina and gives you more energy to do the things you like. As you get back into shape, you will recognize the difference between feeling listless or "out of shape" and feeling physically tired.

"I'm too old."

You're never too old for some type of physical activity. No matter what your level of fitness or your age, you can always find some ways to increase your activity, energy, and sense of well-being. To date, our oldest self-manager has been 99. Fitness is especially important as we age.

"I'm too sick."

It may be true that you are too sick for a vigorous or strenuous exercise program, but you can usually find some ways to be more active. Remember, you can exercise one minute at a time, several times a day. The enhanced physical fitness can help you better cope with your illness and prevent further problems.

"I get enough exercise."

This may be true, but for most people, their jobs and daily activities do not provide enough sustained exercise to keep them fully fit and energetic.

"Exercise is boring."

You can make it more interesting and fun. Exercise with other people. Entertain yourself with a headset and musical tapes or listen to the radio. Vary your activities and your walking routes. You might find exercise time good thinking time.

"Exercise is painful."

The old saying "No pain, no gain" is simply wrong and out-of-date. Recent evidence shows that significant health benefits come from gentle, low-intensity, enjoyable physical activity. You may sweat or feel a bit short of breath, but if you feel more pain when you finish than before you started, take a close look at what you are doing. More than likely you are either exercising improperly or overdoing it for your particular condition. Talk with your instructor, therapist, or doctor. You may simply need to be less vigorous or change the type of exercise that you're doing.

"I'm too embarrassed."

For some, the thought of donning a skin-tight designer exercise outfit and trotting around in public is delightful, but for others it is downright distressing. Fortunately, as we'll describe, the options for physical activity range from exercise in the privacy of your own home to group social activities. You should be able to find something that suits you.

"I'm afraid I might fall."

Many people who are afraid of falling, or who have fallen, decide to limit activity in order to avoid falls. This might seem to make sense in the short run, but before too long, inactivity and the weakness and stiffness that occur actually increase the risk of falling. Maintaining strong and flexible legs and ankles and staying active so that you practise balancing in different positions are important to reduce the risks of falls. If your balance worries you, be sure to read the next section, "Improving Balance," and look in Chapter 7 for the balance exercises marked "BB," and the exercises 26–31 at the end of the exercise section.

"I'm afraid I'll have a heart attack."

In most cases, the risk of a heart attack is greater for those who are not physically active than for those who exercise regularly. But if you are worried about this, check with your doctor. Especially if your illness is under control, it's probably safer to exercise than not to exercise.

"It's too cold, it's too hot, it's too dark, etc."

If you are flexible and vary your type of exercise, you can generally work around the changes in weather that make certain types of exercise more difficult. Consider indoor activities like stationary bicycling or mall walking.

"I'm afraid I won't be able to do it right or be successful. I'm afraid I'll fail."

Many people don't start a new project because they are afraid they will fail or not be able to finish it successfully. If you feel this way about starting an exercise program, remember two things. First, whatever activities you are able to do—no matter how short or "easy"—will be much better for you than doing nothing. Be proud of what you have done, not guilty about what you haven't done. Second, new projects often seem overwhelming—until we get started and learn to enjoy each day's adventures and successes.

Perhaps you have come up with some other barriers. The human mind is incredibly creative. But you can turn that creativity to your advantage by using it to come up with even better ways to refute the excuses and develop positive attitudes about exercise and fitness. If you get stuck, ask others for suggestions, or try some of the self-talk suggestions in Chapter 5.

IMPROVING BALANCE

It is common for people who become weak or who have been inactive for some time to have poorer balance and to worry about falling. Too often, people decide that the best way not to fall is to spend more time sitting and not doing anything active. At first, you might think that if you are not up walking around, you won't be at risk for falling down. However, the effects of being inactive are weakness, stiffness, slower reflexes, and slower muscles. All of these effects actually harm your ability to balance and will eventually increase your risk of falling.

Falls can be caused by personal conditions such as weakness, dizziness, stiffness, poor eyesight, medication effects, loss of sensation, or inner ear problems. Falls can also be caused by external conditions such as poor lighting, uneven surfaces, rugs and carpets, and cluttered floors. Your ability to avoid falls depends on reducing the environmental risks and keeping yourself strong, flexible, and capable of maintaining your balance even when something gets in your way or puts you off balance. Research shows that people who have strong legs and ankles, are flexible, and practise activities that require them to maintain and recover their balance have less fear of falling and actually fall less. If you have fallen or are afraid that you may fall, it is a good idea to talk with your care provider, get your balance checked to make sure there are no vision or inner ear problems that need to be addressed, and make sure your home is safe for you. Exercising to keep yourself strong, flexible, and active also helps protect you from falling.

PREPARING TO EXERCISE

Figuring out how to make the commitment of time and energy to regular exercise is a challenge for everyone. If you have a chronic illness, you have even more challenges. You must take precautions and find a safe and comfortable program. Even with a chronic illness, most people can do some kind of aerobic exercise.

If your illness is not reasonably stable, if you have been inactive for more than six months, or if you have questions about starting an aerobic exercise program, it is best to check with your doctor or therapist first. Take this book with you when you discuss your exercise ideas, or prepare a list of your specific questions.

People with arthritis, for example, should understand how to adapt their exercise to changes in their arthritis and joint problems. People with heart disease or lung disease should generally not "exercise through" potentially serious symptoms such as chest pain, palpitations (irregular heartbeat), shortness of breath, or excessive fatigue. They should notify their physicians of any significant worsening of their usual symptoms or if new symptoms appear. Resumption of exercise should begin only after you get the physician's clearance to do so. Also, don't exercise when you are experiencing flu symptoms, an upset stomach, diarrhea, or other acute illness. Learning how much to push yourself while exercising, without doing "too much," is especially important.

We hope that this chapter will help you gain the knowledge to meet these challenges and enjoy the benefits of physical fitness. Start by identifying your individual needs and limits. If possible, talk with your doctor and other health professionals who understand your kind of chronic illness. Get their ideas about special exercise needs and precautions. Read Chapter 9 of this book. Learn to be aware of your body, and plan activities accordingly.

Respect your body. If you feel acutely ill, don't exercise. If you can't comfortably complete your warm-up period of flexibility and strengthening exercises, then don't try to do more vigorous conditioning exercises. Your personal exercise program should be based on your current level of health and fitness, your goals and desires, your abilities and special needs, and your likes and dislikes. Deciding to improve your fitness, and feeling the satisfaction of success, has nothing to do with competition or comparing yourself to others or even with what you were able to do "before."

OPPORTUNITIES IN YOUR COMMUNITY

Most people who exercise regularly do so with at least one other person. Two or more people can keep each other motivated, and a whole class can build a feeling of camaraderie. On the other hand, exercising alone gives you the most freedom. You may feel that there are no classes that would work for you or there is no buddy with whom to exercise. If so, start your own program; as you progress, you may find that these feelings change.

The Arthritis Society can recommend specific exercise programs in your community. The Heart and Stroke Foundation and Diabetes Society are excellent resources for people with heart disease, stroke, lung disease, or diabetes. Consult the local chapter or branch of the appropriate agency.

Most communities now offer a variety of exercise classes, including special programs for people over 50, adaptive exercises, mall walking, fitness trails, tai chi, yoga, and others. Check with the local Y, community and senior centers, parks and recreation programs, adult education classes, and community colleges. There is a great deal of variation in the content of these programs, as well as in the professional experience of the exercise staff. By and large, the classes are inexpensive, and those in charge of planning are responsive to people's needs.

The hospital in your community may offer medically supervised exercise classes for people with heart or lung disease (cardiac or pulmonary rehabilitation classes). Speak to your physician about enrolling in one of these classes.

Health and fitness clubs usually offer aerobic studios, weight training, cardiovascular equipment, and sometimes a heated pool. For all these services they charge membership fees, which can be high. Ask about low-impact, beginner's, and over-50 exercise classes, both in the aerobic studio and in the pool. Gyms that emphasize weight lifting generally don't have the programs or personnel to help you with a flexible, overall fitness program. These are some qualities you should look for:

1. **Classes designed for moderate- and low-intensity exercise and for beginners.** You should be able to observe classes and participate in at least one class before signing up and paying.

2. **Instructors with qualifications and experience.** Knowledgeable instructors are more likely to understand special needs and be willing and able to work with you.

3. **Membership policies that allow you to pay only for a session of classes or let you "freeze" membership at times when you can't participate.** Some fitness facilities offer different rates depending on how many services you use.

4. **Facilities that are easy to get to, park near, and enter.** Dressing rooms and exercise sites should be accessible and safe, with professional staff on site.

5. **A pool that allows "free swim" times when the water isn't crowded.** Also, find out the policy about children in the pool; small children playing and making noise may not be compatible with your program.

6. **Staff and other members whom you feel comfortable being around.**

One last note: There are many excellent exercise videotapes and DVDs for use at home. These vary in intensity, from very gentle chair exercises to more strenuous aerobic exercise. Ask your doctor, therapist, or voluntary agency for suggestions, or review the tapes yourself.

PUTTING YOUR PROGRAM TOGETHER

The best way to enjoy and stick with your exercise program is to suit yourself! Choose what you want to do, a place where you feel comfortable, and an exercise time that fits your schedule. A woman who wants to have dinner on the table at 6 won't stick with an exercise program that requires her to leave home for a 5 o'clock class. A retired man who enjoys lunch with friends and an afternoon nap is wise to choose an early- or mid-morning exercise time.

Pick two or three activities you think you would enjoy and that wouldn't put undue stress on your body. Choose activities that can be easily worked into your daily routine. If an activity is new to you, try it out before going to the expense of buying equipment or joining a health club. By having more than one exercise, you can keep active while adapting to vacations, seasons, and changing problems with your condition. Variety also helps keep you from getting bored.

Having fun and enjoying yourself are benefits of exercise that often go unmentioned. Too often we think of exercise as serious business. However, most people who stick with a program do so because they enjoy it. They think of their exercise as recreation rather than a chore. Start off with success in mind. Allow yourself time to get used to new experiences and meet new people. You'll probably find that you look forward to exercise.

Some well-meaning health professionals can make it hard for a person with a chronic illness to stick to an exercise program. You may have been told simply to "exercise more on your own." The "how" and "when" of that exercise plan, in fact, may have been left entirely up to you. No wonder so many people never start or give up so quickly! Not many of us would make a commitment to do something we don't fully understand. Experience, practice, and success help us establish a habit. Follow the self-management steps in Chapter 2 to make beginning your program easier.

1. **Keep your exercise goal in mind.** Review "Choose Your Goal and Make a Plan" earlier in this chapter.

2. **Choose exercises you want to do.** Combine activities that move you toward your goal and those recommended by your health professionals. Select exercises and activities from the next two chapters to get started.

3. **Choose the time and place to exercise.** Tell your family and friends about your plan.

4. **Make an action plan with yourself.** Decide how long you'll stick with these particular exercises. Six to eight weeks is a reasonable time commitment for a new program.

5. **Make an exercise diary or calendar, whichever suits you.** A diary or journal will let you record more information. Some people enjoy having a record of what they did and how they felt. For others, a simple calendar on which to note an exercise session is plenty of paperwork. Choose what you like; the point is to have fun and enjoy being active.

6. **Do some self-tests to keep track of your progress.** You will find these at the end of the next two chapters. Record the date and results of the ones you choose.

7. **Start your program.** Remember to begin gradually and proceed slowly, especially if you haven't exercised in a while.

8. **Repeat the self-tests at regular intervals, record the results, and check the changes.**

9. **Revise your program.** At the end of your 6 to 8 weeks, decide what you liked, what worked, and what made exercising difficult. Modify your program and make an action plan for another few weeks. You may decide to change some exercises, the place or time you exercise, or your exercise partner(s).

10. **Reward yourself for a job well done.** Many people who start an exercise program find that the rewards come with improved fitness and endurance. Being able to enjoy family outings, a refreshing walk, or trips to the store, the library, a concert, or a museum are great rewards to look forward to.

Table 6.1 **Advice for Exercise Problems**

Problem	Advice
Irregular or very rapid heartbeat	Stop exercising. Check your pulse. Are the beats regular or irregular? How fast is your heartbeat? Make a note of these and discuss this information with your doctor before exercising again.
Pain, tightness, or pressure in the chest, jaw, arms, neck, or back	Stop exercising. Talk with your doctor. Don't exercise until you have been cleared by your doctor.
Unusual, extreme shortness of breath persisting 10 minutes after you exercise	Notify your doctor and get clearance before exercising again.
Light-headedness, dizziness, fainting, cold sweat, or confusion	Lie down with your feet up, or sit down and put your head between your legs. If it happens more than once, check with your doctor before you exercise again.
Excessive tiredness after exercise, especially if you're still tired 24 hours after you exercise	Don't exercise so vigorously next time. If the excessive tiredness persists, check with your doctor. Talk to your doctor before you exercise again.

KEEPING IT UP

If you haven't exercised recently, you'll undoubtedly experience some new feelings and discomfort in the early days. It's normal to feel muscle tension and possible tenderness around joints, and to be a little more tired in the evenings. Muscle or joint pain that lasts more than two hours after the exercise, or feeling tired into the next day, means that you probably did too much too fast. Don't stop; just exercise less vigorously or for a shorter amount of time the next day.

When you do aerobic exercise, it's natural to feel your heart beat faster, your breathing speed up, and your body get warmer. However, feeling chest pain, excessive shortness of breath, nausea, or dizziness is not what you want. If this happens to you, stop exercising and discontinue your program until you check with your doctor. (See Table 6.1.)

People who have a chronic illness often have additional sensations to sort out. It can be difficult at first to figure out whether it is the illness or the exercise or both that is causing them. Talking to someone else with the illness who has experience starting a new exercise program can be a big help. Once you've sorted out the new sensations, you'll be able to exercise with confidence.

Expect setbacks. During the first year, people average two to three interruptions in their exercise schedule, often because of minor injuries or illnesses unrelated to their exercise. You may find yourself sidelined or derailed temporarily. Don't be discouraged. Try a different activity or simply rest. When you are feeling better, resume your program, but begin at a lower, more gentle level. As a rule of thumb, it will take you the same amount of time to get back into shape as you were out. For instance, if you missed three weeks, it may take at least that long to get back to your previous level. Go slowly. Be kind to yourself. You're in this for the long haul.

Think of your head as the coach and your body as your team. For success, all parts of the team need attention. Be a good coach. Encourage and praise yourself. Design "plays" you feel your team can execute successfully. Choose places that are safe and hospitable. A good coach knows his or her team, sets good goals, and helps the team succeed. A good coach is loyal. A good coach does not belittle, nag, or make anyone feel guilty. Be a good coach to your team.

Besides a good coach, everyone needs an enthusiastic cheerleader or two. Of course, you can be your own cheerleader, but being both coach and cheerleader is a lot to do. Successful exercisers usually have at least one family member or close friend who actively supports their exercise habit. Your cheerleader can exercise with you, help you get other chores done, praise your accomplishments, or just consider your exercise time when making plans. Sometimes cheerleaders pop up by themselves, but don't be bashful about asking for a hand.

With exercise experience you develop a sense of control over yourself and your chronic illness. You learn how to alternate your activities to fit your day-to-day needs. You know when to do less and when to do more. You know that a change in symptoms or a period of inactivity is usually only temporary and doesn't have to be devastating. You know you have the tools to get back on track.

Give your exercise plan a chance to succeed. Set reasonable goals and enjoy your success. Stay motivated. When it comes to your personal fitness program, sticking with it and doing it your way makes you a definite winner.

Suggested Further Reading

Dahm, Diane, and Jay Smith, editors. *Mayo Clinic Fitness for Everybody.* Rochester, Minn.: Mayo Clinic Health Information, 2005.

Fredrikson, Eric. *How to Avoid Falling: A Guide for Active Aging and Independence.* Toronto: Firefly Books, 2004.

Moffat, Marilyn, and Steve Vickery. *Book of Body Maintenance and Repair.* American Physical Therapy Association. New York: Henry Holt & Co., 1999.

Nelson, Miriam E., and Sarah Wernick. *Strong Women Stay Young,* rev. ed. New York: Bantam Books, 2000.

Prudden, Bonnie. *Pain Erasure: The Bonnie Prudden Way.* New York: Ballantine Books, 1980.

Sayce, Valerie. *Exercise Beats Arthritis: An Easy-to-Follow Program of Exercises,* 3rd ed. Boulder, Colo.: Bull Publishing, 1998.

White, Martha. *Water Exercise: 78 Safe and Effective Exercises for Fitness and Therapy.* Champaign, Ill.: Human Kinetics, 1995.

EXERCISING FOR FLEXIBILITY AND STRENGTH: Warm-Up/Cool-Down

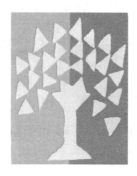

7

You can use the exercises in this chapter in several ways: to get in shape for more vigorous aerobic exercise, to keep active on days when you don't do aerobic exercise, and as part of your warm-up and cool-down routines. Choose exercises to build a strengthening and flexibility program for the whole body. You can also choose specific exercises to improve your balance.

The exercises are arranged in order from the head and neck down to the toes. Most of the upper-body exercises may be done either sitting or standing. Exercises done lying down can be performed on the floor or on a firm mattress. We have labeled the exercises that are particularly important for good posture "VIP" (Very Important for Posture). Exercises to improve balance by strengthening and loosening legs and ankles are marked "BB" (Better Balance). There is also a final section of Balance Exercises that are designed to help you practice balance skills.

You might enjoy creating a routine of exercises that flow together. Arrange them so that you don't have to get up and down too often. Exercising to gentle, rhythmic music can also add to your enjoyment. At the end of the chapter you will also find a reference for an exercise CD designed to go with this book.

These helpful tips apply to all the exercises that follow:

- **Move slowly and gently.** Do not bounce or jerk.

- To loosen tight muscles and limber up stiff joints, stretch just until you feel tension, hold for 10 to 30 seconds, and then relax.

- Don't push your body until it hurts. Stretching should feel good, not painful.

- Start with no more than 5 repetitions of any exercise. Take at least *2 weeks* to increase to 10 repetitions.

- Always do the same number of exercises for your left side as for your right.

- Breathe naturally. Do not hold your breath. Count out loud to make sure you are breathing easily.

- If you feel increased symptoms that last more than 2 hours after exercising, do fewer repetitions next time, or eliminate an exercise that seems to be causing the symptoms. Don't quit exercising.

- All exercises can be adapted for individual needs. The following exercises are designed to include both sides of the body and a full range of motion. If you are limited by muscle weakness or joint tightness, go ahead and do the exercise as completely as you can. **The benefit of doing an exercise comes from moving toward a certain position, not from being able to complete the movement perfectly.** In some cases you may find that after a while you can complete the movement. Other times, you will continue to perform your own version.

NECK EXERCISES

1. Heads Up (VIP)

This exercise relieves jaw, neck, and upper back tension or pain, and is the start of good posture. You can do it while driving, sitting at a desk, sewing, reading, or exercising. Just sit or stand straight and gently slide your chin back. Keep looking forward as your chin moves backward. You'll feel the back of your neck lengthen and straighten. To help, put

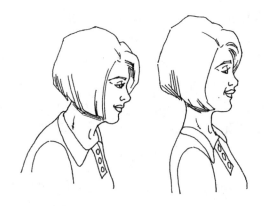

your finger on your nose and then draw straight back from your finger. (Don't worry about a little double chin—you really look much better with your neck straight!)

Clues for finding the correct position:

1. Ear over shoulder, not out in front.

2. Head balanced over neck and trunk, not in the lead.

3. Back of neck more vertical, not leaning forward.

4. Bit of double chin.

2. Neck Stretch

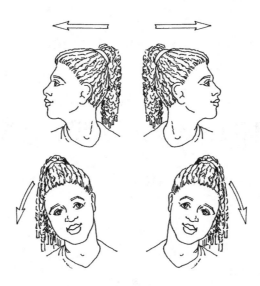

In heads-up position (Exercise 1) and with your shoulders relaxed:

1. Turn slowly to look over your right shoulder. Then turn slowly to look over your left shoulder.

2. Tilt your head to the right and then to the left. Move your ear toward your shoulder. Do not move your shoulder up to your ear.

Don't do these exercises if they cause neck pain, or pain or numbness in your arms or hands.

HAND AND WRIST EXERCISES

A good place to do hand exercises is at a table that supports your forearms. Do them after washing dishes, after bathing, or when taking a break from handwork. Your hands are warmer and more limber at these times.

3. Thumb Walk

Holding your wrist straight, form the letter "O" by lightly touching your thumb to each fingertip. After each "O," straighten and spread your fingers. Use the other hand to help if needed.

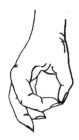 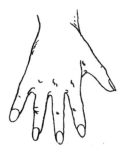

SHOULDER EXERCISES

4. Good Morning Stretch

Start with hands in gentle fists, palms turned away from you and wrists crossed. Breathe in and extend fingers while you uncross your arms and reach up as high as you can. Breathe out and relax.

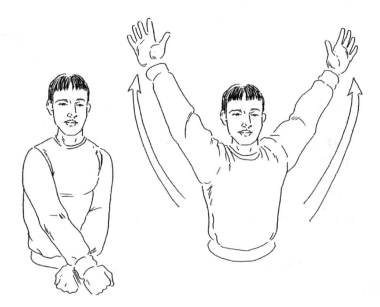

5. Wand Exercise

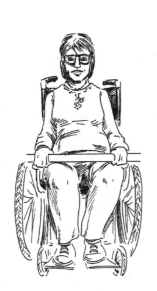
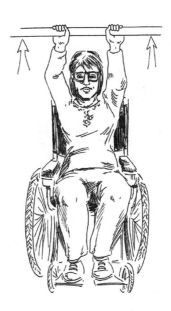

If one or both of your shoulders are tight or weak, you may want to give yourself a "helping hand." This shoulder exercise and the next allow the arms to help each other.

Use a cane, yardstick, or mop handle as your wand. Place one hand on each end and raise the wand as high overhead as possible. You might try this in front of the mirror. This wand exercise can be done standing, sitting, or lying down.

6. Pat and Reach

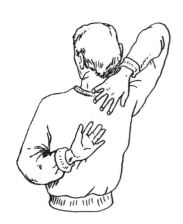

This double-duty exercise helps increase flexibility and strength for both shoulders. Raise one arm up over your head, and bend your elbow to pat yourself on the back. Move your other arm to your back, bend your elbow, and reach up toward the other hand. Can your fingertips touch? Relax and switch arm positions. Can you touch on that side? For most people, one position will work better than the other.

7. Shoulder Blade Pinch (VIP)

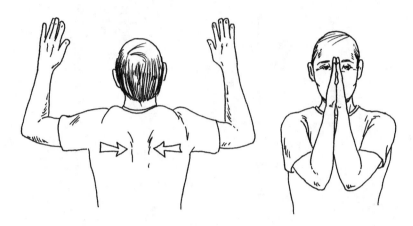

This is a good exercise to strengthen the middle and upper back and to stretch the chest. Sit or stand with your head in heads-up position (Exercise 1) and your shoulders relaxed. Raise your arms out to the sides with elbows bent. Pinch your shoulder blades together by moving your elbows as far back as you can. Hold briefly, then slowly move your arms forward to touch elbows. If this position is uncomfortable, lower your arms or rest your hands on your shoulders.

BACK AND ABDOMINAL EXERCISES

8. Knee to Chest Stretch

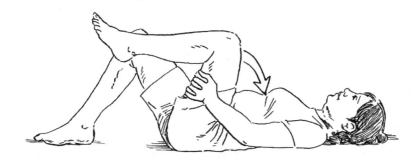

For a low back stretch, lie on the floor with knees bent and feet flat. Bring one knee toward your chest, using your hands to help. Hold your knee near your chest for 10 seconds and lower the leg slowly. Repeat with the other knee. You can also tuck both legs at the same time if you wish. Relax and enjoy the stretch.

9. Pelvic Tilt (VIP)

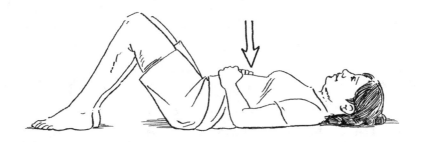

This is an excellent exercise for the low back. Lie on your back with knees bent, feet flat. Place your hands on your abdomen. Flatten the small of your back against the floor by tightening your stomach muscles and your buttocks. It helps to imagine bringing your pubic bone to your chin, or trying to pull your tummy in enough to zip a tight pair of trousers. Hold the tilt for 5 to 10 seconds. Relax. Arch your back slightly. Relax and repeat the pelvic tilt. Keep breathing. Count the seconds out loud. Once you've mastered the pelvic tilt lying down, practise it sitting, standing, and walking.

10. Back Lift (VIP)

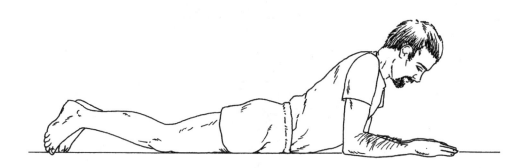

1. This exercise improves flexibility along your spine. Lie on your stomach and rise up onto your forearms. Keep your back relaxed, and keep your stomach and hips down. If this is comfortable, straighten your elbows. Breathe naturally and relax for at least 10 seconds. If you have moderate to severe low back pain, do not do this exercise unless it has been specifically prescribed for you.

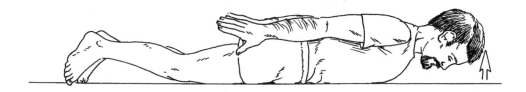

2. To strengthen back muscles, lie on your stomach with your arms at your side or over-head. Lift your head, shoulders, and arms. Do not look up. Keep looking down with your chin tucked in. Count out loud as you hold for a count of 10. Relax. You can also lift your legs, instead of your head and shoulders, off the floor

Lifting both ends of your body at once is a fairly strenuous exercise. It may not be helpful for a person with back pain.

11. Low Back Rock and Roll

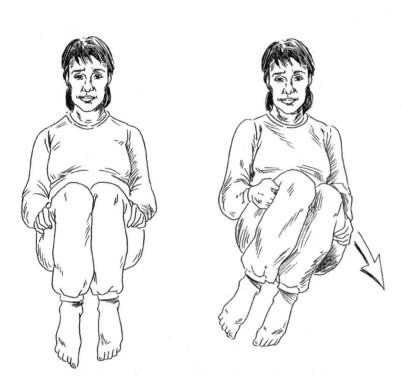

Lie on your back and pull your knees up to your chest with your hands behind the thighs. Rest in this position for 10 seconds, then gently roll the knees from one side to the other, rocking your hips back and forth. Keep your upper back and shoulders flat on the ground.

12. Curl-Up

A curl-up, as shown here, is a good way to strengthen abdominal muscles. Lie on your back, knees bent, feet flat. Do the pelvic tilt (Exercise 9). Slowly curl up to raise your head and shoulders. Uncurl back down, or hold for 10 seconds and slowly lower. Breathe out as you curl up, and breathe in as you go back down. Do not hold your breath. If you have neck problems, or if your neck hurts when you do this exercise, try the next one instead. Never tuck your feet under a chair or have someone hold your feet!

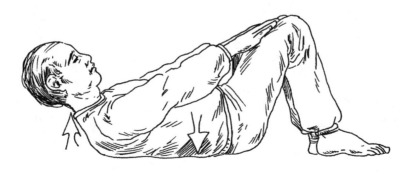

13. Roll-Out

This is another good abdominal strengthener, and it is easy on the neck. Use it instead of the curl-up, or, if neck pain is not a problem, do them both.

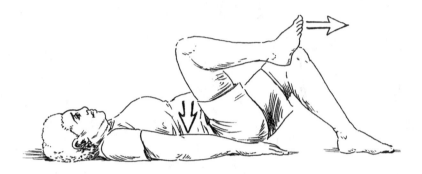

1.   Lie on your back with knees bent and feet flat. Do the pelvic tilt (Exercise 9), and hold your lower back firmly against the floor.

2.   Slowly and carefully, move one leg away from your chest as you straighten your knee. Move your leg out until you feel your lower back start to arch. When this happens, tuck your knee back to your chest. Reset your pelvic tilt and roll your leg out again. Breathe out as your leg rolls out. Do not hold your breath. Repeat with the other leg.

You are strengthening your abdominal muscles by holding your pelvic tilt against the weight of your leg. As you get stronger, you'll be able to straighten your legs out farther and move both legs together.

HIP AND LEG EXERCISES

14. Straight Leg Raises

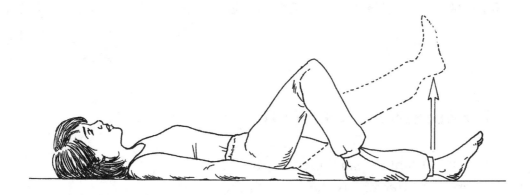

This exercise strengthens the muscles that bend the hip and straighten the knee. Lie on your back, knees bent, feet flat. Straighten one leg. Tighten the muscle on the top of that thigh, and straighten the knee as much as possible. Keeping the knee straight, raise your leg one to two feet (about 50 cm) off the ground. Do not arch your back. Hold your leg up and count out loud for 10 seconds. Relax. Repeat with the other leg.

15. Hip Hooray

This exercise can be done standing or lying on your back. If you lie down, spread your legs as far apart as possible. Roll your legs and feet out like a duck, then in to be pigeon-toed, and move your legs back together. If you are standing, move one leg out to your side as far as you can. Lead out with the heel and in with the toes. Hold onto a counter for support.

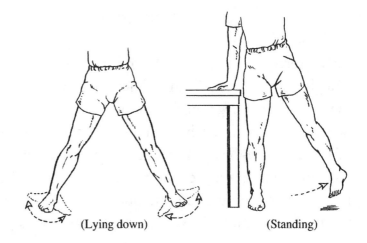

(Lying down)　　　(Standing)

16. Back Kick (VIP) (BB)

This exercise increases the backward mobility and strength of your hip. Hold onto a counter for support. Move the leg up and back, knee straight. Stand tall, and do not lean forward.

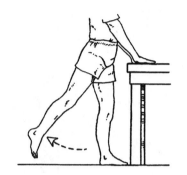

17. Knee Strengthener (VIP)

Strong knees are important for walking and standing comfortably. This exercise strengthens the knee. Sitting in a chair, straighten the knee by tightening up the muscle on top of your thigh. Place your hand on your thigh and feel the muscle work. If you wish, make circles with your toes. As your knee strengthens, see if you can build up to holding your leg out for 30 seconds. Count out loud. Do not hold your breath.

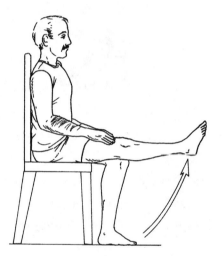

18. Power Knees

This exercise strengthens the muscles that bend and straighten your knee. Sit in a chair and cross your legs at the ankles. Your legs can be almost straight, or you can bend your knees as much as you like. Try several positions. Push forward with your back leg, and press backward with your front leg. Exert pressure evenly so that your legs do not move. Hold and count out loud for 10 seconds. Relax. Change leg positions. Be sure to keep breathing. Repeat.

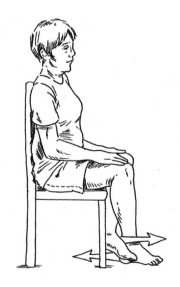

19. Ready-Go (VIP) (BB)

Stand with one leg slightly in front of the other in the position of having your heel on the floor ready to take a step with the front foot. Now tighten the muscles on the front of your thigh, making your knee firm and straight. Hold to a count of 10. Relax. Repeat with the other leg.

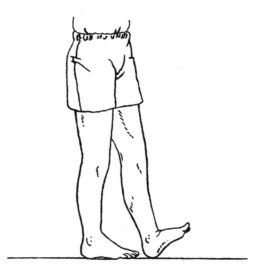

20. Hamstring Stretch

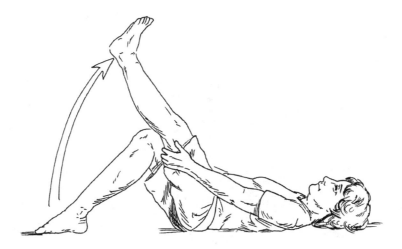

Do the self-test for hamstring tightness (page 131) to see if you need to do this exercise. If you have unstable knees, or "back knee" (a knee that curves backward when you stand up), do not do this exercise.

   If you do have tight hamstrings, lie on your back, knees bent, feet flat. Grasp one leg at a time behind the thigh. Holding the leg out at arm's length, slowly straighten the knee. Hold the leg as straight as you can as you count to 10. You should feel a slight stretch at the back of your knee and thigh.

   Be careful with this exercise. It's easy to overstretch and be sore.

21. Achilles Stretch (BB)

This exercise helps maintain flexibility in the Achilles tendon, the large tendon you feel at the back of your ankle. Good flexibility helps reduce the risk of injury, calf discomfort, and heel pain. The Achilles stretch is especially helpful for cooling down after walking or cycling, and for people who get cramps in the calf muscles. If you have trouble with standing balance or spasticity (muscle jerks), you can do a seated version of this exercise. Sit in a chair with feet flat on the floor. Keep your heel on the floor and slowly slide your foot (one foot at a time) back to bend your ankle and feel some tension on the back of your calf.

Stand at a counter or against a wall. Place one foot in front of the other, toes pointing forward and heels on the ground. Lean forward, bend the knee of the forward leg, and keep the back knee straight, heel down. You will feel a good stretch in the calf. Hold the stretch for 10 seconds. Do not bounce. Move gently.

It's easy to get sore doing this exercise. If you've worn shoes with high heels for a long time, be particularly careful.

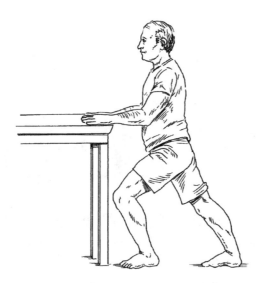

22. Tiptoes (BB)

This exercise will help strengthen your calf muscles and make walking, climbing stairs, and standing less tiring. It may also improve your balance. Hold on to a counter or table for support and rise up on your tiptoes. Hold for 10 seconds. Lower slowly. How high you go is not as important as keeping your balance and controlling your ankles. It is easier to do both legs at the same time. If your feet are too sore to do this standing, start doing it while sitting down. If this exercise makes your ankle jerk, leave it out, and talk to your therapist about other ways to strengthen these calf muscles if needed.

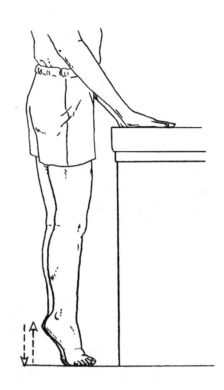

ANKLE AND FOOT EXERCISES

Do these exercises sitting in a straight-backed chair with your feet bare. Have a bath towel and 10 marbles next to you. These exercises are for flexibility, strength, and comfort. This is a good time to examine your feet and toes for any signs of circulation or skin problems, and to check your nails to see if they need trimming.

23. Towel Grabber

Spread a towel out in front of your chair. Place your feet on the towel, with your heels near the edge closest to you. Keep your heels down and your foot slightly raised. Scoot the towel back underneath your feet by pulling it with your toes. When you have done as much as you can, reverse the toe motion and scoot the towel out again.

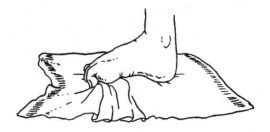

24. Marble Pick-Up

Do this exercise one foot at a time. Place several marbles on the floor between your feet. Keep your heel down, and pivot your toes toward the marbles. Pick up a marble with your toes, and pivot your foot to drop the marble as far as possible from where you picked it up. Repeat until all the marbles have been moved. Reverse the process and return all the marbles to the starting position. If marbles are difficult, try other objects, like jacks, dice, or wads of paper.

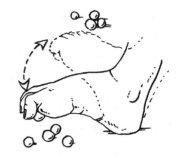

25. Foot Roll

Place a rolling pin (or a large dowel or closet rod) under the arch of your foot, and roll it back and forth. It feels great and stretches the ligaments in the arch of the foot.

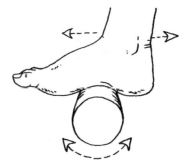

BALANCE EXERCISES

The exercises in this section are designed to let you practise balance activities in a safe and progressive way. The exercises are presented in order of difficulty, so start with the first exercises and work up to the more difficult ones as your strength and balance improve. If you feel that your balance is particularly poor, exercise with someone else close by to give you a supporting hand if needed. Always practise by a counter or stable chair so that you can hold on if you need to. Signs of improving balance are being able to hold a position longer or without extra support, or being able to do the exercise or hold the position with your eyes closed.

26. Beginning Balance

Stand quietly with your feet comfortably apart. Place your hands on your hips and turn your head and trunk as far to the left as possible, and then to the right. Repeat 5 to 10 times. To increase the difficulty, close your eyes and do the same thing.

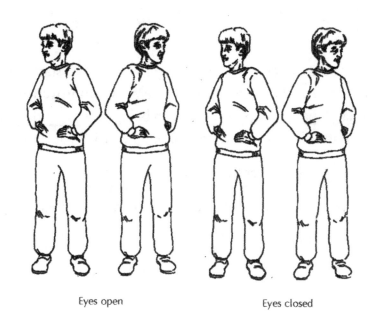

Eyes open   Eyes closed

27. Swing and Sway

Using a counter or back of a stable chair for support, do each of the following 5 to 10 times:

1. Rock back on your heels and then go up on your toes.

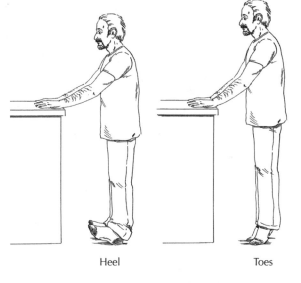

Heel   Toes

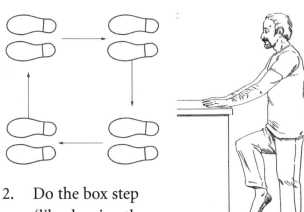

March

2. Do the box step (like dancing the waltz).

3. March in place with eyes open and eyes closed.

28. Base of Support

Do these exercises with stand-by assistance or standing close to a counter for support. The purpose of these exercises is to help you improve your balance by going from a larger to a smaller base of support. Work on being able to hold each position for 10 seconds. When you can do it with your eyes open, practice with your eyes closed.

1. Stand with feet together.

2. Stand with one foot out in front and the other back.

3. Stand heel to toe.

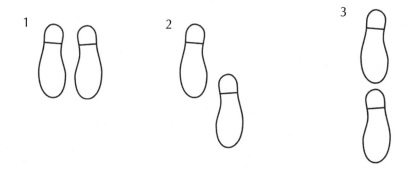

29. Toe Walk

The purpose of this exercise is to increase ankle strength and to give you practice balancing on a small base of support while moving. Stay close to a counter or support. Rise up on your toes and walk up and back along the counter. Once you are comfortable walking on your toes without support and with your eyes open, try with your eyes closed.

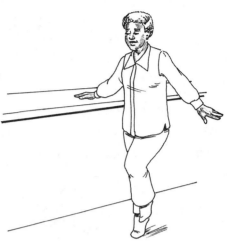

30. Heel Walk

The purpose of this exercise is to increase your lower leg strength and give you practice moving on a small base of support. Stay close to a counter for support. Raise your toes and forefoot and walk up and back along the counter on your heels. Once you are comfortable walking on your heels without support and with your eyes open, try with your eyes closed.

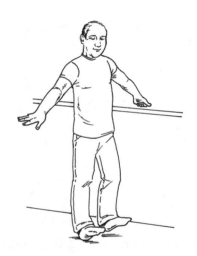

31. One-Legged Stand

Holding onto a counter or chair, lift one foot completely off the ground. Once you are balanced, lift your hand. The goal is to hold the position for 10 seconds. Once you can do this for 10 seconds without holding on, practise it with your eyes closed. Repeat for the other leg.

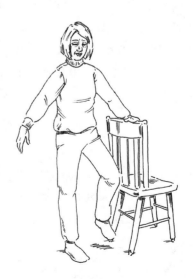

THE WHOLE BODY

32. The Stretcher

This exercise is a whole-body stretch to be done lying on your back. Start the motion at your ankles as explained here, or reverse the process if you want to start with your arms first.

1. Point your toes, and then pull your toes toward your nose. Relax.

2. Bend your knees. Then flatten your knees and let them relax.

3. Arch your back. Do the pelvic tilt. Relax.

4. Breathe in, and stretch your arms above your head. Breathe out, and lower your arms. Relax.

5. Stretch your right arm above your head, and stretch your left leg by pushing away with your heel. Hold for a count of 10. Switch to the other side and repeat.

SELF-TESTS

Whatever our goals, we all need to see that our efforts make a difference. Since an exercise program produces gradual change, it's often hard to tell if the program is working and to recognize improvement. Choose several of these flexibility and strength tests to measure your progress. Not everyone will be able to do all the tests. Choose those that work best for you. Perform each test before you start your exercise program, and record the results. After every four weeks, do the tests again and check your improvement.

1. Arm Flexibility

Do Exercise 6 (pat and reach) for both sides of the body. Ask someone to measure the distance between your fingertips.

Goal: Less distance between your fingertips.

2. Shoulder Flexibility

Stand facing a wall, with your toes touching the wall. One arm at a time, reach up the wall in front of you. Hold a pencil, or have someone mark how far you reached. Also do this sideways, standing about three inches (8 cm) away from the wall.

Goal: To reach higher.

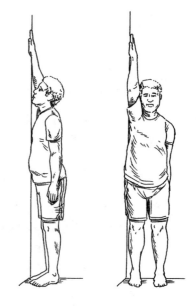

3. Hamstring Flexibility

Do the hamstring stretch (Exercise 20), one leg at a time. Keep your thigh perpendicular to your body. How much does your knee bend? How tight does the back of your leg feel?

Goal: Straighter knee and less tension in the back of the leg.

4. Ankle Flexibility

Sit in a chair with your bare feet flat on the floor and your knees bent at a 90-degree angle. Keep your heels on the floor. Raise your toes and the front of your foot. Ask someone to measure the distance between the ball of your foot and the floor.

Goal: One to two inches (3 to 5 cm) between your foot and the floor.

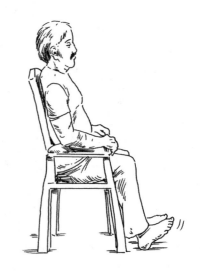

5. Abdominal Strength

Do the curl-up (Exercise 12). Count how many repetitions you can do before you get too tired to do more, or count how many you can do in one minute.

Goal: More repetitions.

6. Ankle Strength

This test has two parts. Stand at a table or counter for support.

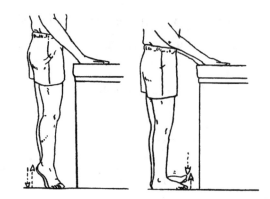

1. Do Exercise 22 (tiptoes) as quickly and as often as you can. How many can you do before you tire?

2. Stand with your feet flat. Put most of your weight on one foot, and quickly tap the floor with the front part of your other foot. How many taps can you do before you tire?

Goal: Ten to fifteen repetitions of each movement.

Suggested Further Reading

Baechle, Thomas R. *Fitness Weight Training*. Chanpgian, Ill.: Human Kinetics Publishers, 2005.

Blahnik, Jay. *Full Body Flexibility*. Champaign, IL: Human Kinetics, 2004.

Copeland, Glenn. Healthy Feet: *The Foot Doctor's Complete Guide for Men and Women*. Key Porter, 2004.

Knopf, Karl. *Stretching for 50 +*. Berkeley, Calif.: Ulysses Press, 2004.

Knopf, Karl. *Strength Training for 50 Plus*. Berkeley, Calif.: Ulysses Press, 2006.

Moccandanza, Roberto. *Stretching Basics.* New York: Sterling Publishing Co., 2004.

Stark, Steven. *The Stark Reality of Stretching: An Informed Approach for All Activities and Every Sport.* Vancouver: Stark Reality Corp., 2000.

Torkelson, Charlene. *Get Fit While You Sit: Easy Workouts from Your Chair.* Alameda, Calif.: Hunter House, 1999.

EXERCISING FOR ENDURANCE:
Aerobic Activities

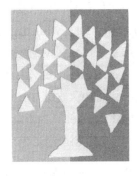

8

How much is enough? One of the biggest problems with endurance (aerobic) exercise is that it is easy to overdo, even for those who don't have a chronic illness. Inexperienced and misinformed exercisers think they have to work very hard for exercise to do any good. Exhaustion, sore muscles, painful joints, and shortness of breath are the results of jumping in too hard and too fast. As a result, some people may discontinue their exercise programs indefinitely, thinking that exercise is just not meant for them.

There is no magic formula for determining how much exercise you need. The most important thing to remember is that some is better than none. If you start slowly and increase your efforts gradually, it is likely that you will maintain your exercise program as a lifelong habit. Generally it is better to begin your conditioning program by underdoing rather than overdoing. Here are some rough guidelines to help you decide how much exercise is enough for you.

Several studies suggest that the upper limit of benefit is about 200 minutes of moderate-intensity aerobic exercise per week. Doing more than that doesn't gain you much (and it increases your risk of injury). On the other hand, doing 100 minutes of exercise per week gets you about 90 per cent of the gain, while 60 minutes of aerobic exercise per week yields about 75 per cent of the gain. Sixty minutes is just 15 minutes of mild aerobic exercise four times a week!

Let's take a closer look at some general guidelines for the frequency, duration, and intensity of aerobic exercise.

- **Frequency:** Three or four times a week is a good choice for aerobic exercise. Taking every other day off gives your body a chance to rest and recover. We recommend that you rest at least one day per week.

- **Time:** Start with just a few minutes, and gradually increase the duration of your aerobic activity to about 30 minutes a session. You can safely increase the time by alternating intervals of brisk exercise with intervals of rest or easy exercise. For example, after 3–5 minutes of brisk walking, do 1–2 minutes of easy strolling, then another 3–5 minutes of brisk walking. Eventually, you can build up to 30 minutes of activity. Then gradually eliminate rest intervals until you can maintain 20–30 minutes of brisk exercise. If 30 minutes seems too long, consider sessions of 10–15 minutes each, to accumulate 30 minutes of moderate physical activity on most days of the week. Either way appears to improve health significantly.

- **Intensity:** Safe and effective endurance exercise should be done at no more than moderate intensity. High-intensity exercise increases the risk of injury and causes discomfort, so not many people stick with it. Exercise intensity is measured by how hard you work. For a trained runner, completing a mile in 12 minutes is probably low-intensity exercise. For a person who hasn't exercised in a long time, a brisk 10-minute walk may be of moderate to high intensity. For others with severe physical limitations, a slow walk may be of moderate intensity. The trick, of course, is to figure out what is moderate intensity for you. There are several easy ways to do this.

TALK TEST

Talk to another person or yourself, or recite poems out loud while you exercise. Moderate-intensity exercise allows you to speak comfortably. If you can't carry on a conversation because you are breathing too hard or are short of breath, you're working too hard. Slow down. The talk test is an easy way to regulate exercise intensity.

If you have lung disease, the talk test might not work for you. If that is the case, try the perceived-exertion test.

PERCEIVED EXERTION

Another way to monitor intensity is to rate how hard you're working on a scale of 0 to 10. Zero, at the low end of the scale, is lying down, doing no work at all. Ten is equivalent to working as hard as possible, very hard work that you couldn't do longer than a few seconds. Of course, you never want to exercise that hard. A good level for your aerobic exercise routine is between 3 and 6 on this scale. At this level, you'll usually feel warmer, that you're breathing more deeply and faster than usual, that your heart is beating faster than normal, but you should not be feeling pain.

Remember, these are just rough guidelines on frequency, duration, and intensity, not a rigid prescription. Listen to your own body. Sometimes you need to tell yourself (and maybe others) that enough is enough. More exercise is not necessarily better, especially if it gives you more pain or discomfort. As *Walking* magazine says, "Go for the smiles, not the miles."

HEART RATE

Unless you're taking heart-regulating medication (such as the beta-blocker propranolol), monitoring your heart rate while exercising is one way to measure exercise intensity. The faster the heart beats, the harder you're working. (Your heart also beats fast when you are frightened or nervous, but here we're talking about how your heart responds to physical activity.) Endurance exercise at moderate intensity raises your heart rate to a range between 60 and 80 percent of your safe maximum heart rate. The safe maximum heart rate declines with age, so your safe exercise heart rate gets lower as you get older. You can follow the general guidelines of Table 8.1, "Age–Exercise Heart Rate," or calculate your individual exercise heart rate. Either way, you need to know how to take your pulse.

Take your pulse by placing the tips of your middle three fingers at your wrist below the base of your thumb. Feel around in that spot until you feel the pulsations of blood pumping with each heartbeat. Count how many beats you feel in 15 seconds. Multiply this number by 4 to find out how fast your heart is beating in one minute. Start by taking your pulse whenever you think of it, and you'll soon learn the difference between your resting and exercise heart rates.

How to calculate your own exercise heart rate range:

1. Subtract your age from 220:

    Example: 220 – 60 = 160   *You*: 220 – _____ = _____

2. To find the lower end of your exercise heart rate range, multiply your answer in step 1 by 0.6:

    Example: 160 × 0.6 = 96   You: _____ × 0.6 = _____

Table 8.1 **Age–Exercise Heart Rate**

Age	Exercise Pulse (Beats per Minute)	Exercise Pulse (15 second count)
30	114–152	28–38
40	108–144	27–36
50	102–136	25–34
60	96–128	24–32
70	90–120	22–30
80	84–112	21–28
Over 80	78–104	19–26

3. To find the upper end of your exercise heart rate range, which you should not exceed, multiply your answer in step 1 by 0.8:

Example: 160 × 0.8 = 128   *You*: _____ × 0.8 = _____

The exercise heart rate range in our example is from 96 to 128 beats per minute. What is yours?

Most people count their pulse for 15 seconds, not a whole minute. To find your 15-second pulse, divide both the lower-end and upper-end numbers by 4. The person in our example should be able to count between 24 (96 ÷ 4) and 32 (128 ÷ 4) beats in 15 seconds while exercising.

The most important reason for knowing your exercise heart rate range is so that you can learn not to exercise too vigorously. After you've done your warm-up and 5 minutes of endurance exercise, take your pulse. If it's higher than the upper rate, don't panic. Slow down a bit. Don't work so hard.

At first, some people have trouble keeping their heart rate within the "ideal" heart rate range. Don't worry about that. Keep exercising at the level with which you're most comfortable. As you get more experienced and stronger, you will gradually be able to do more vigorous exercise while keeping your heart rate within your "goal" range. But don't let the target heart rate monitoring become a burden. Recent studies have shown that even low-intensity exercise can provide significant health benefits. So use the "ideal" heart rate range as a rough guide, but don't worry if you can't reach the lower end of that range. The important thing is to keep exercising!

If you are taking medicine that regulates your heart rate, have trouble feeling your pulse, or think that keeping track of your heart rate is a bother, use one of the other methods to monitor your exercise intensity.

HOW MUCH IS ENOUGH? THE FIT FORMULA

The results of your aerobic exercise program depend on how often you exercise (F = Frequency), how hard you work (I = Intensity), and how long you exercise each day (T = Time). In much the same way a doctor prescribes medicine to have a certain effect, you can select your own "exercise dose" to get the result you want. Your exercise dose comes from how you combine the frequency, intensity, and time of your exercise. A bigger dose gives you different benefits than a smaller dose.

- **Frequency:** Three to five days a week. Three days a week is the starting minimum. As you gain endurance and strength, you can do aerobic exercise more often. If you exercise more vigorously, three days is enough. If your aerobic exercise is a comfortably paced walk, you could build up to five or even seven days a week.

- **Intensity:** No more than moderate intensity. Moderate intensity is being able to carry on a conversation while you exercise, a perceived-exertion level of no more than 6, or an exercise heart rate of no more than 75 per cent of your age-predicted maximum heart rate.

- **Time:** Minimum of 30 minutes of accumulated low to moderate physical activity. For health benefits, the activity may be accumulated in three 10-minute bouts during the day. To improve cardiovascular fitness, it may be necessary to exercise a bit longer each time.

People who are beginning an exercise program will find Health Canada's recommendations useful.

WHEN TO WARM UP AND COOL DOWN

Warm-Up

If you are going to exercise at an intensity that causes you to breathe harder or your heart to beat faster, it is important to warm up first. A warm-up means that you do at least 5 minutes of a low-intensity activity to allow your heart, lungs, and circulation to gradually increase their work. If you are going for a brisk walk, warm up with 5 minutes of slow walking first. If you are riding a stationary bike, warm up on the bike with 5 minutes of no resistance and at no more than 60 rpm (revolutions per minute). In an aerobic exercise class, you will warm up with a gentle routine before getting more vigorous. Warming up reduces the risk of injuries, soreness, and irregular heartbeat.

Cool Down

A cool-down period is important if you have exercised at an intensity that required you to breathe harder and your heart to beat faster, or if you felt warmer or perspired. Repeating the 5-minute warm-up activity or taking a slow walk helps your muscles gradually relax and your heart and breathing to slow down. Gentle stretching and flexibility exercises during the cool-down can be effective for increasing motion because your muscles and joints are warm and more easily stretched. Also, stretching gently now helps reduce the muscle soreness and stiffness that may follow vigorous exercise.

ENDURANCE (AEROBIC) EXERCISES

Many activities can be aerobic. We will examine in detail a few of the more common ones, including walking, swimming, stationary bicycling, and low-impact aerobics.

Walking

Walking can condition your heart and lungs, strengthen bones and muscles, relieve tension, control weight, and generally make you feel good. Walking is easy, inexpensive, safe, and accessible. You can walk by yourself or with company, and you can take your exercise with you wherever you go. Walking is safer and puts less stress on the body than jogging or running. It's an especially good choice if you are older, have been sedentary, or have joint problems.

Most people with a chronic illness can walk as a fitness exercise. If you walk to shop, visit friends, and do household chores, then you'll probably be able to walk for exercise. Using a cane or walker need not stop you from getting into a walking routine. If you are in a wheelchair, use crutches, or experience more than mild discomfort when you walk a short distance, you should consider some other type of aerobic exercise, or consult a physician or therapist for help.

Be cautious the first two weeks of walking. If you haven't been doing much for a while, 10 minutes of walking may be enough. Build up your time with intervals of strolling. Each week increase the brisk walking interval by no more than 5 minutes until you are up to 20 or 30 minutes. Follow the frequency, duration, and intensity guidelines, and read these tips on walking before you start.

Walking Tips

- **Choose your ground.** Walk on a flat, level surface. Walking on hills, uneven ground, soft earth, sand, or gravel is hard work and often leads to hip, knee, or foot pain. Fitness trails, shopping malls, school tracks, streets with sidewalks, and quiet neighborhoods are good places to get started.

- **Always warm up and cool down with a stroll.** It's important to walk slowly for 3 to 5 minutes to prepare your circulation and muscles for a brisk walk, and to finish up with the same slow walk to let your body slow down gradually. Experienced walkers know they can avoid shin and foot discomfort if they begin and end with a stroll.

- **Set your own pace.** It takes practice to find the right walking speed. To find your speed, start walking slowly for a few minutes, then increase your speed to a pace that is slightly faster than normal for you. After 5 minutes, monitor your exercise intensity by checking your pulse, or using the perceived-exertion or talk method. If you are above the range or feel out of breath, slow down. If you are below the range, try walking a little faster. Walk another 5 minutes and check your intensity again. If you are still below your exercise range, keep walking at a comfortable speed and simply check your intensity in the middle and at the end of each walk.

- Increase your arm work. You can also raise your heart rate into the "ideal" or target exercise range by increasing arm work. (Remember that many people with lung disease may want to avoid arm exercises, since they can cause more shortness of breath than other exercises.) Bend your elbows a bit and swing your arms more vigorously. Alternatively, carry a one- or two-pound weight (0.75 kg) in each hand. You can purchase hand weights for walking; hold a can of food in each hand; or put sand, dried beans, or pennies in two small plastic beverage bottles or socks. The extra work you do with your arms increases your intensity of exercise without forcing you to walk faster than you find comfortable.

Shoes

It's not necessary to spend a lot of money on shoes. Wear shoes of the correct length and width with shock-absorbing soles and insoles. Make sure they're big enough in the toe area: The "rule of thumb" is a thumb width between the end of your longest toe and the end of the shoe. You shouldn't feel pressure on the sides or tops of your toes. The heel counter should hold your heel firmly in the shoe when you walk.

Wear shoes with a continuous crepe or composite sole in good repair. Shoes with leather soles and a separate heel don't absorb shock as well as the newer athletic and casual shoes. Shoes with laces or Velcro let you adjust width as needed and give more support than slip-ons. If you have problems tying laces, consider Velcro closures or elastic shoelaces.

Many people like shoes with removable insoles that can be exchanged for more shock-absorbing ones. Insoles are available in sporting goods stores and shoe stores. When you shop for insoles, take your walking shoes with you. Try on the shoe with the insole to make sure there's still enough room inside for your foot to be comfortable. Insoles come in sizes and can be trimmed with scissors for a final fit. If your toes take up extra room, try the three-quarter insoles that stop just short of your toes. If you have prescribed inserts in your shoes already, ask your doctor about insoles.

Possible Problems

If you have pain around your shins when you walk, you may not be spending enough time warming up. Try some ankle exercises before you start walking. Start your walk at a slow pace for at least 5 minutes. Keep your feet and toes relaxed.

Another common problem is sore knees. Fast walking puts stress on knee joints. To slow your speed and keep your heart rate up, try doing more work with your arms (see above). Do the knee strengthener and ready-go (Chapter 7, Exercises 17 and 19) in your warm-up to reduce knee pain.

Cramps in the calf and heel pain can be avoided by doing the Achilles stretch (Chapter 7, Exercise 21) before and after walking. A slow walk to warm up is also helpful. If you have circulatory problems in your legs, and experience cramps or pain in your calves while walking, alternate intervals of brisk and slow walking at whatever pace you can tolerate. Slow down and give your circulation a chance to catch up before the pain is so intense that you have to stop. As you will see, such exercises may even help you to gradually walk farther with less cramping or pain. If this doesn't help, check with your physician or therapist for suggestions.

Maintain good posture. Remember the heads-up position in Chapter 7, and keep your shoulders relaxed to help reduce neck and upper back discomfort.

Swimming

Swimming is another good endurance exercise. The buoyancy of the water lets you move your joints through their full range of motion and strengthen your muscles and cardiovascular system with less stress than on land. Since swimming involves the arms, it can lead to excessive shortness of breath in people with lung disease. However, for people with asthma, swimming may be the preferred exercise, as the moisture helps reduce shortness of breath. People with heart disease who have severely irregular heartbeats and have had an implantable "defibrillator" (AICD) permanently attached to the heart should avoid swimming. For most people with chronic illness, however, swimming is excellent exercise. It uses the whole body. If you haven't been swimming for a while, consider a refresher course.

To make swimming an endurance exercise, you will eventually need to swim continuously for 20 minutes. Use the frequency, duration, and intensity guidelines set out at the beginning of this chapter to build up your endurance. Try different strokes, modifying them or changing strokes after each lap or two. This lets you exercise all joints and muscles without overtiring any one area.

Swimming Tips

- The breast stroke and crawl normally require a lot of neck motion and may be uncomfortable if you have neck pain. To solve this problem, use a mask and snorkel so that you can breathe without twisting your neck.

- Chlorine can be irritating to eyes. Consider a good pair of goggles. You can even have swim goggles made in your eyeglass prescription.

- A hot shower or soak in a hot tub after your workout helps reduce stiffness and muscle soreness. Remember not to work too hard or get too tired. If you're sore for more than two hours, go easier next time.

- Always swim where there are qualified lifeguards, if possible, or with a friend. Never swim alone.

Aquacise

If you don't like to swim or are uncomfortable learning strokes, you can walk laps in the pool or join the millions who are "aquacising"—exercising in water.

Aquacise is comfortable, fun, and effective as a flexibility, strengthening, and aerobic activity. The buoyancy of the water takes weight off the hips, knees, feet, and back. Because of this, exercise in water is generally better tolerated than walking by people who have pain in the hips, knees, feet, and back. Exercising in a pool allows you a degree of privacy in doing your own routine, since no one can see you much below shoulder level.

Getting Started

Joining a water exercise class with a good instructor is an excellent way to get started. The YMCA-YWCA and local Parks and Recreation departments offer classes at different levels of intensity, and for many, you don't need swimming skills, as the class is taught in shallow water. Aquasize classes are taught by certified instructors with your safety in mind. Canadians are fortunate to enjoy a high national standard of both swim and fitness instruction, which is adopted at the provincial level.

You can find these programs, such as *Waterworks* (which is developed, but not taught by, the Arthritis Society), offered at your community pool. Most aquatic programs offer a "Nifty Fifties" or a low intensity session geared toward seniors and those with mobility impairments. Contact your local recreation department.

If you have access to a pool and want to exercise on your own, there are many water exercise books available. One we recommend is *Hydrorobics*, by Joseph A. Krasevec and Diane C. Grimes (Human Kinetics Publishers, 1985). It contains a lot of good ideas for exercise in the water.

Water temperature is always a concern when people talk about water exercise. The Arthritis Society recommends a pool temperature of 84°F (29°C), with the surrounding air temperature in the same range. Except in warm climates, this means a heated pool. If you're just starting to aquacize, find a pool with these temperatures. If you can exercise more vigorously and don't have the condition known as Raynaud's phenomenon or other type of cold sensitivity, you can probably aquacize in cooler water. Many pools where people swim laps are about 80–83°F (27–28°C). It feels quite cool when you first get in, but starting off with water walking, jogging, or another whole-body exercise helps you warm up quickly.

The deeper the water you stand in, the less stress there is on joints; however, water above mid-chest can make it hard to keep your balance. You can let the water cover more of your body just by spreading your legs apart or bending your knees a bit.

Aquacise Tips

- Wear something on your feet to protect them from rough pool floors and to provide traction in the pool and on the deck. Choices vary from terry cloth slippers with rubber soles (they stretch in water, so buy a size smaller than your shoe size) to footgear especially designed for water exercise. Some styles have Velcro tape to make them easier to put on. Beach shoes with rubber soles and mesh tops also work well.

- If you are sensitive to cold or have Raynaud's phenomenon, wear a pair of disposable latex surgical gloves. Boxes of gloves are available at most pharmacies. The water trapped and warmed inside the glove seems to insulate the hand. If your body gets cold in the water, wear a T-shirt and/or full-leg Lycra exercise tights for warmth.

- If the pool does not have steps, and it is difficult for you to climb up and down a ladder, suggest that pool staff position a three-step kitchen stool in the pool by the ladder rails. This is an inexpensive way to provide steps for easier entry and exit, and it is easy to remove and store when not needed.

- Wearing a flotation belt or life vest adds extra buoyancy, to take weight off hips, knees, and feet. That makes exercising more comfortable for these joints.

- You can regulate how hard you work in the water by the way you move. To make the work easier, move slowly. Another way to regulate exercise intensity is to change how much water you push when you move. For example, when you move your arms back and forth in front of you under water, it is hard work if you hold your palms facing each other and clap. It is easier if you turn your palms down and slice your arms back and forth with only the narrow edge of your hands pushing against the water.

- If you have asthma, exercising in water helps to avoid the worsening of asthma symptoms that occurs during other types of exercise. This is probably due to the beneficial effect of water vapor on the lungs. Remember, though, that for many people with lung disease, exercises involving the arms can cause more shortness of breath than leg exercises. You may want to focus most of your aquacizing, therefore, on exercises involving mainly the legs.

- If you have had a stroke, or have another condition that may affect your strength and balance, make sure that you have someone to help you in and out of the pool. Finding a position close to the wall or staying close to a buddy who can lend a hand if needed are ways to add to your safety and security. You may even wish to sit on a chair in fairly shallow water as you do water exercises. Ask the instructor to help you design the best exercise program, equipment, and facilities for your specific needs.

Stationary Bicycling

Stationary bicycles offer the fitness benefits of bicycling without the outdoor hazards. They're preferable for people who don't have the flexibility, strength, or balance to be comfortable pedalling and steering on the road. Some people with paralysis of one leg or arm can exercise on stationary bicycles with special attachments for their paralyzed limb. Indoor use of stationary bicycles may also be preferable to outdoor bicycling for people who live in a cold or hilly area.

The stationary bicycle is a particularly good alternative exercise. It doesn't put excess strain on your hips, knees, and feet; you can easily adjust how hard you work; and weather doesn't matter. Use the bicycle on days when you don't want to walk or do more vigorous exercise, or when you can't exercise outside.

Make It Interesting

The most common complaint about riding a stationary bike is that it's boring. If you ride while watching television, reading, or listening to music, you can become fit without

---

Stationary-Bicycle Checklist

- The bicycle is steady when you get on and off. The resistance is easy to set and can be set to zero. The seat is comfortable.

- The seat can be adjusted for full knee extension when the pedal is at its lowest point.

- Large pedals and loose pedal straps allow the feet to move slightly while pedaling.

- There is ample clearance from the frame for the knees and ankles.

- The handlebars allow good posture and comfortable arm position.

---

becoming bored. One woman keeps interested by mapping out tours of places she would like to visit, and then charts her progress on the map as she rolls off the miles. Other people set their bicycle time for the half hour of soap opera or news that they watch every day. There are also videocassettes of exotic bike tours that put you in the rider's perspective. Book racks that clip on to the handlebars make reading easy.

Riding Tips

- Bicycling uses different muscles than walking. Until your leg muscles get used to pedalling, you may be able to ride only a few minutes. Start off with no resistance. Increase resistance slightly every two weeks. Increasing resistance has the same effect as bicycling up hills. If you use too much resistance, your knees are likely to hurt, and you'll have to stop before you get the benefit of endurance.

- Pedal at a comfortable speed. For most people, 50–60 revolutions per minute (rpm) is a good place to start. Some bicycles tell you the rpm, or you can count the number of times your right foot reaches its lowest point in a minute. As you get used to bicycling, you can increase your speed. However, faster is not necessarily better. Listening to music at the right tempo makes it easier to pedal at a consistent speed. Experience will tell you the best combination of speed and resistance.

- Set your goal for 20 to 30 minutes of pedalling at a comfortable speed. Build up your time by alternating intervals of brisk pedalling with less exertion. Use your heart rate, or the perceived-exertion talk test to make sure you aren't working too hard. If you're alone, try singing songs as you pedal. If you get out of breath, slow down.

- Keep a record of the times and distances of your "bike trips." You'll be amazed at how much you can do.

- On bad days, maintain your exercise habit going by pedalling with no resistance, at a lower rpm, or for a shorter period of time.

Other Exercise Equipment

If you have trouble getting on or off a stationary bicycle, or don't have room for a bicycle where you live, you might try a restorator or arm crank. Ask your therapist or doctor, or call a medical supply house.

A restorator is a small piece of equipment with foot pedals that can be attached to the foot of a bed or placed on the floor in front of a chair. It allows you to exercise by pedaling. Resistance can be varied, and placement of the restorator lets you adjust for leg length and knee bend. A restorator can be a good alternative to an exercise bicycle for people who have problems with balance, weakness, or paralysis. People with other chronic illnesses, such as lung disease, may find the restorator to be an enjoyable first step in getting an exercise program started.

Arm cranks are bicycles for the arms. They are mounted on a table. People who are unable to use their legs for active exercise can improve their cardiovascular fitness and upper-body strength by using the arm crank. It's important to work closely with a therapist to set up your program, because using only your arms for endurance exercise requires different intensity monitoring than using the bigger leg muscles. As mentioned previously, many people with lung disease may find arm exercises to be less enjoyable than leg exercises since they may experience shortness of breath.

There is a wide variety of exercise equipment in addition to what we've mentioned so far. These include treadmills, self-powered and motor-driven rowing machines, cross-country skiing machines, mini-trampolines, and stair-climbing machines. Most are available in both commercial and home models. If you're thinking about exercise equipment, have your objectives clearly in mind. For cardiovascular fitness and endurance, you want equipment that will help you exercise as much of your body at one time as possible. The motion should be rhythmical, repetitive, and continuous. The equipment should be comfortable, safe, and not stressful on joints. If you're interested in a new piece of equipment, try it out for a week or two before buying it.

Exercise equipment that requires you to use weights usually does not improve cardiovascular fitness unless individualized "circuit training" can be designed. A weight-lifting program alone builds strength, but it can put excessive stress on joints, muscles, tendons, and ligaments. Most people will find that the flexibility and strengthening exercises in this book will help them safely achieve significant increases in strength as well as flexibility. Be sure that you consult with your doctor or therapist if you prefer to add strengthening exercises involving weights or weight machines to your program.

LOW-IMPACT AEROBICS

Most people find low-impact aerobic dance a fun and safe form of exercise. "Low impact" means that one foot is always on the floor and there is no jumping. However, low impact does not necessarily mean low intensity, nor do the low-impact routines protect all joints. If you participate in a low-impact aerobics class, you'll probably need to make some modifications based on your condition.

Getting Started

Start off by letting the instructor know who you are, that you may modify some movements to meet your needs, and that you may need to ask for advice. It's easier to start off with a newly formed class than it is to join an ongoing class. If you don't know people, try to get acquainted. Be open about why you may sometimes do things a little differently. You'll be more comfortable and may find others who also have special needs.

Most instructors use music or count to a specific beat and do a set number of repetitions. You may find that the movement is too fast or that you don't want to do as many repetitions. Modify the routine by slowing down to half-time, or keep up with the beat until you start to tire, and then slow down or stop. If the class is doing an exercise that involves arms and legs and you get tired, try resting your arms and do only the leg movements, or just walk in place until you are ready to go again. Most instructors will be able to instruct you in "chair aerobics" if you need some time off your feet.

Some low-impact routines use a lot of arm movements done at or above shoulder level to raise the heart rate. Remember that for people with lung disease, hypertension, or shoulder problems, too much arm exercise above shoulder level can worsen shortness of breath, increase blood pressure, or cause pain, respectively. Modify the exercise by lowering your arms or taking a rest break.

Being different from the group in a room walled with mirrors takes courage, conviction, and a sense of humor. The most important thing you can do for yourself is to choose an instructor who encourages everyone to exercise at her or his own pace and a class where people are friendly and having fun. Observe classes, speak with instructors, and participate in at least one class session before making any financial commitment.

Aerobics Studio Tips

- **Wear shoes.** Many studios have cushioned floors and soft carpet that might tempt you to go barefoot. Don't! Shoes help protect the small joints and muscles in your feet and ankles by providing a firm, flat surface on which to stand.

- **Protect your knees.** Stand with knees straight but relaxed. Many low-impact routines are done with bent, tensed knees and a lot of bobbing up and down. This can be painful and is unnecessarily stressful. Avoid this by remembering to keep your knees relaxed (aerobics instructors call this "soft" knees). Watch in the mirror to see that you keep the top of your head steady as you exercise. Don't bob up and down.

- **Don't overstretch.** The beginning (warm-up) and end (cool-down) of the session will have stretching and strengthening exercises. Remember to stretch only as far as you comfortably can. Hold the position and don't bounce. If the stretch hurts, don't do it. Ask your instructor for a less stressful substitute, or choose one of your own.

- **Change movements.** Do this often enough that you don't get sore muscles or joints. It's normal to feel some new sensations in your muscles and around your joints when you start a new exercise program. However, if you feel discomfort doing the same movement for some time, change movements or stop for a while and rest.

- **Alternate kinds of exercise.** Many exercise facilities have a variety of exercise opportunities: equipment rooms with cardiovascular machines, pools, and aerobic studios. If you have trouble with an hour-long aerobics class, see if you can join the class for the warm-up and cool-down and use a stationary bicycle or treadmill for your aerobic portion. Many people have found that this routine gives them the benefits of both an individualized program and group exercise.

SELF-TESTS FOR ENDURANCE/AEROBIC FITNESS

For some people, just the feelings of increased endurance and well-being are enough to demonstrate progress. Others may need proof that their exercise program is making a measurable difference. You may wish to try one or both of these endurance/aerobic fitness tests before you start your exercise program. Not everyone will be able to do both tests, so pick one that works best for you. Record your results. After four weeks of exercise, do the test again and check your improvement. Measure yourself again after four more weeks.

Distance Test

One of the least expensive pieces of equipment is a pedometer. Because distance can be difficult to set, the best pedometers measure the steps you take. If you get in the habit of wearing a pedometer, it is easy to motivate yourself to add a few extra steps each day. You will be surprised at how these add up.

Find a place to walk, bicycle, swim, or water-walk where you can measure distance. A running track works well. On a street you can measure distance with a car. A stationary bicycle with an odometer provides the equivalent measurement. If you plan on swimming or water walking, you can count lengths of the pool.

After a warm-up, note your starting point and bicycle, or swim, or walk as briskly as you comfortably can for 5 minutes. Try to move at a steady pace for the full time. At the end of 5 minutes, mark your spot or note the distance or number of laps, and immediately take your pulse and rate your perceived exertion from 0 to 10. Continue at a slow pace for 3 to 5 more minutes to cool down. Record the distance, your heart rate, and your perceived exertion.

Repeat the test after several weeks of exercise. There may be a change in as soon as 4 weeks. However, it often takes 8 to 12 weeks to see improvement.

Goal: To cover more distance, to lower your heart rate, or to lower your perceived exertion.

Time Test

Measure a given distance to walk, bike, swim, or water-walk. Estimate how far you think you can go in 1 to 5 minutes. You can pick a number of blocks, actual distance, or lengths in a pool.

Spend 3 to 5 minutes warming up. Start timing and begin moving steadily, briskly, and comfortably. At the finish, record how long it took you to cover your course, your heart rate, and your perceived exertion.

Repeat after several weeks of exercise. You may see changes in as soon as 4 weeks. However, it often takes 8 to 12 weeks for a noticeable improvement.

Goal: To complete the course in less time, at a lower heart rate, or at a lower perceived exertion.

Suggested Further Reading

Fortmann, Stephen P., and Prudence E. Breutrose. *The Blood Pressure Book: How to Get It Down and Keep It Down,* 2nd ed. Boulder, Colo.: Bull Publishing, 2001.

Karpay, Ellen. *The Everything Total Fitness Book.* Avon, MA: Adams Media Corporation, 2000.

Krasevec, Joseph A., and Grimes, Diane C. *Hydrorobics.* Human Kinetics, 1985.

Nelson, Miriam E, Alice H. Lichtenstein, and Lawrence Lindner. *Strong Women, Strong Hearts: Proven Strategies to Prevent and Reverse Heart Disease Now.* New York: G.P. Putnam's Sons, 2005.

Sayce, Valerie, and Ian Faser. *Exercise Beats Arthritis: An Easy-to-Follow Program of Exercises,* 3rd ed. Boulder, Co.: Bull Publishing; Berkeley, Calif.: Publishers Group West, 1998.

Schwartz, Anna L. *Cancer Fitness: Exercise Programs for Cancer Patients and Survivors.* New York: Fireside Books, Simon & Schuster, 2004.

EXERCISING TIPS FOR PEOPLE WITH SPECIFIC CHRONIC ILLNESSES

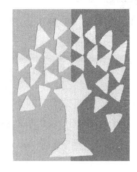

9

UNTIL NOW, OUR SUGGESTIONS HAVE BEEN APPLICABLE TO NEARLY EVERYONE WITH A CHRONIC ILLNESS. Here are some specific recommendations to help you answer any questions you may still have about exercise and your particular chronic health problem.

HEART DISEASE

If you have heart disease, you probably have had one or more of the following conditions:

1. Myocardial infarction (heart attack)

2. Coronary bypass surgery

3. Coronary "balloon" angioplasty

4. Angina pectoris (chest pain or discomfort)

It is important for you to understand, however, that exercise can be both safe and beneficial for many people who have experienced these conditions. It is also important for you to work closely with your doctor to design an exercise program that is safe and beneficial for you. When you visit with your doctor, ask to have your blood pressure checked in each arm to ensure your circulation is equal or close to being equal, in each arm. Remember that exercise not only has been shown to improve the quality of one's life but also may improve the length of one's life. Following are some general exercise guidelines for people with heart disease.

Should I Limit My Exercise Because of My Heart Disease?

Restrictions on conditioning activities may be necessary for some people with heart disease because of one or more of three conditions:

1.   Evidence of an ongoing restriction to blood flow to the heart muscle (ischemia).

2.   Presence of frequent and dangerous irregular heartbeats (arrhythmias).

3.   Decreased pumping strength of the heart muscle.

Your doctor will be able to tell you if you have any of these conditions by examining you and performing tests such as an electrocardiogram (EKG), exercise treadmill test, echocardiogram, or coronary angiogram (see Chapter 16).

If you do not have any of the above conditions, it is safe for you to begin the conditioning program outlined in this book, with common sense as your only restriction. For example, common sense would tell you that you shouldn't try to run a marathon during your first week of conditioning.

One word of caution: Strengthening activities, such as weight lifting or rowing, are generally quite safe but can lead to increased blood pressure, especially for those people with preexisting high blood pressure. Straining (holding your breath as you lift or row) can put unnecessary stress on the heart. If you and your doctor think weight lifting should be part of your conditioning program, remember to breathe out as you are lifting. One way of being sure to breathe is to sing or talk while you are exercising.

If you have any of the three conditions (ischemia, arrhythmias, or decreased pumping strength of the heart muscle), your doctor may wish to place one or more of the following restrictions on your activity.

Begin your conditioning program in a supervised setting, such as a cardiac rehabilitation program at your local hospital or community centre. Even those people with heart disease who don't have any of the three conditions listed above may prefer the supervision and structure of a rehabilitation program.

Once you are cleared for activity by your physician, always keep the intensity of your activity well below the level that produces symptoms, such as chest pain or severe shortness of breath. For example, if you get chest pain during an exercise treadmill test when your heart is beating at 130 beats per minute, you should never let your heart get above 115 beats per minute. Some people can easily judge the intensity of their activity so that it always stays below their "danger zone," but other people find it difficult to do so. For them, it may be easier to wear a heart rate monitor (available at fitness stores and most "Healthy Heart" programs) so that they can check their heart rate as they exercise. If you prefer, remember that you can monitor the intensity of your exercise by two other methods—the talk test and your perceived exertion (see page 134).

If your heart disease is severe, your doctor may want to change your treatment before giving you clearance to exercise. For example, if you have severely limited blood flow to the heart muscle, your doctor may want to treat you with a medicine that suppresses the arrhythmias, or may either want to treat you with special medicines or recommend that you have bypass surgery or "balloon" angioplasty to improve the blood flow to the heart muscle before clearing you for conditioning activities.

Activities that cause you to strain, such as weight lifting and rowing, may be harmful for people whose hearts have decreased pumping strength, and they should be avoided. Safer and more beneficial conditioning activities include light calisthenics, walking, swimming, and stationary bicycling.

Exercising in the recumbent position (lying down)—such as when you swim or pedal a special "recumbent" stationary bicycle—can help improve the efficiency of the heart's pumping action, except for people with severely damaged hearts (those who have had "heart failure," for example). You may or may not find such exercise to be less taxing for you.

Finally, always remember that if you develop new or different symptoms, such as chest pain, shortness of breath, or rapid or irregular heartbeat while at rest or while exercising, you should temporarily discontinue your conditioning activities and contact your physician.

LUNG DISEASE

Exercise training has been found to increase endurance, reduce symptoms, and reduce hospital visits for people with chronic lung disease. Remember, your exercise routine should begin at a very low intensity. Gradually begin to increase your activity, moving from short bouts of exercise to relatively longer ones. With time you'll notice that the shortness of breath at a given level of exertion will start to decrease. Work with your doctor to plan the safest, most beneficial exercise program for you. A few important points to remember:

- **Use your medicine, particularly your inhaler, before you exercise.** It will help you exercise longer and with less shortness of breath.

- **If you become severely short of breath with only minimal exertion, your doctor may want to change your medicines,** or even have you use supplemental oxygen before you begin your conditioning activities.

- **Take plenty of time to warm up and cool down during conditioning activities.** This should include exercises such as pursed-lip breathing and diaphragmatic, or abdominal, breathing (see page 44). The best exercise is probably a daily routine of low intensity, which you can add to gradually. Remember that when exercising, mild shortness of breath is normal. Remember also that before you begin to exercise you will experience a normal "anticipatory" increase in your heart rate and breathing rate. This is normal, but can be intimidating and fatiguing for some people. This makes it even more important to follow a gradual warm-up routine that includes pursed-lip breathing techniques. Be sure to avoid your "trouble zones" of shortness of breath by keeping the duration and intensity of your exercise well below those levels causing severe shortness of breath.

- **Concentrate on your breathing, making sure you breathe in deeply and slowly.** Use pursed-lip breathing when you breathe out (see page 44). Practise so that you take two or three times as much time breathing out as you do breathing in. For example, if you are walking briskly and notice that you can take 2 steps while you're breathing in, you should breathe out through pursed lips over 4 to 6 steps. Breathing out slowly will help you exchange air in your lungs better and will probably increase your endurance.

- **Remember that arm exercises may cause shortness of breath sooner than leg exercises.**

- **Cold and dry air can make breathing and exercise more difficult.** This is why swimming is an especially good activity for people with chronic lung disease.

- **Strengthening exercises such as calisthenics, light weight lifting, and rowing may be helpful,** particularly for people who have become weakened or deconditioned from medications, such as steroids.

• **Using a restorator** (see page 144) **is especially appropriate for some people with lung disease who have a low level of endurance or are fearful of exerting themselves.** The restorator allows a person to remain seated and to start and stop at his or her pleasure. It's a good device to build confidence and get accustomed to exertion in a secure atmosphere.

A Special Note for Those with Severe Lung Disease

Many people with severe lung disease believe that it is impossible to exercise. Getting across a room may take a great deal of effort. If this sounds like you, exercise is especially important. Here are some tips.

Move slowly. When crossing a room or going to the bathroom, many people with lung disease hurry up to get there before their breath runs out. It is much better to slow down. Move slowly, breathing as you go. At first, this will take a real effort, as the tendency is to speed up. With a little practice, you will find that you can go farther with less effort. If you are afraid to try this alone, have someone walk with you, carrying a chair (a folding "cane chair" might be useful), so that you can sit down if needed. Remember, slow and steady is always better. Don't forget to breathe as you walk.

Anyone with lung disease who can get out of bed can exercise 10 minutes a day. Here is how you do it. Every hour, get up from what you are doing and walk slowly across the room or around your chair for 1 minute. Doing this 10 times a day will give you your 10 minutes of exercise.

After you have done this for a week or two and are feeling a little stronger, then walk 2 minutes every hour. You have just doubled your exercise and are now up to 20 minutes a day. When this feels comfortable (in another week or two), change your pattern to walking 3–4 minutes every other hour. Again, wait a week or two and try 5 minutes 3 or 4 times a day. Next, try 6–7 minutes 2 or 3 times a day. You now have the basic idea. Most people with severe lung disease can build up to walking 10 to 20 minutes, once or twice a day, within a couple of months.

The rules are the same as for any other exercise:

1. **Start with what you can do now.** A minute an hour is great!

2. **Add to your program very gradually,** every week to two.

3. **If you ever feel worse after you finish than before you started, cut back on the amount of time you exercise.**

4. **Move slowly.**

5. **Remember to breathe while exercising.**

STROKE

Physical activity, especially physical therapy, is a cornerstone in the recovery of a person who has had a stroke. Strengthening and flexibility exercises help people regain the use of arms and legs that have been affected. Before beginning the conditioning program described in preceding chapters, check with your doctor to make sure your blood pressure is under control. (See the section on hypertension, on page 287.)

If you have weakness or poor balance from your stroke, some activities may cause you to strain, lose your balance, or fall. It may be wise to use a walker, cane, or stick with a partner while you are exercising. You may also wish to sit or alternate sitting and standing during your conditioning, especially if you have weakness in your legs. You may find a restorator helpful with your program. If an arm is affected, you may prefer to do leg exercises. If both a leg and arm are affected, it is probably best to begin with seated exercise. Remember, while a conditioning program can increase your strength, vigour, and endurance, it may not bring improvement to a severely weakened or paralyzed limb. If you have a prescribed exercise program already, talk with your therapist for ideas to combine your therapeutic exercise with a conditioning exercise program.

CLAUDICATION

Exercise for people with claudication in their legs is generally limited only by the leg pain that develops during exercise. The good news is that conditioning exercises can help improve endurance and reduce leg pain for most people. The bad news is that people with claudication sometimes find it impossible to do any type of leg exercises, which keeps them from getting the benefit of a conditioning program. In this case, they usually need to have bypass surgery on the vessels in their affected leg.

To gradually improve endurance and lessen leg pain, daily short periods of leg exercise (walking, bicycling, etc.) should be performed just short of the point of leg pain. When the discomfort starts, rest, slow down, or change activities until it subsides. Then the short period of exercise should be repeated, again to the point of some discomfort, but not severe pain. This cycle of exercise and rest should initially be repeated for 5–10 minutes and, with time, gradually increased to 30–60 minutes. Many people find that they can gradually increase the length of time they can walk comfortably or exercise with this method. Remember, arm exercises won't usually cause leg pain, so be sure to include them as an important part of your conditioning program.

Other methods that may help delay calf pain when you walk are to wear "rocker-bottom" shoes or to walk more slowly and use more arm swing.

HYPERTENSION

Before beginning a conditioning program, a person with high blood pressure should check with a doctor to make sure that his or her blood pressure is under control. This generally means that it consistently runs somewhere around 160/90 or less. The first blood pressure number (160) is the systolic blood pressure. This part of the blood pressure reading will normally go up during vigorous exercise, but for someone with hypertension it should never be allowed to go above 200. The second blood pressure reading is the diastolic blood pressure, which generally does not increase during exercise.

You should avoid exercises that can potentially worsen your hypertension, such as those causing you to strain while holding your breath (isometrics, weight lifting, and rowing, for example). Also, exercising with arms overhead will cause increased blood pressure and heart rate and should be avoided. Include endurance exercises that rhythmically contract and relax muscles in your program. These are generally not harmful, but can actually be of benefit because they help lower both your blood pressure and your weight.

To be safe, you may want to monitor your own blood pressure at the beginning, middle, and end of your exercise time as you begin to establish your program. (Blood pressure monitors can be purchased in most pharmacies and are generally easy to use. Instructions are provided, of course.) If your blood pressure is ever higher than 200/110, temporarily discontinue your conditioning exercises until you speak with your physician about the need for possible changes in your hypertension treatment plan.

OSTEOARTHRITIS

Since osteoarthritis begins as primarily a problem with joint cartilage, an exercise program should include taking care of cartilage. Cartilage needs joint motion and some weight bearing to stay healthy. In much the same way that a sponge soaks up and squeezes out water, joint cartilage soaks up nutrients and fluid and gets rid of waste products by being squeezed when you move the joint. If the joint is not moved regularly, cartilage deteriorates. If the joint is continually compressed, as the hips and knees are by long periods of standing, the cartilage can't expand and soak up nutrients and fluid.

Any joint with osteoarthritis should be moved through its full range of motion several times daily to maintain flexibility and to take care of the cartilage. Judge your activity level so that pain is not increased. If hips and knees are involved, walking and standing should be limited to two to four hours at a time, followed by at least an hour off your feet to give the cartilage time to decompress. Using a cane on the opposite side of the painful hip or knee will reduce joint stress and often get you over a rough time. Good posture, strong muscles, and good endurance, as well as shoes that absorb the shocks of walking, are important ways to protect cartilage and reduce joint pain. Knee-strengthening exercises (Exercises 17, 18, and 19 in Chapter 7) performed daily can help reduce knee pain and protect the joint.

OSTEOPOROSIS

Regular exercise plays an important part in preventing osteoporosis and strengthening bones already showing signs of disease. Endurance and strengthening exercises are the most effective for strengthening bone. Flexibility and back and abdominal strengthening exercises are important for maintaining good posture. Look for the VIP exercises in Chapter 7. You can help yourself with a regular exercise program that includes some walking and general flexibility and strengthening of your back and stomach muscles.

If you have osteoporosis, or think that you may be at risk for this condition, here are some exercise precautions to remember:

- **No heavy lifting.**

- **Avoid falls.** Be careful on pool decks, waxed floors, icy sidewalks, or cluttered surfaces.

- **Don't bend down to touch your toes when standing.** This puts unnecessary pressure on your back. If you want to stretch your legs or back, lie on your back and bring your knees up toward your chest.

- **Sit up straight, and don't slouch.** Good sitting posture puts less pressure on the back.

- **If your balance is poor or you feel clumsy, consider using a cane or walking stick** when you're in a crowd or on unfamiliar ground.

RHEUMATOID ARTHRITIS

People with rheumatoid arthritis should pay special attention to flexibility, strengthening, and the appropriate use of their joints. Maintaining good posture and joint motion will help joints, ease pain, and avoid tightness. Arthritis pain and long periods spent sitting or lying down can quickly lead to poor posture and limited motion, even in the joints not affected by arthritis. Be sure to include hand and wrist exercises in your daily program. A good time to do these is after washing dishes or during a bath, when hands are warm and limber.

Rheumatoid arthritis sometimes affects the bones in the neck. It is best to avoid extreme neck movements and not to put pressure on the back of the neck or head.

Stiffness in the morning can be a big problem. Flexibility exercises before getting up or during a hot bath or shower seem to help. A favourite way to get loosened up is to "stretch like a cat and then shake like a dog." Also, gentle flexibility exercises in the evening before bed have been shown to reduce morning stiffness.

DIABETES

Regular exercises can be an important part of controlling blood glucose levels and improving health for everyone with diabetes. However, people who are taking medication to control diabetes should discuss any change in exercise habits with their doctor or nutritionist, because changes in activity levels often require changes in medication and eating schedules.

Exercise is beneficial for people with diabetes in several ways. Mild to moderate aerobic exercise decreases the need for insulin and helps control blood glucose levels by increasing the sensitivity of body cells to insulin and lowering blood glucose levels both during and after exercise. This type of regular exercise also is essential for losing weight and reducing cardiovascular risk factors such as high blood lipid levels and high blood pressure.

The exercise program recommended for people with diabetes is generally the same as the conditioning program described earlier. Mild to moderate aerobic exercise for no more than 40 minutes performed as part of a general conditioning program in the morning or early afternoon is a safe and effective way to help control diabetes and stay healthy.

Additional considerations for exercise with diabetes are to begin an exercise program only when your diabetes is well under control, keep in touch with your doctor to make changes in medication and diet if needed, and coordinate eating, medication, and exercise to avoid hypoglycemia (low blood sugar). If you have problems with sensation or poor circulation, be sure to check your skin regularly and protect yourself from blisters and abrasions. It is especially important to inspect your feet and practise good skin and nail hygiene regularly. Shoe inserts can be tailored to help protect the soles of the feet.

Suggested Further Reading

Lam, Paul, and Horstman, Judith. *Overcoming Arthritis: How to Relieve Pain and Restore Mobility through a Unique Tai Chi Program*. New York: DK Publishing, 2002.

Nelson, Miriam E, Alice H. Lichtenstein, and Lawrence Lindner. *Strong Women, Strong Hearts: Proven Strategies to Prevent and Reverse Heart Disease Now*. New York: G.P. Putnam's Sons, 2005.

Sayce, Valerie, and Ian Fraser. *Exercise Beats Arthritis: An Easy-to-Follow Program of Exercises*. Boulder, Colo.: Bull Publishing, 1998; Melbourne, Australia: Fraser Publications, 1987.

Schwartz, Anna. *Cancer Fitness: Exercise Programs for Patients and Survivors*. New York: Fireside, Simon & Schuster, 2004.

Silver, David S. *Playing through Arthritis: How to Conquer Pain and Enjoy Your Favorite Sports and Activities*. New York: McGraw-Hill, 2003.

Vedral, Joyce L. *Bone Building and Body Shaping Workout*. New York: Simon & Schuster, 1998.

White, Martha. *Water Exercise: 78 Safe and Effective Exercises for Fitness and Therapy*. Champaign, Ill.: Human Kinetics, 1995.

Websites with Exercising Tips

http://www.arthritis.ca/tips

www.osteoporosis.ca

http://www.ncpad.org/index.php.
> The National Center on Physical Activity and Disability website offers information about exercise and physical activity for a great many chronic conditions.

http://medlineplus.gov.
> This site contains information and links for many conditions, including information about physical activity and exercise. It is a service of the National Library of Medicine and the National Institutes of Health.

Other Resources

Public libraries have a good selection of magazines available. Some recommended good reads are: *Arthritis Today*; Johns Hopkins Medical Letter *Health After 50*; *Mayo Clinic Health Letter*, Tufts University *Health & Nutrition Letter*, University of California, Berkeley, *Wellness Letter*.

Medical research journals available at your library: *Best Practices Quarterly,* Sport Medicine Council of British Columbia; *Applied Physiology, Nutrition and Metabolism/Physiologie appliquée, nutrition et métabolisme; The Physician and Sportsmedicine; Canadian Journal of Public Health/Revue Canadienne de santé publique.*

COMMUNICATING 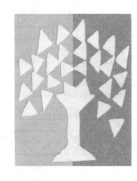 10

Y OU JUST DON'T UNDERSTAND! How often has this statement, expressed or unexpressed, summed up a frustrating verbal exchange? The goal in any communication between people is that the other person understands what you are trying to say. Feeling that you are not understood leads to frustration, and a prolonged feeling of frustration can lead to depression, anger, and helplessness. These are not good feelings for anyone, especially people with long-term health problems. When communication breaks down, not only do we experience these negative emotions, but we may also experience other physical symptoms. For example, the heart rate can speed up, and cholesterol and blood sugar levels can rise. We become more prone to headaches, body aches, and digestive problems, as well as becoming more sensitive to pain. The worry caused by conflict and misunderstanding can make us irritable, unable to concentrate, and therefore more likely to have accidents. Clearly, poor communication is bad for our physical, mental, and emotional health.

Poor communication is the biggest factor in poor relationships, whether they be between spouses, other family members or friends, coworkers, or doctors and patients. Even in casual relationships, poor communication causes frustration. How often have you been angry and frustrated as a customer, and how often is this because of poor communication?

When you have a long-term condition, good communication becomes a necessity. Your health care team, in particular, must "understand" you. As a self-manager, it is in your best interest to learn the skills necessary to make your communications as effective as possible.

In this chapter, we discuss ways to improve the communication process. Specifically, these are ways to express feelings in a positive way and to minimize conflict—how to ask for help, how to say no, as well as how best to listen, how to recognize body language and different styles of communication, and how to get more information from the other person.

While reading this chapter, keep in mind that communication is a two-way street. As uncomfortable as you may feel about expressing your feelings and asking for help, chances are that others are also feeling this way. It may be up to you to make sure the lines of communication are open. Be careful not to get caught in being uncomfortable with others because "they should know. . . ."

EXPRESSING YOUR FEELINGS

Having a long-term condition brings about many feelings, some of them not pleasant. Here are some hints on how to express these feelings in a positive and constructive manner.

Start by taking a few moments to review exactly what the situation is that is bothering you and what you are feeling. For example, John and Steve had agreed to go together to a sporting event. When John came to pick up Steve, he was not ready and was not sure he wanted to go, as he was having some trouble with his arthritic knees. The following conversation took place.

John: *Why do you always spoil my plans? At least you could have called and I could have asked my son to go with me.*

Steve: *You just don't understand. If you had pain like I do, you wouldn't be so quick to criticize. You don't think of anyone but yourself.*

John: *Well, I can see that I should just go by myself.*

In the above situation, neither John nor Steve had stopped to think about what was really bothering him or how he felt about it. Rather, they each blamed the other for an unfortunate situation.

The following is the same conversation but with both people using thoughtful communications.

John: *When we have made plans and then at the last minute you are not sure you can go, I feel frustrated and angry. I don't know what to do—go on without you, stay here and change our plans, or just not make future plans.*

Steve: *When this arthritis acts up at the last minute, I am also confused. I keep hoping I can go and so don't call you because I don't want to disappoint you and I really want to go. I keep hoping that my knees will get better as the day wears on.*

John: *I understand.*

Steve: *Let's go to the game. You can let me off at the gate before parking so I won't have to walk as far. Then I can do the steps slowly and be in our seats when you arrive. I do want us to keep making plans. In the future, I will let you know sooner if I think my arthritis is acting up.*

John: *Sounds good to me. I really do like your company and also knowing how I can help. It is just that being caught by surprise makes me angry.*

John and Steve talked about the specific situation and how they felt about it. Neither blamed the other. Unfortunately, we are often in situations where the other person uses blaming communications, or we are caught not listening and revert to blaming communications. Even in this situation, thoughtful communication can be helpful. Look at the following example.

Jan: *Why do you always spoil my plans? At least you could have called. I am really tired of trying to do anything with you.*

Sandra: *I understand. When this asthma acts up at the last minute, I am confused. I keep hoping I can go and so don't call you because I don't want to disappoint you and I really want to go. I keep hoping that I will get better as the day wears on.*

Jan: *Well, I hope that in the future you will call. I don't like being caught by surprise.*

Sandra: *I understand. If it is OK with you, let's go shopping now. I can walk a short way and rest in the coffee shop with my book while you continue to shop. I do want us to keep making plans. In the future, I will let you know sooner if I think my asthma is acting up.*

In this last example, only Sandra is using thoughtful communication. Jan continues to blame. The outcome, however, is still positive, with both people accomplishing what they want. The following are some suggestions for accomplishing good communications and creating supportive relationships.

1. **Always show respect and regard for the other person.** Try not to preach or be demanding, and avoid demeaning or blaming comments such as when Jan says, "Why do you always spoil my plans?" The use of the word "you" is a clue that your communication might be blaming.

2. **Be clear.** Describe a specific situation or your observations using the facts. Avoid words like "always" or "never." For example, Sandra said, "When this asthma acts up at the last minute, I am confused. I keep hoping I can go and so don't call you because I don't want to disappoint you and I really want to go. I keep hoping that I will get better as the day wears on."

3. **Test your assumptions verbally by asking for clarification.** Jan did not do this. She assumed that Sandra was being rude by not calling her, rather than asking Sandra why she hadn't called earlier to let her know how she was feeling. Remember that assumptions are often the place where good communications break down. One sign that you are making assumptions is when you are thinking "he or she should know. . . ."

4. **Be open and honest about your feelings.** Sandra did this when she talked about wanting to go, not wanting to disappoint Jan, and hoping that her asthma would get better.

5. **Accept the feelings of others and try to understand them.** This is not always easy. Sometimes you need to think about what has been said. Rather than answer immediately, remember that it is always acceptable to use "I understand" or "I don't fully understand. Could you explain some more?"

6. **Be tactful and courteous.** You can do this by avoiding sarcasm and blaming.

7. **Work at using humour, but at the same time know when to be serious.**

8. **Be careful not to make yourself a victim by not expressing your needs and feelings and then expecting others to act the way you think they "should" act.** Also, you should not have to apologize all the time for your feelings, but if what you've said or done has hurt the other person, then you should apologize.

9. **Finally, become a good listener.**

"I" MESSAGES

Many of us are uncomfortable expressing our feelings. This discomfort can be acute. This is especially so when it seems we may be critical of the person we're talking to.

If emotions are high, attempts to express frustration can be laden with "you" messages that suggest blame. These messages are aimed at the other person, causing the other person to feel as though he or she is under attack. Suddenly, the other person is on the defensive, and protective barriers go up. The person trying to express feelings, in turn, feels greater anxiety when faced with these defensive barriers, and the situation escalates to anger, frustration, and bad feelings.

The use of "I," however, doesn't strike out or blame. It is another form of communication that helps to express how you feel, rather than how the other person makes you feel. Here are some examples of "I" messages:

"You" message:	Why are you always late? We never get anywhere on time.
"I" message:	I get really upset when I'm late. It's important to me to be on time.
"You" message:	There's no way you can understand how lousy I feel.
"I" message:	I'm not feeling well. I could really use a little help today.

Watch out for hidden "you" messages. These are "you" messages with "I feel . . ." stuck in front of them. Here's an example:

"You" message:	You always walk too fast.
HIDDEN "You" message:	I feel angry when you walk so fast.
"I" message:	I have a hard time walking fast.

The trick to "I" messages is to avoid the use of the word "you," and, instead, report your personal feelings using the word "I." Of course, like any new skill, "I" messages take practice. Start by really listening, both to yourself and to others. Take some of the "you" messages you hear and turn them into "I" messages in your head. By playing this word game in your head, you'll be surprised at how fast it becomes a habit in your own expressions.

EXERCISE—"I" MESSAGES

Change the following statements into "I" messages. (Watch out for "hidden you" messages!)

You expect me to wait on you hand and foot!

Doctor, you never have enough time for me. You're always in a hurry.

You hardly ever touch me anymore. You haven't paid any attention to me since my heart attack.

You didn't tell me the side effects of all these drugs you're giving me or why I have to take them, doctor.

There are some cautions to note when using "I" messages. First, they are not a panacea. Sometimes the listener has to have time to hear them. This is especially true if "you" messages and blaming have been the more usual ways of communicating. Even if at first using "I" messages seems ineffective, continue to use them and refine your skill.

Also, some people may use "I" messages as a means of manipulation. If used in this way, problems can escalate. To be used effectively, "I" messages must report honest feelings.

When using "I" statements seems difficult, try using this format: "when (here put a specific situation) I (state your feelings)." For example, "When you do not call, I worry."

One last note: "I" messages are an excellent way to express positive feelings and compliments! "I really appreciate the extra time you gave me today, doctor."

MINIMIZING CONFLICT

While learning how to express our feelings through the use of "I" messages instead of "you" messages goes a long way to help reduce conflict in our relationships, there are other communication techniques that can also help.

When a discussion seems to be getting off the topic and emotions start to run high, try to shift the focus of the conversation. That is, bring the focus of the discussion back to what you agreed to talk about in the first place, and away from what is starting to happen between you. For example, you might say something like, "We're both getting upset now and drifting away from the topic we agreed to discuss." Or, "I feel like we are bringing up other things than what we agreed to talk about, and I'm getting upset. Can we discuss these other things later and just talk about what we originally agreed on?"

Another tactic that prevents conflict or upset is to ask for time to think about things and respond later, when your emotions are not so intense. For example, you might say, "I think I understand your concerns, but I need more time to think about it before I can respond." Or, "I hear what you are saying, but I am too frustrated to respond now. I need to find out more information about this before I can answer you."

Also, make sure you understand each other's viewpoints, concerns, or feelings by summarizing what you heard and asking for clarification. You may also try switching roles. Try arguing the other person's position as thoroughly and thoughtfully as possible. This will help you to understand all the sides of an issue, as well as to respect and value the other's point of view. It will also help you to develop tolerance and empathy for others.

Lastly, you may not always find the perfect solution to a problem, or reach total agreement on an issue, but you can work toward an acceptable compromise. Find something that you can both agree to try for awhile. For example, you can do it your way this time, and the other person's way the next time. Agree to part of what you want, and part of what the other person wants. Or, decide what you'll do, and what the other person will do in return. These are all forms of compromise that can help you through those difficult times in a relationship when you feel as though you never completely agree.

ASKING FOR HELP

Problems with communication around the subject of help are pretty common. For some reason, many people feel awkward about asking for help or in refusing help. Although this is probably a universal problem, it can come up more often for people dealing with long-term health conditions.

It may be emotionally difficult for some of us to ask for needed help. Maybe it's difficult for us to admit to ourselves that we are unable to do things as easily as in the past. When this is the case, try to avoid hedging your request: "I'm sorry to have to ask this . . ." "I know this is asking a lot . . ." "I hate to ask this, but . . . " Hedging tends to put the other person on the defensive: "Gosh, what's he going to ask for that's so much, anyway?" Be specific about what help you are requesting. A general request can lead to misunderstanding, and the person can react negatively to insufficient information, which then leads to a further breakdown in communication. But a specific request is more likely to lead to the desired goal or a positive result.

General request:	I know this is the last thing you want to do, but I need help moving. Will you help me?
Reaction:	Uh . . . well . . . I don't know. Um . . . can I get back to you after I check my schedule? (probably next year!)
Specific request:	I'm moving next week, and I'd like to move my books and kitchen stuff ahead of time. Would you mind helping me load and unload the boxes in my car Saturday morning? I think it can be done in one trip.
Reaction:	I'm busy Saturday morning, but I could give you a hand Friday night, if you'd like.

People with health problems also sometimes deal with offers of help that are not needed or desired. In most cases, these offers come from people who are dear to you and genuinely want to be helpful. A well-worded "I" message allows you to refuse the help tactfully, without embarrassing the other person. "Thank you for being so thoughtful, but today I think I can handle it myself. I'd like to be able to take you up on your offer another time, though."

SAYING NO

Suppose, however, you are the one being asked to help someone. Responding readily with yes or no may not be advisable. Often, we need more information before we can respond to the request.

If the request lacks enough information for us to respond, often our first feelings are negative. The example we just discussed about helping a person move is a good one. "Help me move" can mean anything from moving furniture up stairs to picking up the pizza for the hungry troops. Again, using skills that get at the specifics will aid the communication process. It is important to understand what the specific request is before responding. Asking for more information or paraphrasing the request will often help clarify the request, especially if prefaced by a phrase such as "Before I answer . . . " (this will hopefully prevent the person whose request you are paraphrasing from thinking that you are going to say yes).

Once you know what the specific request is and have decided to decline, it is important to acknowledge the importance of the request to the other person. In this way, the person will see that you are rejecting the request rather than the person. Your turn-down should not be a put-down. "You know, that's a worthwhile project you're doing, but I think it's beyond my capabilities this week." Again, specifics are the key. Try to be clear about the conditions of your turn-down: Will you always turn down this request, or is it just that today or this week or right now is a problem?

ACCEPTING HELP

Many times our family or friends offer help. We often hear "How can I help?" Our reaction is often "I don't know" while we are thinking "they should know. . . ." Instead, be prepared to accept help by having a specific answer. For example, "It would be great if we could go to the movies once a month" or "Could you please take out the garbage? I can't lift it." Just remember that most people cannot read your mind, so you'll need to tell them what help you want and thank them for it.

LISTENING

This is probably the most important communication skill. Most of us are much better at talking than we are at listening. We need to actually listen to what the other person is saying and feeling. Most of us are already preparing a response, instead of just listening. There are several levels involved in being a good listener.

1. **Listen to the words and tone of voice, and observe body language** (see next section). Sometimes it is difficult to begin a conversation if there is a problem. There may be times when the words being used don't tell you there is something bothering this person. Is the voice wavering? Does he or she appear to be struggling to find "the right

words"? Do you notice body tension? Does he or she seem distracted? If you pick up on some of these signs, this person probably has more on her or his mind than words are expressing.

2. **Acknowledge having heard the other person.** Let the person know you heard them. This may be a simple "uh huh." Many times the only thing the other person wants is acknowledgment, or just someone to listen, because sometimes merely talking to a sympathetic listener is helpful.

3. **Acknowledge the content of the problem.** Let the other person know you heard both the content and emotional level of the problem. You can do this by restating the content of what you heard. For example, "You are planning a trip." Or you can respond by acknowledging the emotions: "That must be difficult" or "How sad you must feel." When you respond on an emotional level, the results are often startling. These responses tend to open the gates for more expression of feelings and thoughts. Responding to either the content or emotion can help communication along by discouraging the other person from simply repeating what has been said.

4. **Respond by seeking more information** (see page 169). This is especially important if you are not completely clear about what is being said or what is wanted. There is more than one useful method for seeking and getting information.

Body Language and Conversational Styles

As mentioned earlier, part of listening to what others are saying includes observing how they say it. Even when we say nothing, our bodies are talking; sometimes they are even shouting. Research shows that more than half of what we communicate is conveyed through our body language rather than our words. Therefore, if we want to improve our communication skills, we must also become aware of body language, facial expressions and tone of voice. These should match what we say in words; otherwise we end up sending mixed messages and creating more misunderstandings. For example, if you want to make an assertive statement, look at the other person and keep your expression friendly. Stand tall and confident; relax your legs and arms and breathe. You may even lean forward to show your interest. Try not to sneer or bite your lips; this might indicate discomfort or doubt.

Also, don't move away or slouch, as these communicate disinterest and uncertainty, which contradicts what you are trying to assert to the other person.

When you notice that the body language and words of others don't seem to match, gently point this out to that person, and ask for clarification to avoid misunderstandings. For example, you might say, "Dear, I hear you saying that you would like to go with me to the family picnic, but you look tired and you're yawning as you speak. Would you rather stay home and rest, while I go alone?"

In addition to reading people's body language, it is helpful to recognize and appreciate that we all express ourselves differently. Many factors influence our conversational style; it varies according to where we were born, how we were raised, our occupation, our cultural background, and especially our gender. For example, women tend to ask more personal questions to show interest and to form relationships, whereas men are more likely to interrupt, offer opinions or suggestions, and state facts in conversations. Men tend to discuss problems just to find solutions, whereas women want to share their feelings and experiences more. No one style is better or worse, just different. By acknowledging and accepting these differences, we can reduce some of the misunderstanding, frustration, and resentment we feel in our communications with others.

GETTING MORE INFORMATION

Getting more information from another person is a bit of an art, requiring special consideration. It can involve techniques that may be simple or more subtle.

Ask for more. This is the simplest way to get more information. "Tell me more" will probably get you more, as will "I don't understand . . . please explain," "I would like to know more about . . . ," "Would you say that another way?" "How do you mean?" "I'm not sure I got that," and "Could you expand on that?"

Paraphrase. This is a good tool if you want to make sure you understand what the other person meant (not just what he or she said, but meant). Paraphrasing can either help or hinder effective communication, though, depending on the way the paraphrase is worded. It is important to remember to paraphrase in the form of a question, not a statement. For example, assume another person says:

Well, I don't know. I'm really not feeling up to par. This party will be crowded, there'll probably be smokers there, and I really don't know the hosts very well, anyway.

If we were to paraphrase this as a statement rather than a question, it might look like this:

Obviously, you're telling me you don't want to go to the party.

Paraphrased as a question:

Are you saying that you'd rather stay home than go to the party?

The response to the first paraphrase might be anger:

No, I didn't say that! If you're going to be that way, I'll stay home for sure.

Or the response might be no response—a total shutdown of the communication, because of either anger or despair ("he just doesn't understand"). People don't like to be told what they meant.

On the other hand, the response to the second paraphrase using a question might be:

That's not what I meant. Now that I am using oxygen, I'm just feeling a little nervous about meeting new people. I'd appreciate it if you'd stay near me during the party. I'd feel better about it, and I might have a good time.

As you can see, the second paraphrase promotes further communication, and you have discovered the real reason the person was expressing doubt about the party. You obtained more information from the second paraphrase and no new information from the first one.

Be specific. If you want specific information, you must ask specific questions. We often automatically speak in generalities. For example:

Doctor:	*How have you been feeling?*	*Patient:*	*Not so good.*

The doctor doesn't have much in the way of information about the patient's condition. "Not so good" isn't very useful. Here's how the doctor gets more information:

Doctor:	*Are you still having those sharp pains in your left arm?*	*Patient:*	*Yes. A lot.*

Doctor: How often?   *Patient: A couple of times a day.*

Doctor: How long do they last?   *Patient: A long time.*

Doctor: About how many minutes
would you say?

. . . and so on.

Physicians have been trained in ways to get specific information from patients, but most of us have not been trained to ask specific questions. Again, simply asking for specifics often works: "Can you be more specific about . . . ?" "Are you thinking of something particular?" If you want to know "why," be specific about what the topic is. If you ask a specific question, you will be more likely to get a specific answer.

Simply asking "Why?" can unnecessarily prolong your attempt to get specific information. In addition to being a general rather than a specific word, "why" makes a person think in terms of cause and effect, and he or she may respond at an entirely different level than you had in mind.

Most of us have had the experience where a three-year-old just keeps asking "Why?" over and over and over again, until the information the child wants is finally obtained (or the parent runs from the room, screaming). The poor parent doesn't have the faintest idea what the child has in mind and answers, "Because . . ." in an increasingly specific order until the child's question is answered. Sometimes, however, the direction the answers take is entirely different from that of the child's question, and the child never gets the information he or she wanted. Rather than "why," begin your responses with "who," "which," "when," or "where." These words promote a specific response.

One last note about getting information: Sometimes we do not get the correct information because we do not know what question to ask. For example, you may be seeking legal services from a senior centre. You call and ask if they have a lawyer, and hang up when the answer is no. If, instead, you had asked where you might get low-cost legal advice, you may have gotten two or three referrals.

COMMUNICATING WITH MEMBERS OF YOUR HEALTH CARE TEAM

The key to making the health care system work better involves our ability to develop good communication with members of our health care team. This, however, can be a challenge because many of us feel intimidated or afraid to talk freely with our providers. Some professionals use unfamiliar medical words that we just don't understand or that confuse us. And we often hesitate to ask what these words mean. Also, many of us are afraid to share personal things about ourselves because we don't really know and trust our providers. These fears block communication.

Providers share the responsibility for poor communication because they often feel too busy or important to take the time to talk with and know their patients. They may be hurried and may ignore our questions or how their actions might offend us.

While we do not have to become best friends with our providers, we should expect that they are attentive, caring, and able to explain things clearly to us, especially if we have an ongoing health condition. As a person with a chronic health problem, the relationship you have with your provider must be looked on as a long-term one requiring regular work, much like a business partnership or even a marriage.

Your provider will probably know more intimate details about you than anyone else, except perhaps your spouse or your parents. You, in turn, should feel comfortable expressing your fears, asking questions that you may think are "stupid," and negotiating a treatment plan to satisfy you both, without feeling "put down" or that your provider is just not interested.

There are two things to keep in mind that will help to open, and keep open, the lines of communication with the members of your health care team. How do they feel? Too often, we expect our providers to act like warmhearted computers— gigantic brains, stuffed with knowledge about the human body, and especially your human body, able to analyze the situation and produce a diagnosis, prognosis, and treatment on demand—and be warm, caring persons who make you feel as though you're the only person they care about or take care of.

Actually, most providers wish they were just that sort of person, but no one provider can be all things to all patients. Providers are human, too. They get headaches, they get tired, and they get sore feet. They have families who demand their time and attention, and they have to fight bureaucracies as formidable as those the rest of us face.

Most doctors and other health care professionals received gruelling training and entered the health care system because they wanted to make sick people well. It is frustrating for them not to be able to cure someone with a chronic condition like emphysema or arthritis. They must take their satisfaction from improvements rather than cures, or even from maintenance of existing conditions rather than declines. Undoubtedly, you have been frustrated, angry, or depressed from time to time about your illness, but bear in mind that your doctor has probably felt similar emotions about his or her inability to make you well. In this, you are truly partners.

Second, in this partnership between you and your providers, the biggest threat to a good relationship and good communication is time. If you or your provider had a fantasy about the best thing to happen in your relationship, it would probably involve more time for you both—more time to discuss things, more time to explain things, more time to explore options. When time is short, the resulting anxiety can bring about rushed messages, often "you" messages, and messages that are just plain misunderstood—with no time to correct them.

Most doctors and other providers are usually on very tight schedules. This fact becomes painfully obvious to you when you have had to wait in the doctor's office because of an emergency that has delayed your appointment. Doctors try to stay on schedule, and sometimes patients and doctors alike feel rushed as a consequence. One way to help you to get the most from your visit with the doctor or other provider is to take **P.A.R.T.**

Prepare	**Ask**	**Repeat**	**Take Action**

Prepare

Before visiting or calling your doctor, prepare your "agenda." What are the reasons for your visit? What do you expect from your doctor?

Take some time to make a written list of your most important concerns or questions. But be realistic. If you have 13 different problems, it isn't likely that your doctor can adequately deal with that many concerns in one visit. Identify your main concerns or problems. Writing them down also helps you remember them. Have you ever thought to yourself, after you walked out of the doctor's office, "Why didn't I ask about . . . ?" or "I forgot to mention . . . ." Making a list beforehand helps you ensure that your main concerns get addressed.

Mention your main concerns right at the beginning of the visit. Don't wait until the end of the appointment to bring up concerns, because there won't be the time to properly deal with them. Give your list to the doctor. If the list is long, expect that only two or three items will be addressed this visit, and let your doctor know which items are the most important to you. Studies show that doctors allow an average of 18 seconds for the patient to state his or her concerns before interrupting with focused questioning. Preparing your questions in advance will help you use your 18 seconds well.

As an example of bringing up your concerns at the beginning of the visit, when the doctor asks, "What brings you in today?" you might say something like "I have a lot of things I want to discuss this visit" (looking at his or her watch and appointment schedule, the doctor immediately begins to feel anxious), "but I know that we have a limited amount of time. The things that most concern me are my shoulder pain, my dizziness, and the side effects from one of the medications I'm taking" (the doctor feels relieved because the concerns are focused and potentially manageable within the appointment time available).

Try to be as open as you can in sharing your thoughts, feelings, and fears. Remember, your physician is not a mindreader. If you are worried, try to explain why: "I am worried that what I have may be contagious," or "My father had similar symptoms before he died," and so on. The more open you are, the more likely it is that your doctor can help you. If you have a problem, don't wait for the doctor to "discover" it. State your concern immediately. For example, "I am worried about this mole on my chest."

Give your physician feedback. If you don't like the way you have been treated by the physician or someone else on the health care team, let your physician know. If you were unable to follow the physician's advice or had problems with a treatment, tell your physician so that adjustments can be made. Also, most physicians appreciate compliments and positive feedback, but patients are often hesitant to praise their doctors. So, if you are pleased, remember to let your physician know it.

Preparing for a visit involves more than just listing your concerns. You should be prepared to concisely describe your symptoms to the doctor (when they started, how long they last, where they are located, what makes them better or worse, whether you have had similar problems before, whether you have changed your diet, exercise, or medications in a way that might contribute to the symptoms, etc.). Bring a list of all the medications (both prescription and nonprescription) and other things you are taking, or bring the containers and show them to the doctor. If a treatment has been tried, you should be prepared to report the effect of the treatment. And if you have previous records or test results that might be relevant to your problems, bring them along. Be sure to tell your doctor about the trends (are you getting better or worse, or are you the same?) and tempo (is it faster or slower?) of your problem, not just how you feel today. For example, "In general I am slowly getting better, although today I do not feel well." In treating a chronic condition, the trends and tempo are very important.

Ask

Another key to effective doctor-patient communication is asking questions. Getting understandable answers and information is one of the cornerstones of self-management. You need to be prepared to ask questions about diagnosis, tests, treatments, and follow-up.

1. **Diagnosis:** Ask your doctor what's wrong, what caused it, if it is contagious, what the future outlook (or prognosis) is, and what can be done to prevent it in the future.

2. **Tests:** Ask your doctor if any medical tests are necessary, how they will affect your treatment, how accurate they are, and what is likely to happen if you are not tested. If you decide to have a test, find out how to prepare for the test and what it will be like. Also ask how you will get the results and when.

3. **Treatments:** Ask about your treatment options including lifestyle change, medications, surgery. Inquire about the risks and benefits of treatment and the consequences of not treating.

4. **Follow-up:** Find out if and when you should call or return for a follow-up visit. What symptoms should you watch for, and what should you do if they occur?

You may wish to take some notes on important points during the visit or consider bringing along someone to act as a second listener. Another set of eyes and ears may help you later recall some of the details of the visit or instruction. You can also bring a tape recorder so you can listen to the conversation again with your complete attention. This can also be shared with others to get their reactions.

Repeat

It is extremely helpful to briefly repeat back to the doctor some of the key points from the visit and discussion. These might include diagnosis, prognosis, next steps, and your treatment recommendations and instructions. This is to double-check that you clearly understood the most important information. Repeating back also gives the doctor a chance to quickly correct any misunderstandings and miscommunications. If you don't understand or remember something the physician said, admit that you need to go over it again. For example, you might say, "I'm pretty sure you told me some of this before, but I'm still confused about it." Don't be afraid too ask what you may consider a "stupid" question. These questions can often indicate an important concern or misunderstanding.

Take Action

When the visit is ending, you need to clearly understand what to do next. When appropriate, ask your physician to write down instructions or recommend reading material for more information on a particular subject.

If, for some reason, you can't or won't follow the doctor's advice, let the doctor know. For example, "I didn't take the aspirin. It gives me stomach problems," or "My insurance doesn't cover that much physical therapy, so I can't afford it," or "I've tried to exercise before, but I can't seem to keep it up." If your doctor knows why you can't or won't follow advice, alternative suggestions can sometimes be made to help you overcome the barrier. If you don't share the barriers to taking actions, it's difficult for your doctor to help.

Also, before you leave the office, make sure you understand the next steps. For example, should you return for another visit? If so, why and when? Also, if there were tests taken, can you phone for the results? Are there any danger signs to watch for and report to your doctor?

Asking for a Second Opinion

Many people find it uncomfortable to ask their doctor for a second opinion about their diagnosis or treatment. Especially if you have had a long relationship with your doctor or simply like him or her, you may worry that asking for another opinion might be interpreted by the doctor as questioning his or her competence. It is a rare doctor whose feelings will be hurt by a sincere request for another opinion. If your condition is medically complicated or difficult, the doctor may have already consulted with another doctor (or more than one) about your case, at least on an informal basis.

Even if your condition is not particularly complicated, asking for a second opinion is a perfectly acceptable, and often expected, request. Doctors prefer a straightforward request, and asking in the form of a nonthreatening "I" message will make this task simple:

> *I'm still feeling confused and uncomfortable about this treatment. I feel another opinion might help me feel more reassured. Can you suggest someone I could consult?*

In this way, you have expressed your own feelings without suggesting that the doctor is at fault. You have also confirmed your confidence in him or her by asking that he or she suggest the other doctor. (Remember, however, that you are not bound by his or her suggestion; you may choose anyone you wish for a second opinion.)

Give Positive Feedback to Your Providers

Your providers need to know how satisfied you are with your care. If you do not like the way you have been treated by any of the members of your health care team, let this person know. In the same way, if you are pleased with your care, also let your providers know. Everyone appreciates compliments and positive words of feedback, especially members of your health care team. They are human, and your praise can help nourish and console these busy, hardworking professionals. Letting them know that you appreciate their efforts is one of the best ways to improve your relationship with them, plus it makes them feel good!

Good communication skills help make life easier for everyone, especially when long-term health problems enter the picture. The skills discussed in this chapter, though brief, will hopefully help smooth the communication process. In summary, the box on the next page gives examples of some words that can help or hinder.

WORKING WITH THE HEALTH CARE SYSTEM

Today many of the frustrations we have with members of our health care team might be frustrations with provincial or federal health care delivery systems. It may feel as if we get less time with the doctor or other members of our health care team, and we spend more and more time waiting. Also, when some of us were growing up, things seemed much easier. Before universal medicare, we went to the doctor, received a bill, and that was it. Now, we may have to wait for third-party approval for some procedures. Additionally, what one person qualifies for in one province may not be covered for someone else in another province.

WORDS THAT HELP	WORDS THAT HINDER
Right now, at this time, at this point, today	Never, always, every time, constantly
I	You
Who, which, where, when	Obviously . . .
How do you mean, please explain, tell me more, I don't understand	Why

In many countries, health care has become more complex, and in many cases, it has become big business. There are many more types of health care providers working with many more patients. They play supporting roles in these organizations and share in the same frustrations. It has become impossible for one provider to know everything about his or her patients, and patients often see more than one provider. In addition, there are many more tests to take and other health professionals with whom to consult, such as registered dietitians and physical therapists; and, of course, there are many more drugs. All of this means that health care may be better and more thorough, but getting that care is much more complicated.

If you are unhappy with the provincial or federal health care system, don't just steam and get mad—do something about it. Find out who is in charge, whether it is a politician or an administrator, and find out how decisions are made. Then share your feelings in a constructive way by letter, phone, or e-mail. The problem is that the people who make the decisions tend to isolate themselves from the patients, so it is easier to express our feelings to the receptionist, nurse, or doctor. Unfortunately, these people have little or no power in the system. Sometimes they can tell you who to call or write, but if not, contact your MLA or MNA and ask for the contact person in the ministry or department you are dealing with. You will be a part of making the health care system more responsive to patient needs.

The following are a few hints for working with the health care system. Not all of these problems and suggestions will apply to all systems, but most do.

- **"I hate the phone system."** Or, "I hate it when I call and all I get is an automated message." Often, when we call for an appointment or information, we are routed through an automated phone system. This is frustrating, and unfortunately there is not much we can do about it. However, phone systems tend not to change too often, so if we can memorize the numbers or keys to press, we can move more quickly from one part of the system to another without wasting time. Sometimes, pressing the pound key, #, or 0 will get us to a real person. Once you do get through, ask if there is a way to do this faster next time. Is there another number? Is there a "best" time of the day to call?

- **"It takes too long to get an appointment."** As our systems get busier, this is often a problem. Ask for the first available appointment. Take it. Then ask how you can learn about cancellations. In some systems they will be happy to call you to fill in a spot. In others, you may have to call them once or twice a week to check on cancellations. Ask the person making the schedule what you can do to get an earlier appointment by taking a cancellation. He or she might also give you a telephone number so that you can reach him or her directly. No matter how frustrated you are, though, be nice. The scheduler has power and can see to it whether or not you get the appointment you want.

- **"I have so many doctors; I do not know who to ask for what."** One of those doctors has to be in charge, so your job is to find out which one. Ask each doctor who is in charge of coordinating your care. When you get a name, it is most likely your primary care doctor or GP. Call him or her up to confirm that he or she is doing the coordination. Ask how you can help. Also, be sure to let this person know when someone else orders a test or new medication; this is just what he or she wants and needs to help you. Keeping the doctor informed of these events is especially important when there is no electronic medical record.

- **"So what is an electronic medical record?"** More and more of your medical information is being put on a secure computer that can be accessed by any of your providers—as long as they are in the same system. You should know what information is on the system. Sometimes it is just test results; other times it is test results and medication information; and sometimes it is everything that is known about you. It is important to understand that an electronic medical record is just like a paper record: It does no good if your providers don't read it. For example, when you have a test, the doctor ordering the test will be informed when the test results are ready. However, your other doctors will not know anything about it unless you tell them to read the results. In short, learn about the medical records system that contains your information so you can help all your providers use it more effectively.

Your health records may be accessible through the Information and Privacy Office of your hospital. You will be asked to fill out two or three forms. It might be helpful for you to name another person who is entitled to access your health records, in case you are not able to represent yourself in the future. Find out more about this in chapter 12.

- **"I have to wait too long in the waiting room or the examination room."** Emergencies happen sometimes, and this can cause a wait. More often, you are at the mercy of an inefficient system. Before leaving home, call your doctor and ask how long you will have to wait. Then respond that you will be there, but not until about 15 minutes before you are expected to be seen by the doctor. You can also show up and ask about the wait. Go to the visit prepared to wait; bring a book or something else to do while you wait. Or, rather than getting upset, let the receptionist know that you are going to step out for a little while to run a short errand nearby, or for a cup of coffee or some shopping, and that you will return within a specified amount of time.

- **"I don't have enough time with the doctor."** This is a system problem. The doctor is usually told how much time he or she has with each patient. When making the appointment, ask for the amount of time you want, especially if this is more than 10 or 15 minutes, but be prepared to make a case for more time. You can also ask for the last appointment in the day. You may have to wait a while, but at least the doctor will not be rushed by having to see another patient.

  Remember—if you request more time than is allotted, you make other people wait. While this may not seem like much at first glance, it could be. A doctor often sees 30 patients a day. If each one takes 5 extra minutes, this means that the doctor has to work an extra two and a half hours that day. That little bit of extra time really adds up.

- **"I can't get my doctor on the phone. She won't call back."** Ask your doctor(s) how to best communicate directly with them. This might be by email, or they may give you their private number or a number of a nurse practitioner with whom they work. The more a doctor trusts you not to abuse the privilege of having personal contact information, the more likely you are to be able to establish direct communication.

If you are given this privilege, use it wisely. Usually one does not call the doctor directly for a medication refill. Learn and use the system for doing this. If you do need to contact the doctor about medications, send a message through the nurse or send a note and return envelope two to three weeks before your prescription runs out. Save the minor concerns and questions for the next visit. In other words, contact your doctor directly only for the important things.

By the way, a medical emergency is certainly important, but it is best not to waste time trying to contact your doctor; rather, call 911 (in Canada), go to a hospital emergency department, or call the rescue squad for emergencies.

Parting Words of Advice

- **If something in the health care system is not working for you, ask how you can help to make it work better.** Very often, if you learn the mysteries of the system, you can solve or at least partially solve your problems.

- **Be nice—or at least as nice as possible.** Getting labeled as a difficult patient will just make life more difficult for you.

If you think that things should not be this way and that it is not fair to place this burden on the patient, we wholeheartedly agree. Health systems should change to be more responsive and patient friendly. A few health care systems are already doing this. In the meantime, we offer these suggestions to help you deal better with a difficult situation.

Suggested Further Reading

Beach, Wayne A. *Conversation About Illness.* Hillsdale, N.J.: Lawrence Erlbaum, 1996.

Beck, Aaron. *Love Is Never Enough: How Couples Can Overcome Misunderstandings, Resolve Conflicts, and Solve Relationship Problems Through Cognitive Therapy.* New York: Harper & Row, 1988.

Dector, Michael. *Navigating Canada's Health Care.* Toronto: Penguin Canada, 2006.

Feldman, William. *Take Control of Your Health: The Essential Roadmap to Making the Right Health Care Decisions.* Toronto: Key Porter Books, 2007.

McKay, Matthew, Martha Davis, and Patrick Fanning. *Messages: The Communication Skills Book.* Oakland, Calif.: New Harbinger, 1995.

Rosenberg, Marshall. *Getting Past the Pain Between Us: Healing and Reconciliation Without Compromise.* Encinitas, CA: Puddle Dancer Press, 2003.

Talking with Your Doctor: Communication Basics for Cancer Patients. Workshop kit. Health Canada, 2000.

SEX AND INTIMACY

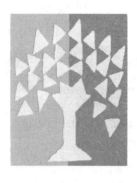

11

COUPLES WHO LIVE WITH A CHRONIC HEALTH PROBLEM FACE A CHALLENGE IN KEEPING THIS IMPORTANT PART OF THEIR RELATIONSHIP ALIVE AND WELL. Fear of injury or of bringing about a health emergency can dampen desire in one or both partners. Likewise, fear of increasing symptoms can frustrate couples, even if the symptoms occur only during sex itself. Sex, after all, is supposed to be joyful and pleasurable, not scary or uncomfortable!

For humans, sex is more than the act of sexual intercourse; it is also the sharing of physical and emotional sensuality. There is a special intimacy when we make love. Believe it or not, having a chronic health problem might actually improve your sex life by causing you to experiment with new types of physical and emotional stimulation for you and your partner. This process of exploring sensuality with your partner can open communication and strengthen your relationship as well. Additionally, natural "feel-good" hormones, called "endorphins," are released in our bloodstreams when we have sex.

For many people with chronic conditions, it is intercourse itself that is most difficult to sustain, because of the physical demands it places on our bodies. Intercourse brings about increased heart rate and breathing and can tax someone with limited energy or breathing or circulatory problems. Therefore, it is helpful to spend more time on sensuality or foreplay and less on actual intercourse. By concentrating on ways to arouse your partner and give pleasure while in a comfortable position, your intimate time together can last longer and be very satisfying. Many people enjoy climax without intercourse; others may wish to climax with intercourse. For some, climax may not be as important as sharing pleasure, and they are satisfied without an orgasm. No matter how or if climax is reached, uncomfortable symptoms can be minimized if we concentrate on foreplay and sensuality

187

rather than intercourse itself. There are many ways to enhance sensuality during sexual activity. In sex, as in most things, our minds and bodies are linked. By recognizing this, we can increase the sexual pleasure we experience through both physical and cognitive stimulation.

Emotional concerns can also be a serious factor for someone with health problems. Someone who has had a heart attack or a stroke is often concerned that sexual activity will bring on another attack. People with breathing difficulties worry that sex is too strenuous and will bring on an attack of coughing and wheezing, or worse. Their partners may fear that sexual activity might cause these problems, or even death, and that they would be responsible.

One of the most subtle and devastating barriers to fulfilling sexuality is the damage that has been caused to a person's self-image and self-esteem. Many report that they believe they are physically unattractive as a result of their disease—their paralysis, their shortness of breath, their weight gain from medications, or the changing shape of their joints—a sense of not being a whole, functioning being. This causes them to avoid sexual situations, and they "try not to think about it." This often leads to depression, and depression leads to lack of interest in sex, and that leads to depression . . . a vicious cycle. Depression can be treated and you can feel better. For more on depression and how to help yourself overcome it, see Chapter 4.

Even good sex can get better. Thankfully, there are ways you and your partner can explore sensuality and intimacy, as well as some ways to overcome fear during sex.

OVERCOMING FEAR DURING SEX

Anyone who has experienced a chronic condition has experienced fear that it will get worse, or even that an episode could be life-threatening. Health problems can really get in the way of the activities that we want and need to do. When sex is the activity that fear affects, we have a difficult problem: Not only are we denying ourselves an important, pleasurable part of life, but we probably feel guilty about denying our partner the same. Our partner may even feel more fearful and guilty than we do—afraid that he or she might hurt us during sex and guilty for maybe feeling resentful. This dynamic can cause serious problems in a relationship, and the resulting stress and depression can even produce more symptoms. We don't have to allow this to happen!

Remember the real estate maxim "The three most important things to consider when buying a house are location, location, and location"? Well, for successful sexual relationships, the three most important things are communication, communication, and communication! The most effective way to address the fears of both partners is to confront them and find ways to alleviate them through effective communication and problem solving. Without effective communication, learning new positions and ways to increase sensuality are not going to be enough. This is particularly important for people who may worry about how their health problem may make them look physically to others. Often, they find that their partner is far less concerned about their looks than they are.

When you and your partner are comfortable with talking about sex, you can go about finding solutions to the problems your chronic health problem imposes on you. To start with, you can share what kinds of physical stimulation you prefer and which positions you find most comfortable. Then you can share the fantasies you find most arousing. It's difficult to dwell on fears when your mind is occupied with a fantasy!

To get this process started, you and your partner may find some help with communication skills in Chapter 10 and problem-solving techniques in Chapter 2. Remember, if these techniques are new, give them time and practice. As we find with any new skill, it takes patience to learn to do them well.

SENSUALITY WITH TOUCH

The largest sensual organ of our bodies is the skin. It is rich with sensory nerves. The right touch on almost any area of our skin can be very erotic. Fortunately, sexual stimulation through touch can be done in just about any position. It can be further enhanced with the use of oils, flavored lotions, feathers, fur gloves—turn your imagination loose on this one! Just about any part of the skin can be an erogenous zone, but the most popular are the mouth (of course!), ear lobes, neck, breasts (for both genders), navel area, hands (fingertips if you are giving pleasure, palms if you are receiving pleasure), wrists, small of the back, buttocks, toes, and insides of the thighs and arms. Experiment with the type of touch—some find a light touch arousing, others prefer a firm touch. It is not necessary to limit yourself to your hands, either. Many people become very aroused when touched with the lips, tongue, or sex toys.

SENSUALITY WITH FANTASY

What goes on in our minds can be extremely arousing. If it weren't, there would be no strip clubs, pornography, or even romance novels. Most people engage in sexual fantasy at some time or another. There are probably as many sexual fantasies as there are people, and any is

OK to mentally indulge in. If you discover a fantasy that you and your partner share, you can play it out in bed, even if it is as simple as a particular saying you or your partner like to hear during sex. Engaging the mind during sexual activity can be every bit as arousing as the physical stimulation. It is also useful when symptoms during sex interfere with your enjoyment.

OVERCOMING SYMPTOMS DURING SEX

Some people are unable to find a sexual position that is completely comfortable, or they find pain, shortness of breath, or fatigue during sex to be so distracting that it interferes with their enjoyment of sex or their ability to have an orgasm. This situation can pose some special problems. If you are unable to climax, you may feel resentful of your partner if he or she is able to climax, and your partner may feel guilty about it. If you avoid sex because you are frustrated, your partner may become resentful and you may feel guilty. Your self-esteem may suffer. Your relationship with your partner may suffer. Everything suffers.

One thing you can do to help deal with this situation is to time the taking of medication to be at peak effectiveness when you want to have sex. Of course, this would involve planning ahead! The type of medication may be important, too. If you take a narcotic-type pain reliever, for example, or one containing muscle relaxants or tranquilizers, you may find that your sensory nerves are dulled along with your pain. Obviously, it would be counterproductive to dull the nerves that will give you pleasure. Your thinking may also be muddled due to the medication, making it more difficult to focus. Some medications can also make it difficult for a man to achieve an erection. Ask your doctor or pharmacist about possible timing or alternatives if this is a problem for you.

Another way to deal with uncomfortable symptoms is to become the world's best expert at fantasy! To be really good at something, you have to train for it, and this is no exception. The idea here is to develop one or more sexual fantasies that you can indulge in when needed, making it vivid in your mind. Then, during sex, you can call up your fantasy and concentrate on it. By concentrating on the fantasy, or on picturing you and your partner making love while you actually are, you are keeping your mind consumed with erotic thoughts rather than your symptoms. However, if you have not had experience in visualization and imagery techniques, generally used for relaxation exercises such as those in Chapter 5, you will need to practice several times a week to learn it well. All of this practice need not be devoted to your chosen sexual fantasy, however. You can start with any guided imagery tape or script such as the one in Chapter 5, working to make it more vivid each time you practice. Start with just picturing the images. When you get good at that, add and dwell on colors; then, in your mind, look down to your feet as you walk; then listen to the sounds around you; then concentrate on the smells and tastes in the image and feel your skin being touched by a breeze or mist; and, finally, feel yourself touch things in the image. Work on one of the senses at a time. Become good at one before going on to another. Once proficient at imagery, you can invest your own sexual fantasy and picture it, hear it, smell it, and feel it. You can even begin your fantasy by picturing yourself setting your symptoms aside. The possibilities are limited only by your imagination!

Learning to call on this level of concentration can also help you focus on the moment. Really focusing on your physical and emotional sensations during sex can be powerfully erotic. If your mind wanders (this is normal), gently bring it back to the here and now. **IMPORTANT:** *Do not try to overcome chest pain in this way. Chest pain should not be ignored, and a physician should be consulted right away.*

If you decide that you wish to abstain from sexual activity because of your chronic health problem, or if it is not an important part of your life, that's OK—but it is important to your relationship with your partner that he or she be in agreement with your decision. Good communication skills are essential in this situation, and you may even benefit from both of you discussing the situation with a professional therapist present. Someone trained to deal with important interpersonal situations can help facilitate the discussion.

SEXUAL POSITIONS

In order to minimize symptoms during sex, as well as to minimize fear of pain or injury for both partners, it is important to find positions that are comfortable for both partners. Generally, comfortable positions can be found through experimentation. Everybody is different; no one position is good for everyone. We encourage you to experiment with different positions, possibly before you and your partner are too aroused for you to want to change to a more comfortable position. Experiment with placement of pillows or with using a sitting position on a chair.

No matter which position you try, it is often helpful to do some warm-up exercises before sex. Look at some of the stretching exercises from Chapter 7. Exercise can help your sex life in other ways, as well. Becoming more fit is an excellent way to increase comfort and endurance during sex. Walking, swimming, bicycling, and so on can benefit you in bed as well as anywhere else by reducing shortness of breath, fatigue, and pain. Also, learn your limits and pace yourself, just as you would with any other physical activity.

During sexual activity, it may be advisable to change positions periodically if your symptoms come on or increase when you stay in one position too long. This can be done in a playful fashion, whereby it becomes fun for both of you instead of a chore. Stopping to rest is OK!

SPECIAL CONSIDERATIONS

There are specific issues that are of concern for people with certain health problems. People who are recovering from a heart attack or stroke, for example, are often afraid to resume sexual relations for fear of not being able to perform or of bringing on another attack or even death. It is even more common for their partners to refrain because of this fear. Fortunately, this is a myth, and sexual relations can be resumed as soon as you feel ready to do so. With stroke, in particular, there may be residual paralysis or weakness requiring a little more attention to finding the best positions for support and comfort and the most sensitive areas of the body to caress. There may also be concerns about bowel and bladder control that require consideration. The Heart and Stroke Foundation of Canada (www. heartandstroke.ca) has guides to sexuality for those with heart disease or stroke. They also offer information and advice about sildenafil (Viagra) and similar drugs and the risk for men with erection difficulty. Your pharmacist will also be a helpful resource.

People with diabetes sometimes report problems with sexual function. Men may have difficulty achieving or maintaining an erection, which can be caused by medication side effects or other medical conditions associated with diabetes. Women and men can have reduced feeling (neuropathy) in the genital area. Women's most common complaint is inadequate vaginal lubrication. For people with diabetes, the most effective ways to prevent or lessen these problems is to maintain tight management of blood sugar, exercise, keep a positive outlook, and generally take care of themselves. Lubricants can help with sensitivity for both men and women. If you are using condoms, be sure to use a water-based lubricant; petroleum-based lubricants destroy latex. The use of a vibrator can be very helpful for those with neuropathy, and concentrating on the most sensual parts of the body for stimulation can help make sex pleasurable. There are new therapies for men with erectile problems. According to the Canadian Diabetes Association (www.diabetes.ca), a recognized drug such as sildenafil may be useful to men with diabetes. A common misconception about sildenafil is that you take the pill and instantly have an erection. An erection only occurs with arousal, so take your time and relax. You may feel that talking about sexual issues won't help, or you are the only one with sexual problems. You are not alone; talking does help, and your doctor or an information referral specialist at the Canadian Diabetes Association will help you. They are trained to assist you and take away the awkwardness related to these sensitive issues.

Chronic or recurring pain can put a big damper on sexual interest. It can be difficult to feel sexy when you are hurting or are afraid that sex will make you hurt. People with pain as the predominant symptom of arthritis, migraine headaches, bowel disease, or other disorder often have the challenge of having to overcome pain in order to become sexually aroused or to have an orgasm. This is one area where concentration and focus, as discussed earlier in this chapter, are most helpful skills. Learning to focus on the moment or on sexual fantasy can distract you from the pain and allow you to concentrate on sex and your partner. Time your pain medication to have maximum effect during sex, find a comfortable position, take it slow and easy, relax, and enjoy extended foreplay. The Arthritis Society (www.arthritis.ca) can offer resources and guides for those with joint or back pain.

No matter what your chronic health problem, your doctor should be your first consultant on solutions to sexual problems caused by your condition. Sometimes something as simple as changing medication or its timing can make a difference. It's unlikely that your problem is unique; your doctor has probably heard about it before and may have some solutions. Remember, this is just another problem associated with your chronic condition, just like fatigue, pain, and physical limitations, and it is a problem that can be addressed. Chronic health problems need not end sex. Through good communication and planning, satisfying sex can prevail. By being creative and willing to experiment, both the sex and the relationship can actually be better.

MADE IN CANADA

For the past thirty years Sue Johanson has been talking about sex. She now has a website with every episode of her television show, Talk Sex With Sue Johanson, available for viewing at your leisure. (www.talksexwithsue.com) Johanson, a Canadian, is a gently-aged registered nurse who speaks plainly about all sexual matters. The shows are not just about the mechanics of sex; she has online articles about couples' communication along with coping with illness and age. An excellent selection of books is listed on the website, and most are available from the public library in your town.

Suggested Further Reading

Carlton, Lucille. *In Sickness and in Health: Sex, Love and Chronic Illness.* Miami, Fla.: National Parkinson Foundation, 1996.

Herbert, Lauren Andrew. *Sex and Back Pain: Advice on Restoring Comfortable Sex Lost to Back Pain.* Impacc USA, 1997.

Johanson, Sue. *Sex, Sex, and More Sex.* Penguin Canada, 2004.

Klein, Marty. *Ask Me Anything: A Sex Therapist Answers the Most Important Questions for the '90s.* San Francisco: Pacifica Press, 1996.

Klein, Marty, and Riki Robbins. *Let Me Count the Ways: Discovering Sex Without Intercourse.* New York: J. P. Tarcher, 1999.

Ornstein, Robert, and David Sobel. *Healthy Pleasures.* Reading, Mass.: Addison Wesley Longman, Inc., 1990.

Saul, David. *Sex for Life: The Lover's Guide to Male Sexuality.* Vancouver: Apple Publishing Company Ltd., 1999.

Seidman, David. *The Longevity Sourcebook.* Los Angeles: Lowell House, 1997.

Silverberg, Cory, Miriam Kaufman, and Fran Odette. *The Ultimate Guide to Sex and Disability: For All of Us Who Live with Disabilities, Chronic Pain and Illness.* San Francisco: Cleis Press, 2003.

Taguchi, Yosh. *Private Parts: A Doctor's Guide to the Male Anatomy.* Montreal: McClelland & Stewart.

Ulrich, Kathy, and Chandler, Vicki. *Loving With Back Pain: Good Sex With a Bad Back.* Wondersight LLC, 1996.

MAKING YOUR WISHES KNOWN: Advance Directives for Health Care

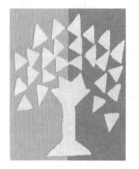

12

I T HAS BEEN SAID THAT LIFE IS THE GREATEST RISK FACTOR FOR DYING. All of us have feelings about our own death and the death of loved ones. Death may be feared, welcomed, accepted, or, all too often, pushed aside to be thought about at a different time. Somewhere, in the back of our minds, most of us have ideas about how and when we would like to die. For some of us, life is so important that we feel everything should be done to sustain it. For others, life is important only so long as we can be active participants. For many people, the issue isn't really death but, rather, dying. We have all heard about the eighty-year-old who died skiing. This may be considered a "good" death. On the other hand, we may have a friend or family member who spent years in a nursing home unaware of his or her surroundings. This is usually not what we would wish for ourselves.

While none of us can have absolute control over our own death, this, like the rest of our lives, is something we can help manage. That is, we can have input, make decisions, and probably add a great deal to the quality of our death. Proper management can lessen the negative impacts of our death on our survivors. This chapter deals with information to help you better manage some of the legal issues of death—specifically advance directives for health care, otherwise known as enduring power of attorney for health care, and in Quebec, the mandate for health care. While each province has different regulations, this information should be useful wherever you live. The information in this chapter deals with specific legal documents that differ from province to province. However, the issues discussed are universal. As you read, take what is useful to you and skip over the rest. Let us start with some definitions.

At any time in your life you may appoint another person as a power of attorney. This is commonly used when parents go on vacation so someone can take care of any emergency that might occur with the children. When you add an enduring power of attorney, it comes into action when you become mentally incompetent, through traumatic injury or end-stage illness. Some provinces have Representation Agreements, which outline your wishes for your health and personal care: whether you want to remain at home and who is responsible for making care decisions for you, right down to details about hairdressing or barber appointments. It is important to become familiar with the acts and regulations that apply in your jurisdiction, and then sort out what is best for you and your circumstances. This is your opportunity to communicate your wishes for your future health care. An enduring power of attorney for health care is a document in which you appoint someone else to act as your agent concerning health care. In other words, it allows someone else to make decisions for you. It does not give the person the right to act in other ways, such as handling your financial matters. This document is activated only when for some reason you are unable to make decisions yourself (e.g.,being in a coma or mentally incompetent).

Besides naming someone as your agent, the enduring power of attorney can give guidelines to your agent about your wishes concerning health care. You do not have to give guidance to your agent. However, many people wish to do so. This guidance can indicate almost anything you want done for your care; it may range from the use of aggressive life-sustaining measures to the withholding of life-sustaining measures.

To complete an enduring power of attorney for health care means making many decisions.

First, you must decide who will be your agent. This can be a friend or member of the family. It cannot be the physician who is providing your care. There are some considerations to be made in choosing your agent. This person should generally be available in the geographic area where you live. If the agent is not available to make decisions for you, he or she is not much help. Just to be on the safe side, you can also name a back-up agent who would act in your behalf if your primary agent were not available. **Second, you must be sure that this person thinks like you think or at least would be willing to carry out your wishes. Third, the person must be someone who you feel would be able**

to carry out your wishes. Sometimes a spouse or child is not the best agent because this person is too close to you emotionally. For example, if you wished not to be resuscitated in the case of a severe heart attack, your agent has to be able to tell the doctor not to resuscitate. This could be very difficult or impossible for a family member to decide then and there. Be sure the person you choose as your agent is up to this task and would not say "do everything you can" at this critical time. **Finally, you want your agent to be someone who will not find this job too much of an emotional burden.** Thus, the person has to be comfortable with the role, as well as willing and able to carry out your wishes.

In review, look for these characteristics in an agent:

- Someone who is likely to be available should they need to act on your behalf.

- Someone who understands your wishes and is willing to carry them out.

- Someone who is emotionally prepared and able to carry out your wishes.

- Someone who will not be emotionally burdened by carrying out your wishes.

As you can see, finding the right agent is a very important task. This may mean talking to several people. These may be the most important interviews that you ever conduct. We will talk more about discussing your wishes with family, friends, and doctor later.

The other major decision is what you want to put in your enduring power of attorney for health care. In other words, what are your directions to your agent? Some forms give several general statements of desires concerning medical treatment.

For example:

I do not want my life to be prolonged and I do not want life-sustaining treatment to be provided or continued: (1) if I am in an irreversible coma or persistent vegetative state; or (2) if I am terminally ill and the application of life-sustaining procedures would serve only to artificially delay the moment of my death; or (3) under any other circumstances where the burdens of the treatment outweigh the expected benefits. I want my agent to consider the relief of suffering and the quality as well as the extent of the possible extension of my life in making decisions concerning life-sustaining treatment.

I want my life to be prolonged and I want life-sustaining treatment to be provided unless I am in a coma or vegetative state which my doctor reasonably believes to be irreversible. Once my doctor has reasonably concluded that I will remain unconscious for the rest of my life, I do not want life-sustaining treatment to be provided or continued.

I want my life to be prolonged to the greatest extent possible without regard to my condition, the chances I have for recovery, or the cost of the procedures.

If you use a form containing such suggested general statements, all you need to do is initial the statement that best applies to you.

Other forms make a "general statement of granted authority," in which you give your agent the power to make decisions. However, you do not write out the details of what these decisions should be. In this case, you are trusting your agent to follow your wishes. Since these wishes are not explicitly written, it is very important that you have discussed them in detail with your agent.

All forms also have a space in which you can write out any specific wishes. You are not required to give specific details but may wish to do so.

Knowing what details to write is a little complicated because none of us knows the exact circumstances in which the agent will have to act. However, you can get some idea by asking your doctor what he thinks are the most likely developments for someone with your condition. Then you can direct your agent on how to act. Your specific directions can discuss outcomes, specific circumstances, or both. If you discuss outcomes, then the statement should focus on which types of outcomes would be acceptable and which would not—for example, "resuscitate if I can continue to fully function mentally." The following are some of the more common specific circumstances encountered with major chronic diseases.

- **Alzheimer's disease and other neurologic problems are diseases that can leave you with little or no mental function.** As we said earlier, these are generally not life-threatening, at least not for many years. However, things happen to these patients that can be life-threatening, such as pneumonia and heart attacks. What you need to do is decide how much treatment you want. For example, do you want antibiotics if you get pneumonia? Do you want to be resuscitated if your heart stops? Do you wish a feeding tube if you are unable to feed yourself? Remember, it is your choice as to how you answer each of these questions. You may not want to be resuscitated but may want a feeding tube. If you want aggressive treatment, you may want to use all means possible to sustain life; alternatively, you may not want any special means to be used to sustain life. For example, you may want to be fed but may not want to be placed on life-support equipment.

- **You have very bad lung function that will not improve.** Should you become unable to breathe on your own, do you want to be placed in an intensive care unit on mechanical ventilation (a breathing machine)? Remember, in this case you will not improve. To say that you never want ventilation is very different from saying that you don't want it if it is used to sustain life when no improvement is likely. Obviously, mechanical ventilation can be life-saving in cases such as a severe asthma attack when it is used for a short time until the body can regain its normal function. Here, the issue is not whether to use mechanical ventilation ever but, rather, when or under what circumstances you wish it to be used.

- **You have a heart condition that cannot be improved with angioplasty (cleaning out the arteries) or surgery.** You are in the cardiac intensive care unit. If your heart stops functioning, do you want to be resuscitated? As with artificial ventilation, the question is not "Do you ever want to be resuscitated?" but rather "Under what conditions do you or do you not want resuscitation?"

From these examples you can begin to identify some of the directions that you might want to give in your advance directive or enduring power of attorney for health care. Again, to understand these better or to make them more personal to your own condition, you might want to talk with your physician about what the common problems and decisions are for people with your condition.

In summary, there are several decisions you need to make in directing your agent on how to act in your behalf:

- **Generally, how much treatment do you want?** This can range from the very aggressive—that is, doing many things to sustain life—to the very conservative—which is doing almost nothing to sustain life, except to keep you clean and comfortable.

- **Given the types of life-threatening events that are likely to happen to people with your condition, what sorts of treatment do you want and under what conditions?**

- **If you become mentally incapacitated, what sorts of treatment do you want for other illnesses, such as pneumonia?**

Many people get this far. They have thought through their wishes about dying and have even written them down in an enduringe power of attorney for health care. This is an excellent beginning but not the end of the job. A good manager has to do more than just write a memo. He or she has to see that the memo gets delivered. If you really want your wishes carried out, it is important that you share them fully with your agent, your family, and your doctor. This is often not an easy task. In the following section, we will discuss ways to make these conversations easier.

Before you can have a conversation, all interested parties need to have copies of your enduring power of attorney for health care. Once you have completed the documents, have them witnessed and signed. In some places you can have your enduring power of attorney notarized instead of having it witnessed. Make several copies at any copy center. You will need copies for your agent(s), family members, and doctor. It also does not hurt to give one to your lawyer.

Now you are ready to talk about your wishes. Nobody likes to discuss their own death or that of a loved one. Therefore, it is not surprising that when you bring up this subject the response is often "Oh, don't think about that," or "That's a long time off," or "Don't be so morbid; you're not that sick." Unfortunately, this is usually enough to end the conversation. Your job as a good self-manager is to keep the conversation open. There are several ways to do this. First, plan on how you are going to begin your discussion of this subject. Here are some suggestions.

Prepare your enduring power of attorney, and then give copies to the appropriate family members or friends. Ask them to read it and then set a specific time to discuss it. If they give you one of those responses presented earlier, say that you understand that this is a difficult topic, but that it is important to you that you discuss it with them. This is a good time to practice the "I" messages discussed in Chapter 10—for example, "I understand that death is a difficult thing to talk about. However, it is very important to me that we have this discussion."

You might get blank copies of the enduring power of attorney form for all your family members and suggest that you all fill them out and share them. This could even be part of a family get-together. Present this as an important aspect of being a mature adult and family member. Making this a family project in which everyone is involved may make it easier to discuss. Besides, it will help to clarify everyone's values about the topics of death and dying.

If these two suggestions seem too difficult or, for some reason, are impossible to carry out, you might write a letter or email, or prepare a video or CD that can then be sent to members of your family. Talk about why you feel your death is an important topic to discuss and that you want them to know your wishes. Then state your wishes, providing reasons for the choices you indicate. At the same time, send them a copy of your enduring power of attorney for health care. Ask that they respond in some way or that you set aside some time to talk in person or on the phone with them.

Of course, in deciding on your agent, it is important that you choose someone with whom you can talk freely and exchange ideas. If your chosen agent is not willing to or is unable to talk to you about your wishes, then you have probably chosen the wrong agent. Also, don't be fooled. Just because someone is very close does not mean that he or she really understands your wishes or would be able to carry them out. This is not a topic that should be left to a mutual, unspoken understanding unless you don't mind if they decide differently from what you wish. For this reason, choosing someone who is not as close to you emotionally is sometimes better. Talking with your agent is especially important if you have not written details of your wishes.

TALKING WITH YOUR DOCTOR

From our research, we have learned that, in general, people have a much more difficult time talking to their doctors about their wishes surrounding death than to their families. In fact, only a very small percentage of people who have written enduring powers of attorney for health care, or other advance directives, ever share these with their physician.

There are several reasons why it is important that this discussion take place. First, you need to be sure that your doctor has values that are compatible with your wishes. If you and your doctor do not have the same values, it may be difficult for him or her to carry out your wishes. Second, your doctor needs to know what you want. This allows him or her to take appropriate actions such as writing orders to resuscitate or not to use mechanical resuscitation. Third, your doctor needs to know who your agent is and how to contact this person. If an important decision has to be made and your wishes are to be followed, the doctor must talk with your agent.

It is important to give your doctor a copy of your enduring power of attorney for health care so that it can become a permanent part of your medical record. Again, the problem is often how to start this conversation with the doctor.

As surprising as it may seem, many physicians also find this a very difficult topic to discuss with their patients. After all, they are in the business of helping to keep people alive and well; they don't like to think about their patients dying. On the other hand, most doctors want their patients to have enduring powers of attorney for health care. This relieves them of pressure and worry.

If you wish, plan a time with your doctor when you can discuss your wishes. This should not be a side conversation at the end of a regular visit. Rather, start a visit by saying, "I want a few minutes to discuss with you my wishes in the event of a serious problem or impending death." When put in this way, most doctors will make time to talk with you. If the doctor says that he or she does not have enough time, then ask when you can make another appointment to talk with him or her. This is a situation in which you may need to be a little assertive. Sometimes a doctor, like your family members or friends, might say, "Oh, you don't have to worry about that, let me do it" or "We'll worry about that when the time comes." Again, you will have to take the initiative, using an "I" message to communicate that this is important to you and you do not want to put off the discussion.

Sometimes doctors do not want to worry you. They think they are doing you a favor by not describing all the unpleasant things that might happen to you or the potential treatments in case of serious problems. You can help your doctor by telling him or her that having control and making some decisions about your future will ease your mind. Not knowing or not being clear on what will happen is more worrisome than being faced with the facts, unpleasant as they may be, and dealing with them.

Even knowing all of the above, it is still sometimes hard to talk with your doctor. Therefore, it might also be helpful to bring your agent with you when you have this discussion. The agent can facilitate the discussion and, at the same time, meet your doctor. This also gives everyone a chance to clarify any misunderstandings about your wishes. It opens the lines of communication so that if your agent and physician have to act to carry out your wishes, they can do so with few problems. If somehow you just "can't" talk with your doctor, at least mail him or her a copy of your enduring power of attorney. This way it will become part of your medical records.

When you go the hospital, be sure the hospital has a copy of your enduring power of attorney. If you cannot bring it, be sure your agent knows to give a copy to the hospital. This is important, as your doctor may not be in charge of your care in the hospital.

There is one thing not to do. Do not put your enduring power of attorney in your safe deposit box—no one will be able to get it when it is needed. You might like to seek advice from the community law clinics sponsored by the Canadian Bar Association in many communities. You do not need to consult a lawyer, but do exercise caution and take steps to protect yourself.

Many seniors' and veteran's organizations also sponsor clinics and workshops to help you plan your future health care.

So now you have done all the important things. The hard work is over. However, remember that you can change your mind at any time. Your agent may no longer be available, or your wishes might change. Be sure to keep your enduring power of attorney for health care updated. Like any legal document, it can be revoked or changed at any time. The decisions you make today are not forever.

If you travel from province to province, check with a lawyer or legal advocate in the province in which you are staying to ensure your document is recognized in that province. For those who travel south in the winter months, (snowbirds) get solid legal advice to ensure your wishes are carried out. The USA has very different laws concerning advance directives.

Making your wishes known about how you want to be treated in case of serious or life-threatening illness is one of the most important tasks of self-management. The best way to do this is to prepare a durable power of attorney for health care and share this with your family, close friends, and physician.

A few more notes about preparing for death:

In many parts of Canada, as well as in other parts of the world, both palliative care and hospice care are available. In everyone's life there comes a time when medical care is no longer helpful and we need to prepare for death. Today, we often have several weeks or months, and sometimes years to make these preparations. This is when hospice care is so very useful. The aim of hospice care is to provide the terminally ill patient (someone who is expected to die within months) with the highest quality of life possible. Palliative care is available for those expected to live more than six months. At the same time, hospice professionals help both the patient and the family prepare for death with dignity and also help the surviving family members. Today most hospices are "in home" programs. This means that the patient stays in his or her own home and the services come to them. In some places there are also residential hospices where people can go for their last days.

One of the problems with hospice care is that often people wait until the last few days before death to ask for this care. They somehow see asking for hospice care as "giving up." By refusing hospice care, they often put an unnecessary burden on themselves, friends, and family. The reverse is also often true. Families say they can cope without help. This may be true, but the patient's life and dying may be much better if hospice cares for all the medical things so that family and friends are free to give love and support.

Hospice care can be most useful for the months before death. Most hospices only accept people who are expected to die within six months. This does not mean that you will be thrown out if you "outlive" your time. Six months is a guideline, not a fixed time. The message here is that if you, a family member, or a friend is in the ending stage of illness, find and utilize your local hospice. It is a wonderful final gift.

Across Canada, there are differences in how you put together your enduring power of attorney or a health care directive. You may hear these referred to as "living wills," but this is not a legal document in Canada. An excellent overview of each province is to be found at the CBC website: www.cbc.ca/news/background/wills. The terms are explained in plain language, and resources for each province are listed. You will find workshops offered across Canada by groups such as The Public Guardian and Trustee partnered with local bar associations and community groups. These are your best resource for this information. If you discover that you have a complex situation, then you will need to consult a lawyer experienced in estates and wills.

Here are resources for across Canada

Resources

British Columbia
The Canadian Centre for Elder Law Studies
A Division of the British Columbia Law Institute
Telephone: 604-822-0633
E-mail: ccels@bcli.org
www.ccels.ca

Representation Agreement Resource Centre
Centre for Quality of Life Planning
Telephone: 604-408-7414
E-mail: info@rarc.bc
www.rarc.ca

Alberta
Department of Justice
Enduring Power of Attorney and Personal Directive
www.justice.gov.ab.ca./dependent_adults/enduring_powers_of_attorney

Saskatchewan
Department of Justice
Enduring Power of Attorney, Health Care Directive
www.justice.gov.sk.ca

Manitoba
Advanced Health Care Directive
www.gov.mb.ca/laws/statutes

Ontario
Advocacy Centre for the Elderly
www.advocacycentreelderly.org

Quebec
Curateur public du Quebec
My Mandate in Case of Incapacity
www.curateur.gouv.qc.ca

Newfoundland and Labrador
Advance Health Care Directive
www.hoa.gov.nl.ca

New Brunswick
Public Legal Information and Information Service of New Brunswick
Telephone: 506-453-5369
E-mail: pleisnb@web.ca
www.legal-info-legale.nb.ca

Nova Scotia
Medical Consent Act

Prince Edward Island
Consent to Treatment and Health Care Directive
Ministry of Health

Northwest Territories
Enduring Power of Attorney
Department of Justice

Yukon
Enduring Power of Attorney
A Lawyer is required for this matter

The Canadian Bar Association branch office in your community.

Suggested Further Reading

Stolp, Hans. *When a Loved One Dies.* Hampshire, UK: O'Books, 2005.

HEALTHY EATING

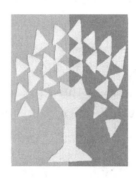

13

EVELOPING HEALTHY EATING HABITS IS IMPORTANT FOR EVERYONE. We know that a well-balanced eating plan not only gives us more energy and endurance to carry out our daily activities, but also makes us feel good and helps reduce our risk for certain health problems. While food alone cannot prevent or cure a chronic health condition, learning to make healthier food choices at each meal can help us strengthen our immune system, manage symptoms more effectively, prevent complications, and feel more in control of our health.

Changing our eating habits, though, can be challenging. The way we eat and prepare our foods are habits that have developed over years and, for many of us, represent an important part of our cultural customs and family traditions. Therefore, suddenly trying to change everything about the way we eat is not realistic, and could become frustrating and unpleasant. If we really want to make healthful, permanent changes in our eating habits, then it is important to do this little by little over time.

In this chapter, we offer some suggestions to help you begin making changes in your eating habits without losing variety and your enjoyment of food. We have included tips for planning well-balanced meals, making healthier food choices, managing a healthy weight, and minimizing some of the problems commonly associated with eating and weight management. Just like any of the other self-management techniques discussed in this book, healthy eating will help you take control of your health.

WHAT IS HEALTHY EATING?

Healthy eating does not mean that you can never eat your favourite foods again or that you have to "diet" or buy "special" foods. Rather, it means learning to make healthier choices in the foods you eat most of the time, finding new or different ways to prepare these foods, and eating regularly and in moderation.

Depending on your health condition and individual needs, the goals of healthy eating will be different from one person to the next. For example, for people with diabetes, a goal may be to monitor the amount of carbohydrates they eat to help reach and maintain their target blood glucose level.

Blood glucose is the amount of glucose (sugar) in the blood. People whose diabetes is not well managed have high blood glucose. For people with heart disease, the goals might be to reduce cholesterol and the amount and type of fat in the foods they eat. Cholesterol is a substance found in some foods and also produced by the body. An oversupply of cholesterol can lead to atherosclerosis (hardening of the arteries) and heart disease. People with high blood pressure need to increase fruits, vegetables, and low-fat dairy foods, and lower fat intake. For those wanting to lose weight, the goal is to eat less; and so on. (For more information on eating tips for people with specific long-term health conditions, refer to page 224-228 of this chapter.)

All of us, though, can benefit by learning to eat healthier. To start, we can follow these basic principles: Eat a wide variety of foods, eat regular meals at the same times every day, and try to eat the same amount of food at each meal.

Eating a variety of foods is important so that the body gets all the essential nutrients it needs to function well. The nutrients we need are proteins, carbohydrates, fat, vitamins, and minerals. Each plays an important role and can be found in varying amounts in the different food groups. Taking vitamins and food supplements can never replace eating a variety of foods. These "extras" contain only the nutrients we know about. To get all essential nutrients (both known and unknown), we need to eat a variety of foods.

Eating regularly and eating something after you arise in the morning every day provides the body with the fuel it needs to function well throughout the day, and keeps you feeling energetic. For this reason, it is best to space your meals and/or snacks out during the day, remembering to include a morning meal. A morning meal is important because it is the first source of energy for the body after a long night of fasting. Eating breakfast is also one of the secrets that helps with weight loss. Deciding how to space meals will depend on an individual's needs, preferences, and lifestyle. Some people may do well with three regular meals spaced four to five hours apart, while others who cannot eat as much at a meal may need to eat smaller, more frequent meals or snacks during the day.

Eating the same amount at each meal also ensures that the body has an adequate supply of energy to function optimally throughout the day. Skipping meals or eating a large meal with tiny meals can throw your system and energy level off and lead to unplanned and unhealthy snacking. It can also aggravate symptoms or cause other problems, such as irritability or mood swings and low blood glucose, or hypoglycemia. Eating too much can cause problems as well, such as indigestion or increased discomfort or pain from difficulties in breathing when the stomach becomes distended and the diaphragm is crowded. Eating too much at the evening meal can also contribute to weight gain and poor sleep.

Now, you are probably asking yourself, "What is the right amount to eat at each meal?" Well, unfortunately, there is no one simple or right answer to this question for everyone. The amount we should eat depends on many factors, including our age, sex, body size, activity level, and health needs. This is why the suggested number of servings and portion sizes for different food groups are usually given in ranges. The sections from Health Canada's *Eating Well With Canada's Food Guide* on pages 217-223 will provide you with recommendations on the types of food to eat, and outline the number of servings per day required by different age groups. This information is also available at www.healthcanada.ca.

PLANNING A HEALTHY MEAL

By now, most of us know that an eating plan that is low in fat and high in fibre is healthy for everyone. But many of us have difficulty putting this into practice when planning and preparing meals. Therefore, we have provided the following formula and sample food guide to help you plan and prepare healthier meals and snacks.

A Formula For Healthy Meals

This general formula for a healthy meal not only offers variety, but also encourages you to eat more servings of vegetables and fruit (at least five a day), as well as to choose more appropriate portion sizes for the foods we include in our regular meals. This guide assumes three meals a day.

A healthy or well-balanced meal or snack should include:

• One portion of protein-rich foods; making up one-fourth of your meal: Examples of proteins from the accompanying food guide include lean meat, skinless poultry, fish, low-fat or fat-free milk products, or a meat substitute like tofu. Cooked meat portions should be about the size of the palm of your hand and about as thick as your little finger. Consider those choices that are lower in fat and prepare with little or no added salt.

• One or more portions of vegetables that are low in starch or carbohydrates, making up at least half your meal: Portion sizes on these vegetables are not limited, and they can be eaten as often as you like. Examples from the guide include leafy green vegetables,

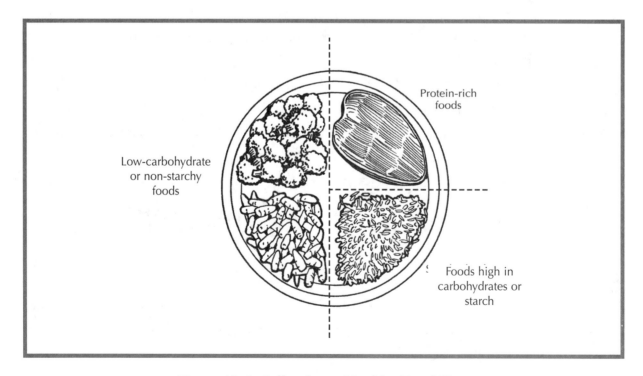

Figure 13.1 **Following a Healthy Food Plan**

tomatoes, broccoli, cucumber, etc. For green vegetables, the darker the green, the more nutrients. *Canada's Food Guide* recommends eating at least one dark green and one orange vegetable each day.

•   One portion of grain products (*Canada's Food Guide* recommends that at least half of your grain portion each day be whole grain- with one of the vegetables that are high in starch or carbohydrates, making up the other one-fourth of your meal: These foods include whole wheat breads, brown rice, pasta, legumes, corn, potatoes, crackers, popcorn, etc. Portion sizes may need to be limited for these foods if you are counting carbohydrates and/or calories. (For portion sizes, see the accompanying food guide.)

•   One portion of fruit or fruit juice: Portion sizes for fruit are also limited if you are counting carbohydrates and/or calories. *Canada's Food Guide* suggests choosing vegetables and fruit more often than juice.

•   Moderate use or avoidance of foods that are high in fat, sugar, and sodium, such as processed foods, salad dressings, lard and other fats, oils, jelly, jam, relish, sweets and candy, salty snacks, alcohol, and soft drinks.

This formula also corresponds well with the Health Canada *Eating Well With Canada's Food Guide*, which suggests we eat the following amounts of different foods each day:

For children 2-3 years old:
4 servings of vegetables and fruits
3 servings of grains
2 servings of milk and alternatives
1 serving of meat and alternatives

For children 4-8 years old:
5 servings of fruits and vegetables
4 servings of grains
2 servings of milk and alternatives
1 serving of meat and alternatives

For children 9-13 years old:
6 servings of fruits and vegetables
6 servings of grains
3-4 servings of milk and alternatives
1-2 servings of meat and alternatives

For females age 14-18:
7 servings of fruit and vegetables
6 servings of grains
3-4 servings of milk and alternatives
2 servings of meat and alternatives

For males age 14-18:
8 servings of fruits and vegetables
7 servings of grains
3-4 servings of milk and alternatives
3 servings of meat and alternatives

For women 19-50 years of age:
7-8 servings of vegetables and fruits
6-7 servings of grains
2 servings of milk and alternatives
2 servings of meat and alternatives

For men 19-50 years of age:
8-10 servings of vegetables and fruits
8 servings of grains
2 servings of milk and alternatives
3 servings of meat and alternatives

For women 51 years or older
7 servings of vegetables and fruits
6 servings of grains
3 servings of milk and alternatives
2 servings of meat and alternatives

For men 51 years or older
7 servings of vegetables and fruits
7 servings of grains
3 servings of milk and alternatives
3 servings of meat and alternatives

The chart on pages 213-214 tells you a little more about proteins, carbohydrates, and fats.

Reading Food Labels

Most of us have eaten foods that come from a can, box, package, or some other type of container. These containers list a great deal of information, including a panel labeled "Nutrition Facts." With the exception of foods prepared in the store, or those from small manufacturers, Health Canada requires all companies to provide nutrition information on most food packages. If the package is too small to list all the nutritional contents, the manufacturer usually includes a telephone number or address where you can call or write for this information.

Reading and understanding these Nutrition Facts will help you learn how to make healthier choices and to find out the amounts and kinds of nutrients in them. The parts of the label that are going to help you manage your condition and to eat healthy food are the (1) serving size; (2) calories; (3) total carbohydrates; (4) total fat, cholesterol, and trans fats; and (5) sodium.

PROTEINS perform numerous functions in the body. They are the building blocks for the body's muscles, are part of our red blood cells and the enzymes and hormones that help regulate bodily functions, and help the body's immune system to fight infection and build or repair damaged tissues. Enzymes are proteins that aid the chemical reactions within our bodies. Protein also provides some energy for the body to do its work, although providing energy is the main job of carbohydrates. Protein is comprised of smaller units called amino acids. Our bodies produce some of the amino acids it needs, while others we must get from food. Animal foods like meat, fish, poultry, eggs, and milk and soy foods like tofu are considered complete proteins because they provide us with all the amino acids that the body needs. Other proteins from plants like legumes (dried beans, peas, and lentils), grains, nuts, and seeds are called incomplete proteins because they are missing one or more of the amino acids that the body needs. However, whenever you eat a bit of a complete protein with an incomplete one, or two complementary incomplete proteins like rice and beans, these form a complete protein that the body can use. In addition, plant proteins are very beneficial since they contain dietary fibre, have no cholesterol, and with a few exceptions are low in fat. Nuts and seeds are high in fat, but healthful kinds of fat. Plant proteins also supply us with phytochemicals, which are substances that have been shown to be protective against diseases such as cancer and heart disease.

CARBOHYDRATES are the major source of energy for the body's muscles and metabolic functions. They should make up the majority of the foods and calories we eat each day. Carbohydrates are sometimes classified as starches (complex carbohydrates-and sugars (simple carbohydrates-and are found in a wide variety of foods, primarily foods from plants. The only animal foods that contain any carbohydrates are milk and yogurt. Starchy carbohydrate-containing foods include grains, rice, pasta, bread, legumes (dried beans, peas, and lentils), and root vegetables (potatoes, carrots, winter squash, etc.). Sugars are found in fruits and some dairy products, as well as table and brown sugar, honey, syrups, and jellies. When you choose whole grains, fruits, and vegetables you get the full complement of all the vitamins, minerals, phytochemicals, and fibre that were put there originally by nature. White and other refined flours and white rice do not contain fibre and have also been stripped of many of their nutrients as well as phytochemicals.

(continues on next page)

FAT is essential for our bodies to function properly and be healthy. Every one of us needs a small amount each day to help build, strengthen, and repair body tissue. Unfortunately, most of us get way too much fat and too much of the wrong kind of fat. Fat can be divided into "good" and "bad" fats, relative to their effects on our health. "Bad" fats, also known as saturated fats, can increase your blood cholesterol and risk of heart disease. They are found mostly in animal foods like red meat; processed meats like bacon; poultry; whole milk; dairy foods, including cream cheese, butter, and sour cream; and palm and coconut oils. Another kind of "bad" fat is called trans fats; these are found in many processed snack and dessert foods. Trans fats are usually listed as "partially hydrogenated" or "hydrogenated" oils on food labels. In contrast, "good" fats, also known as unsaturated fats, can help reduce blood cholesterol and, in addition, help keep your body's cells healthy. Good fats are found in most plant-based oils (soybean, safflower, canola, olive, etc.) and foods like nuts, avocados, and olives. In addition, fatty fish like salmon, mackerel, trout, and tuna are also high in good fats; these are called omega-3 fatty acids, which are helpful in reducing the risk of heart disease.

Fat—just like protein and carbohydrates—can be used to supply the body with energy. But fat contains twice the number of calories per gram as protein or carbohydrates, so fat calories add up quickly. When we eat more calories than we need—and it doesn't matter if they come from protein, carbohydrates, or fat, the extra calories get stored in the body, leading to weight gain and increased risk of several health problems.

VITAMINS AND MINERALS are essential for everyone. They help build strong blood, bones, and muscles and ensure that the body functions the way it should. If we eat a wide variety of whole foods, especially whole grains, a lot of plant-based foods, and lower-fat protein sources, we are more likely to get all the vitamins and minerals that we need. In doing so, it may not be necessary to take a vitamin or mineral supplement. Supplements do not take the place of a good, balanced eating plan. However, if you do choose to take a supplement, select a generic brand (they are usually as good as the higher-priced, brand names) that contains 50% to 100% of the recommended daily allowance; try to stay away from "mega" supplements, unless prescribed and supervised by your doctor. Getting too much of certain vitamins and minerals can be harmful and may cause toxic reactions.

Nutrition Facts to Look for on Food Labels

Nutrition Facts
Per 125 mL (87 g)

Amount Per Serving	% Daily Value
Calories 80	
Fat 0.5 g	1%
Saturated 0 g	0%
+ Trans 0 g	
Cholesterol 0 mg	
Sodium 0 mg	0%
Carbohydrate 18 g	6%
Fibre 2 g	9%
Sugars 2 g	
Protein 3 g	
Vitamin A 2%	Vitamin C 10%
Calcium 0%	Iron 2%

Valeur nutritive
par 125 mL (87 g)

Teneur	% valeur quotiolenne
Calories 80	
Lipides 0.5 g	1%
saturés 0 g	0%
+ trans 0 g	
Cholesterol 0 mg	
Sodium 0 mg	0%
Glucides 18 g	6%
Fibres 2 g	9%
Sucres 2 g	
Proteines 3 g	
Vitamin A 2%	Vitamin C 10%
Calcium 0%	Iron 2%

- The nutrient information is based on one serving size or a specified amount of food, such as 125 mL (87 g), as shown in the sample Nutrition Facts label. All the other nutrition information you read is based on the serving size. This serving size is fixed. You might actually eat more or less. If the specified amount or serving size is not the same as you eat, then you will need to adjust the rest of the nutrition information according to your serving size. For example, if you eat 250 mL (175 g) of rice and the specified amount is 125 mL, then you will need to double the values for everything else listed.

- Calories are given for the specified amount only. The Nutrition Facts table will also include a list of nutrients and the amount of each nutrient in the specified quantity of food. The % Daily Value listed on the right of the table gives a context for the amount of the nutrient in the specified amount. You can use the Daily Value, which is based on recommendations for healthy eating, to see if a serving of the food contains a lot or a little of a nutrient.

(continues on next page)

Nutrition Facts to Look for on Food Labels

- The total carbohydrates (18 g) listed in the sample label are per specified amount and include the amount of fibre (2 g), as well as sugars (2 g) in or added to the product. This fact is especially important for individuals who are watching or counting carbohydrates. If you are counting carbohydrates for meal planning, the grams of fibre can be subtracted from the total grams of carbohydrates.

- Be aware of the amount of cholesterol (0 mg in the sample table). The recommended total amount is less than 300 mg daily.

- Note the amount of sodium (0 mg in the sample label). The recommended amount is less than 400 mg per serving. Most processed foods tend to be high in sodium, so watch for ingredients that have sodium somewhere in their name. Limit the amount of salt you have in a day to 5 mL (1 teaspoon).

- The amount of total fat (.5 g per 125 mL in this example-includes saturated or "bad" fats and unsaturated or "good" fats. Saturated and trans fats are the "bad" fats. Also, look at the list of ingredients on the package; if you see the words "partially hydrogenated" or "hydrogenated" vegetable oils, then the product contains trans fats. When the food is a processed sweet or snack food, you can assume that it contains trans fats. For individuals watching their fat intake, look for products with less saturated and trans fats, as well as a total fat content of 5 g or less per serving, as in our example. Most Nutrition Facts labels do not list the amount of monounsaturated and polyunsaturated fats, or "good" fats (it's optional to list these according to Health Canada regulations). But you can find out how much mono and poly are in the food by subtracting the saturated and trans fat from the total fat. The leftover amount, in our example .5 g., is "good" fat.

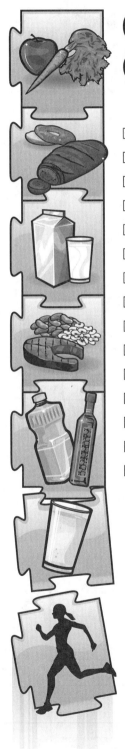

CANADA'S FOOD GUIDE SUGGESTS...

☑ Eat the recommended **amount** and **type** of food each day.

☑ Eat at least one dark green and one orange vegetable each day.

☑ Choose vegetables and fruit prepared with little or no added fat, sugar or salt.

☑ Have vegetables and fruit more often than juice.

☑ Make at least half of your grain products whole grain each day.

☑ Choose grain products that are lower in fat, sugar or salt.

☑ Drink skim, 1% or 2% milk each day.

☑ Select lower fat milk alternatives.

☑ Have meat alternatives such as beans, lentils and tofu often.

☑ Eat at least two Food Guide Servings of fish each week.

☑ Select lean meat and alternatives prepared with little or no added fat or salt.

☑ Include a small amount of unsaturated fat each day.

☑ Satisfy your thirst with water.

☑ Limit foods and beverages high in calories, fat, sugar or salt.

☑ Be active every day.

Source: Health Canada

Beyond the Basics:

Meal Planning for Healthy Eating,
Diabetes Prevention and Management

Meal Plan

TIME							
CARBOHYDRATES (grams / choices)							
GRAINS & STARCHES							
FRUITS							
MILK & ALTERNATIVES							
OTHER CHOICES							
VEGETABLES							
MEAT & ALTERNATIVES							
FATS							

Meal Plan

TIME							
CARBOHYDRATES (grams / choices)							
GRAINS & STARCHES							
FRUITS							
MILK & ALTERNATIVES							
OTHER CHOICES							
VEGETABLES							
MEAT & ALTERNATIVES							
FATS							

Source: Canadian Diabetes Association

WHAT IS ONE FOOD GUIDE SERVING? AN EXAMPLE

FOOD GROUP: MILK & ALTERNATIVES

The Milk & Alternatives group contains milk and yogurt choices with primarily heart health varieties. For the purpose of maintaining a 15g carbohydrate content, most portion sizes are 1 cup.

CHOOSE MORE OFTEN:

Food Item	Serving Size	Available CHO (g)	Protein (g)	Fat (g)	GI
Milk, buttermilk, cultured, low fat	1 cup (250mL)	12	8	2	n/a
Milk, canned, evaporated	½ cup (125mL)	13	9	10	n/a
Milk, canned, evaporated, fat free	½ cup (125mL)	13	8	Trace	n/a
Milk, whole, 3.25%	1 cup (250mL)	11	8	8	34
Milk, 2%	1 cup (250mL)	12	8	5	n/a
Milk, 1%	1 cup (250mL)	12	8	2	n/a
Milk, goat	1 cup (250mL)	11	9	10	n/a
Milk, skim	1 cup (250mL)	12	8	Trace	32
Milk, sheep	1 cup (250mL)	13	15	17	n/a
Milk, lactose reduced, 2%	1 cup (250mL)	15	8	5	n/a
Milk, powdered, skim	2 Tbsp (30mL)	15	8	Trace	n/a
Soy milk, fluid	1 cup (250mL)	15	9	5	44
Soy milk, fluid chocolate/strawberry	½ cup (125mL)	14	9	3	n/a
Soy milk, Fibre fortified	1 cup (250mL)	13	7	4	n/a
Soy yogurt, vanilla	⅓ cup (75mL)	15	5	2	n/a
Yogurt, flavoured, low fat, artificially sweetened	1 cup (250mL)	15	8	Trace	14
Yogurt, plain, low fat	¾ cup (175mL)	15	4	2	36
Yogurt, plain, whole milk	¾ cup (175mL)	13	10	4	n/a
Yogurt, drinkable	200mL	15	5	3	38
Yogurt, Mousse, regular	¼ cup (60mL)	15	5	3	n/a
Yogurt, Mousse, low fat	⅓ cup (75mL)	10	6	Trace	n/a
Yogurt Smoothie, regular	118mL	17	6	1	n/a
Yogurt Smoothie, low fat	236mL	16	11	0	n/a

CHO – Carbohydrates
GI – Glycemic Index

Beyond the Basics: Meal Planning for Healthy Eating, Diabetes Prevention and Management
December 20, 2005 – Version 2 – Milk & Alternatives

The
Glycemic Index

 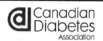

What is the Glycemic Index of food?

The Glycemic Index (GI) is a scale that ranks carbohydrate-rich foods by how much they raise blood glucose levels compared to a standard food. The standard food is glucose or white bread.

Why should I eat foods with a low Glycemic Index?

Eating foods with a low Glycemic Index may help you to:

- Control your blood glucose level
- Control your cholesterol level
- Control your appetite
- Lower your risk of getting heart disease
- Lower your risk of getting type 2 diabetes

Use these meal planning ideas to include the Glycemic Index as part of healthy eating.

- Enjoy vegetables, fruits and low-fat milk products with your meals. These are carbohydrate-rich foods that, in general, have low glycemic index.
- Plan your meals with foods in the **low and medium** Glycemic Index starch choices on the list that follows.
- Try foods such as barley, bulgar, couscous, or lentils, which have a low Glycemic Index.
- Consult a registered dietitian for help with choosing low GI foods, adapting recipes, and other ways to incorporate low GI foods in your meal plan.

If I eat foods with a low Glycemic Index can I eat as much as I want?

No. Using the Glycemic Index to choose foods is only one part of healthy eating.

Healthy eating also means:

- Eating at regular times
- Choosing a variety of foods from all food groups
- Limiting sugars and sweets
- Reducing the amount of fat you eat
- Including foods high in fibre
- Limiting salt, alcohol and caffeine

Remember that checking your blood glucose before and **2 hours after a meal** is the best way to know how your body handles the meal.

Printed September 2008   **Check out the Canadian Diabetes Association website, diabetes.ca, for more information.**

A lot of starchy foods have a high Glycemic Index (GI). Choose medium and low GI foods more often.

LOW GI (55 OR LESS) [*†] Choose most often ✓✓✓	MEDIUM GI (56-69) [*†] Choose more often ✓✓	HIGH GI (70 OR MORE) [*†] Choose less often ✓
BREADS: 100% stone ground whole wheat Heavy mixed grain Pumpernickel	**BREADS:** Whole wheat Rye Pita	**BREADS:** White bread Kaiser roll Bagel, white
CEREAL: All Bran™ Bran Buds with Psyllium™ Oat Bran™	**CEREAL:** Grapenuts™ Puffed wheat Oatmeal Quick oats	**CEREAL:** Bran flakes Corn flakes Rice Krispies™
GRAINS: Barley Bulgar Pasta/noodles Parboiled or converted rice	**GRAINS:** Basmati rice Brown rice Couscous	**GRAINS:** Short-grain rice

OTHER:
Sweet potato
Yam
Legumes
    Lentils
    Chickpeas
    Kidney beans
    Split peas
    Soy beans
    Baked beans
	OTHER:
	Potato, new/white
	Sweet corn
	Popcorn
	Stoned Wheat Thins™
	Ryvita™ (rye crisps)
	Black bean soup
	Green pea soup
		OTHER:
		Potato, baking (Russet)
		French fries
		Pretzels
		Rice cakes
		Soda crackers

One change I will make **now** is:

_____

_____

_____

_____

_____

_____

_____

_____

_____

_____

*expressed as a percentage of the value for glucose   † Canadian values where available

Adapted with permission from: Foster-Powell K, Holt SHA, Brand-Miller JC. International table of glycemic index and glycemic load values Am J Clin Nutr. 2002;76:5-76

111018 08-395 09/08 Q-2M

4 EAT WELL AND BE ACTIVE TODAY AND EVERY DAY

- *Limit foods and beverages high in calories, fat, sugar or salt.*
- *Be active every day.*

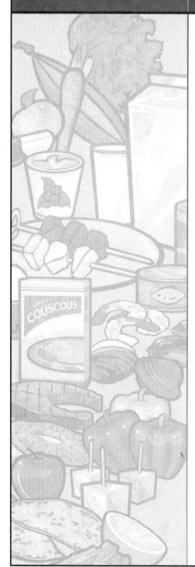

Both eating well and being active are essential to a healthy lifestyle.

Eat well

Follow Canada's Food Guide by eating the recommended amount and type of food each day. People should also limit foods and beverages high in calories, fat, sugar or salt (sodium) such as:

- cakes and pastries
- chocolate and candies
- cookies and granola bars
- ice cream and frozen desserts
- doughnuts and muffins
- french fries
- potato chips, nachos and other salty snacks
- alcohol
- fruit flavoured drinks
- soft drinks
- sports and energy drinks
- sweetened hot or cold drinks

Be active

Follow Canada's Physical Activity Guide recommendations to be active every day and inactive less often. Adults should build 30 to 60 minutes of moderate physical activity, such as walking briskly, into each day. Children and youth need at least 90 minutes of activity every day.

WHAT ARE THE BENEFITS OF EATING WELL AND BEING ACTIVE?

- Better overall health
- A healthy body weight
- More energy
- Lower risk of disease
- Feeling and looking better
- Stronger muscles and bones

Source: Health Canada

5 ADVICE FOR DIFFERENT AGES AND STAGES

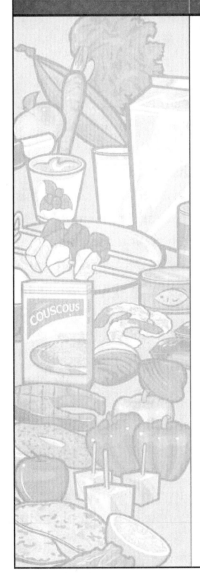

Eating Well with Canada's Food Guide is designed to help make sure most people get enough vitamins, minerals and other nutrients from the healthy eating pattern. Some groups of people, however, need more of certain nutrients or require specific guidance on selecting foods within or in addition to the eating pattern.

Advice for different ages and stages includes:

- Young children need small nutritious meals and snacks each day.

- For young children, nutritious foods that contain fat should not be restricted.

- Women who could become pregnant, as well as those who are pregnant or breastfeeding, need a daily multivitamin containing folic acid.

- Pregnant women need a multivitamin that contains iron.

- Pregnant and breastfeeding women need more calories.

- Men and women over the age of 50 need a daily vitamin D supplement.

Source: Health Canada

EATING TIPS FOR PEOPLE WITH SPECIFIC LONG-TERM CONDITIONS

Please remember that this formula for healthy eating is a general guideline that is applicable to almost everyone; however, each individual may have slightly different needs, depending on age, gender, body size, activity level, health, likes and dislikes, and even the availability or affordability of certain foods. The following are some specific recommendations for people with different long-term health problems.

Diabetes

Nutrition therapy is considered an integral part of diabetes management and treatment, according to the Clinical Practice Guidelines (CPG) of the Canadian Diabetes Association. Meeting your nutritional needs by following the guidelines can also help to control and reduce blood glucose levels when combined with other diabetes-related therapy and treatment. (Excerpts from this guide are found on pages 217-223 of this chapter).

You might find it helpful to visit a diabetes educator or a registered dietician. At this visit, you will learn how to choose carbohydrate foods with a low glycemic index more often than foods with a high glycemic index. Choosing these foods will help you maintain good blood glucose control. Recent research shows nutrition therapy to be an important part of diabetes management. You will find full details on following a healthy diet and balancing food intake with insulin, medications, activity and other diabetes-related therapies in Chapter 19, MANAGING DIABETES. This nutritional information is helpful for everyone to help make healthy decisions when choosing carbohydrate foods.

The Canadian Diabetes Association has a pamphlet, *Just the Basics*, which is full of tips for healthy eating, diabetes prevention, and diabetes management. When used combination with the *Eating Well with Canada's Food Guide*, most people with diabetes will discover they can plan enjoyable meals, while at the same time, help to control their blood glucose levels.

If you have diabetes and have not yet had the opportunity to meet with a registered dietitian, reading the section on Healthy Eating in Chapter 19 will help you with planning nutritious, well-balanced and well-spaced meals.

Circulatory problems, heart disease and high blood pressure, are complications that people with diabetes are at higher risk of developing. Making healthy food choices can help to prevent these complications. Controlling the amount and types of fat that you eat, and the amount of sodium in your food can also help.

Even a small weight loss such as 5% of your initial body weight can make a big difference to your blood glucose levels. By combining exercise and food choices to successfully manage your weight, you not only manage your target blood glucose, but you increase your feeling of well being. (Some tips for reducing fat and increasing fibre in your diet can be found in the boxes on page 226 and 227). Also read the section on Managing a Healthy Weight on page 228 of this chapter.

Heart Disease

For people with heart disease, it is very important to reduce the amount of fat and cholesterol in the foods you eat and to increase your fibre intake. This helps to prevent the narrowing and hardening of the arteries that can cause heart attacks. Reducing fat also helps to control your blood pressure and weight. In the same way, reducing your salt and sodium intake can help to prevent or control high blood pressure (hypertension). Try to limit the salt you add to your food to no more than 1 teaspoon per day. Use herbs and other spices for flavor. The food guide also lists some of the problem foods that are higher in fat, cholesterol, and sodium to help you make healthier choices. The tips mentioned on pages 226 and 227 also provide suggestions for ways to reduce fat and increase fiber in your eating plan. Basically, most of the fat you eat should come from "good" or unsaturated fats, and very little from "bad" saturated fats. Also, you should eat as little as possible of the foods prepared in or with partially hydrogenated or trans fatty acids, also referred to as trans fat.

Lung Disease

For people with lung disease, especially emphysema, it is sometimes necessary to increase the amount of protein you eat. This helps increase your energy, strength, and resistance. Also, people who have difficulty eating enough to maintain an adequate amount of nutrients may need to eat foods that contain more calories than normally recommended. The section on "Common Problems with Gaining Weight" (page 240) lists some suggestions for increasing the amount of nutrients and calories in your eating plan.

If you have specific concerns about your eating plan, consult with your doctor or a registered dietitian to help you identify which tips are appropriate for you, as well as to adjust some of these more general recommendations to meet your unique health needs. (The title "registered dietitian," "professional dietitian" and "dietitian" are protected by law—through provincial legislation—so that only qualified practitioners who have met education qualifications can use the title.) A dietitian is a health professional who has a Bachelor's degree

---

Tips for Reducing Fat in Your Eating Plan

- Eat more skinless poultry and fish, and less red meat with a moderate-size portion (75 g cooked, which is about the size of a deck of cards, or 125 mL [½ cup]).

- Choose leaner cuts of meat.

- Trim off the visible fat and remove the skin from poultry.

- Limit egg yolks to four a week, including eggs in prepared foods.

- Eat small portions of organ meats (liver, kidneys, brains) only occasionally.

- Broil, barbecue, or grill meats instead of frying them.

- Avoid deep-fried foods.

- Skim fat off stews and soups during cooking and refrigerate overnight so the fat is easy to remove the next day.

- Use low-fat or nonfat milk and dairy products (like sour cream, cottage cheese, yogurt, ice cream, and cream cheese).

- Use less butter, margarine, oils, gravy, sauces, spreads, and salad dressings in food preparation (no more than 3–4 teaspoons [15–20 mL] per day).

- For foods that don't need cooking at heats beyond 350 degrees C, use a good quality, non-stick pan with small amounts of cooking oil spray.

- As a cheaper alternative to purchased cooking sprays, simply fill a pump with any unsaturated oil.

Tips for Choosing Healthful Carbohydrates and Increasing Fiber in Your Eating Plan

- Build your meals around vegetables, whole-grain products, and fruits.

- Eat a variety of fruits and vegetables, raw or slightly cooked.

- Eat whole fruit rather than drinking fruit juice.

- Eat low-fat grain products such as whole-wheat breads, brown rice, and corn tortillas instead of white flour pastas, white flour tortillas, and white rice.

- Eat more foods made with oats, barley, and legumes (dried beans, peas, and lentils) at least a few times each week and as meat substitutes.

- Choose shredded wheat, All Bran™, or raisin bran for cold breakfast cereals.

- Eat higher-fibre crackers, such as whole-rye or multigrain crackers and whole-grain flat bread (breads made from unleavened dough and baked in flat, often round loaves.

- Snack on fruit or nonfat yogurt, not sweets, pastries, or ice cream.

- Choose foods with whole wheat or whole grain listed as the first ingredient. Choose breads with as few ingredients in the ingredient list as possible. According to the non-profit web site www.healthiestfoods.org, this is an indicator that the bread is less processed than those with longer ingredient lists.

- Add fibre gradually over a period of a few weeks and drink plenty of water to help move the fibre through your system.

specializing in foods and nutrition, as well as practical training in a hospital or community setting. Dietitians are members of a provincially regulated profession that has public protection as its mandate. As such, they are accountable for their conduct and the care they provide. Typically, dietitians working in hospitals or health care institutions use the term "dietitian," whereas those in community settings might use the term "nutritionist." The term "nutritionist" is not protected by law in all provinces, however, which means that people with varying levels of training and knowledge can call themselves nutritionists. You can contact your provincial regulatory body or check the Dietitians of Canada website (www.dietitians.ca) for a listing of registered dietitians in your area.)

MANAGING A HEALTHY WEIGHT[1]

Reaching and/or maintaining a healthy weight is important for everyone. Your weight can have a considerable impact on your disease symptoms and your ability to exercise or otherwise manage health problems. Therefore, finding a healthy weight and maintaining it are key parts of the self-management process. But what is a healthy weight?

For one thing, a healthy weight does not refer to an "ideal" weight. There is no such thing as an "ideal" weight for an individual. The tables of "ideal" weights are only general guidelines of weight ranges based on population statistics. These tables should not be used to determine a healthy weight. Also, being at a healthy weight does not mean being thin or "skinny" like the popular images portrayed in the media. These body shapes and low weights are unrealistic, if not unachievable or unsustainable, for most of us. Indeed, being too thin can contribute to health problems just as being too heavy can.

A healthy weight is one whereby you reduce your risk of developing health problems, or further complicating existing ones, and feel better both mentally and physically. It should be thought of in terms of a "healthy weight range" because nearly all of us will vary up and down by a kilogram or two, which is all right. Determining a healthy weight range depends on several factors, such as your age, your activity level, your body composition (i.e., how much of your weight is fat), your body fat distribution (i.e., where the fat is on your body), and whether or not you have weight-related medical problems such as high

---

[1] Portions of this chapter have been adapted from two publications: *Thinking About Losing Weight?* Northern California Regional Health Education Center, Kaiser Permanente Medical Care Program, 1990. *The Weight Kit.* Stanford Center for Research in Disease Prevention, Health Promotion Resource Center, Stanford University, 1990.

blood pressure or a family history of such problems. When you take these things into consideration, you may already be at a healthy weight and need only maintain it by eating well and staying active.

If you are not certain whether or not you are within a healthy weight range, you can find out by learning to calculate your Body Mass Index (BMI) and your waist circumference (WC). Your BMI is a measure of body weight based on weight and height, and is related to health. To determine your BMI, Health Canada's website (www.hc-sc.gc.ca/fn-an/nutrition/weights-poids/guide-ld-adult/qa-qr-pub_e.html) recommends using the following formula:

BMI = weight in kilograms divided by height in metres squared.

If your BMI calculates as....

Less than 18.5—this classifies you as being underweight and potentially at risk for health problems such as osteoporosis, undernutrition and eating disorders.

18.5 to 24.9—this classifies you at a healthy weight.

25 to 29.9—this classifies you as being overweight. However, if you are physically active and have a lot of muscle mass, the excess weight may be muscle, not body fat, and so may not be a problem.

30 and up—you are considered obese and it is very likely that you have a large amount of body fat. Extra body fat is associated with increased risk of diabetes, heart disease, high blood pressure, gallbladder disease, and some forms of cancer.

The BMI measurements or values may not be correct for all ethnic populations or for the elderly. Some studies recommend waist circumference (WC) as a better form of measurement for some individuals. Neither is a perfect indicator—a combination of BMI and WC is currently being used by both health and fitness professionals.

The WC is an indicator of waist circumference. Excess fat around the waist and upper body (an "apple" body shape-is associated with greater health risk than fat located more in the hip and thigh area (the "pear" shape).

According to Health Canada, a WC at or above 102 cm for men, and 88 cm for women, is associated with an increased risk of developing health problems such as diabetes, heart disease, and high blood pressure. Even if your BMI is in the "healthy weight" range, a high WC indicates some health risk.

If you are overweight, consider asking your doctor to refer you to a registered dietitian for help in determining a healthy weight range for you, given your condition and treatment needs.

The decision to change weight is a very personal one. To help you decide whether or not you are ready to make any changes, ask yourself the following questions:

Why Change My Weight?

The reasons for losing or gaining weight are different for each individual. The most obvious reason may be your physical health, but there may also be psychological or emotional reasons for wanting to change. Examine for yourself why you want to change.

For example, changing my weight will help me . . .

- Lessen my disease symptoms (e.g., pain, fatigue, shortness of breath) and control blood glucose

- Give me more energy to do the things I want to do

- Feel better about myself

- Change the way others perceive me

- Feel more in control of my disease and/or my life

If you have other reasons, jot them down here:

_____

_____

_____

_____

_____

_____

What Will I Have to Change?

Two ingredients for successful weight management are developing an active lifestyle and making changes in your eating patterns. Let's look closely at what each of these involves.

An active lifestyle implies doing some physical activity that burns calories and helps regulate appetite and metabolism, both important for weight management. Physical activity can also help you develop more strength and stamina, as well as move and breathe more easily. In other words, activity doesn't wear you down or out, but actually boosts your energy level. You will find much more information about exercise and tips for choosing activities that suit your needs and lifestyle in Chapters 6 through 9.

Making changes in your eating habits starts by making small, gradual changes in what you eat. This may mean changing the emphasis on or quantity of certain foods you eat. You will find tips for doing this at the beginning of the chapter.

Here's a quick tip to help you get started; it includes both ingredients for successful weight management, physical activity, and changes in your eating plan. It's called the "200 Plan."

The "200 Plan"

- Every day, eat 100 fewer calories and exercise to use up 100 more calories. This "200 Plan" will help you to take off up to 9 kg in a year.

- What's an easy way to eat 100 fewer calories a day? Cut out one slice of bread, or a medium-size cookie, or the amount of butter or margarine you put on a slice of toast, or half a candy bar.

- What's an easy way to use up 100 more calories a day? Add 20 to 30 minutes to your regular exercise routine, such as walking, bicycling, dancing, or gardening. Take the stairs more, and park farther away from the store.

While most of us are concerned with losing weight and keeping it off, some people with long-term health problems struggle to gain or maintain a healthy weight. If you experience a continual or extreme weight loss because your condition or treatment interferes with your appetite or depletes your body of valuable nutrients, you may need to work at gaining weight.

Things That Will Enable Me to Make the Desired Changes	Things That Will Make it Difficult for Me to Change
Example: I have the support of family and friends.	*Example:* The holidays are coming up and there are too many gatherings to prepare for.

Some common problems associated with making changes in your eating habits and/or weight management are discussed on page 231.

You can also find more information on healthy eating in the references listed at the end of this chapter. Particularly useful are Health Canada's Food Guide for Healthy Eating and the Dietitians of Canada website (www.dietitians.ca), which includes features for helping you track your food choices and activity level, as well as for healthy meal planning.

Am I Ready to Change for Good?

Success is important in weight management. Therefore, the next step is to evaluate whether or not you are ready to make these changes. If you are not ready, you may be setting yourself up for failure and those nasty weight "ups and downs." This is not only discouraging but unhealthy as well. For this reason it is helpful to plan ahead by considering the following types of questions:

- Is there someone or something that will make it easier for you to change?

- Are there problems or obstacles that will keep you from becoming more active or changing the way you eat?

- Will worries or concerns about family, friends, work, or other commitments affect your ability to carry out your plans successfully at this time?

Looking ahead at these factors can help you find ways to build support for desired changes, as well as minimize possible problems you may encounter along the way. Use the chart on page 232 to help you identify some of these factors.

After you have examined these things, you may find that now is not the right time to start anything. If it is not, set a date in the future for a time when you will reevaluate these changes. In the meantime, accept that this is the right decision for you at this time, and focus your attention on other goals.

If you decide that now is the right time, start by changing those things that feel most comfortable to you. You don't have to do it all right away. Remember, slow and steady wins the race.

To help get started, keep track of what you are currently doing. For example, write down your daily routine to identify where you might be able to add some exercise. Or keep a food diary for a week to see what, when, why, and how much you eat. This can help you identify how and where to make changes in your eating habits, as well as how to shop for and prepare meals. The diary may also help you look at the relationship between your eating patterns and emotions or other symptoms. The sample food–mood diary on page 235 may be useful. Next, choose only one or two things to change first. Allow yourself time to get used to these and then add more changes. The goal setting and action planning skills discussed in Chapter 2 will help with this.

COMMON PROBLEMS WITH EATING FOR HEALTH

"I enjoy eating out (or I hate to cook), so how do I know if I'm eating well?"
Whether it's because you don't have time, you hate to cook, or you just don't have the energy to go grocery shopping and prepare meals, eating out may suit your needs. This is not necessarily bad if you know which choices are healthy ones.
Here are tips on eating out:

- **Select restaurants that offer variety and flexibility in types of food and methods of preparation.** Feel free to ask what is in a dish and how it is prepared, especially if you are eating in a restaurant where the dishes are new or different from what you are used to.

- **Plan what type of food you will eat and how much.** (You can bring the leftovers home.)

- **Choose items low in fat, sodium, and sugar or ask if they can be prepared that way.** For example, appetizers might include steamed seafood or raw vegetables without fancy sauces or dips, or bread without butter. You may request salad with dressing on the side, or bring your own oil-free dressing. For an entree, you might try broiled, barbecued, baked, grilled, or steamed dishes. Choose fish or poultry over red meat. Avoid breaded, fried, sauteed, or creamy dishes. Choose dishes whose ingredients are listed. Instead of a whole dinner, consider ordering à la carte, an appetizer for your main dish, or lots of vegetables (without butter or sauces). For dessert, select fruit, nonfat yogurt, or sherbet. You might split an entree or a dessert with someone else.

Food–Mood Diary

Date	Time	What I Ate	Where I Ate	Mood/Feelings

- **Order first so that you aren't tempted to change your order after hearing what others have selected.**

- **If you want fast food,** choose salads with dressing on the side, baked potatoes instead of fries, juice or milk instead of soda, and frozen yogurt instead of ice cream or shakes. To help you navigate their menus, most fast-food restaurants now make information about the nutrition content of their foods readily available, either in-store or by going to the company website.

"I snack while I watch TV (or read)."

If you know this is a problem for you, plan ahead by preparing healthier snacks. For example, rather than eating "junk" food like chips and cookies, munch on fresh fruit, raw vegetables, or air-popped popcorn. Try designating specific areas at home and work as "eating areas" and limit your eating to those areas.

"I eat when I'm bored/depressed/feeling lonely, etc."

Many people find comfort in food. Some people eat when they don't have anything else to do or just to fill in time. Some eat when they're feeling down or bothered. Unfortunately, at these times, you often lose track of what and how much you eat. These are also the times when celery sticks, apples, or popcorn never seem to do the trick. Instead, you start out with a full bag of potato chips and, by the end of an hour, have only crumbs left. To help control these urges, try to:

- **Keep a food–mood diary.** Every day, list what, how much, and when you eat. Note how you are feeling when you have the urge to eat. Try to spot patterns so you can anticipate when you will want to eat without really being hungry. (The sample diary on page 235 can be used for this.)

- **Make a plan for when these situations arise.** If you catch yourself feeling bored, go for a short walk, work on a jigsaw puzzle, or otherwise occupy your mind and hands. This may be a time to practise a distraction technique.

"Healthy food doesn't taste the same as real food. When I eat, I want something with substance, like meat and potatoes! The healthy stuff just doesn't fill me up!"

Just because you are trying to make healthier food choices does not mean that you will never again eat meat and potatoes. It only means that you will make other choices sometimes, change some of the ways you prepare these foods, and change what you buy at the store. Some of these tips are discussed on pages 226 and 227, and additional information is available in the references at the end of this chapter. There are also many excellent books that offer tasty low-fat recipes, as well as Internet sites you can access for new recipe ideas.

"But I LOVE to cook!"

If you love to cook, you are in luck. This is your opportunity to take a new cooking class or to buy a new cookbook on healthy cooking. Again, experiment with different ways to modify your favourite recipes, making them lower in fat, sugar, and sodium.

"I'm living alone now, and I'm not used to cooking for one. I find myself overeating so that food isn't wasted."

This can be a problem, especially if you are not used to measuring ingredients. You may be overeating or eating a "second dinner" to fill time. Or maybe you are one of those people who will eat for as long as the food is in front of you. Whatever the reason, here are some ways to help you to deal with the extra food:

- **Don't put the serving dishes on the table.** Take as much as you feel you can comfortably eat and bring only your plate to the table.

- **As soon as you've finished eating, or even served up your portion, wrap up what you haven't eaten and put it in the refrigerator or freezer.** This way, you have leftovers for the next day or whenever you don't want to cook.

- **Invite friends over for dinner once in a while** so that you can share food and each other's company, or plan a potluck supper with neighbours, relatives, or members of your church, clubs, or other groups you belong to.

COMMON PROBLEMS WITH LOSING WEIGHT

"Gosh, I wish I could lose 2 kg in the next two weeks. I want to look good for...."

Sound familiar? Most everyone who has tried to lose weight wants to lose it quickly. This is a hard pattern to break because, although it may be possible to lose 1-2 kg in one or two weeks, it is not healthy, nor is the weight likely to stay off. Rapid weight loss is usually water loss, which can be dangerous, causing the body to become dehydrated. When this happens you may also experience other symptoms such as light-headedness, headaches, fatigue, and poor sleep. Rather than doing this to yourself, try a different approach—one employing realistic goal setting, action planning, and positive thinking and self-talk. (These are discussed in greater detail in Chapters 2 and 5, respectively.) Here are some approaches to sensible weight loss:

- **Set your goal to lose weight gradually,** just 1 kg a month.

- **Identify the specific steps you will take to lose this weight,** for example, increasing activities and/or changing what you eat.

- **Change your thinking** from "I really need to lose 1 kg right away" to "Losing this weight gradually will help me keep it off for good."

- **Be patient.** You didn't gain weight overnight, so you can't expect to lose it overnight.

"I can lose the first few kilograms relatively painlessly, but I just can't seem to lose those last couple of kilograms."

This can be frustrating and puzzling, especially when you have been eating healthy and staying active. However, it is quite common and usually means that your body has adapted to your new calorie intake and activity level. While your first impulse may be to cut your calorie intake even further, it probably won't help and could be unhealthy. Remember, you want to make changes you can live with.

Ask yourself how much of a difference ½ kg, one kg or even 1.5 kg will really make. If you are feeling good, chances are you don't need to lose more weight. It is not unhealthy to live with a couple of extra kilograms, if you are staying active and eating low-fat foods. You may already be at a healthy weight given your body size and shape. Also, you may be replacing fat with muscle, which weighs more. However, if you decide that these kilograms must go, try the following:

- **Modify your goal** so that you maintain your weight for a few weeks; try to lose ½ kg or so more gradually over the next few weeks.

- **Try adding to your physical activity exercise goals,** especially if the current activity you do has become easy. Increasing your activity level will help you to use more calories and maintain your muscle mass. Less weight will be stored in the form of fat. (Tips for safely increasing your exercise are found in Chapter 6.)

- Again, **be patient and allow your body time** to adjust to your new patterns.

"I always feel so deprived of the foods I love when I try to lose weight."

The key to reaching and maintaining a healthy weight is to make changes you can tolerate, even enjoy. This means they must suit your lifestyle and needs. Unfortunately, when thinking about losing weight, most of us tend to think of all the things we can't eat. Change this way of thinking now! There are probably as many (if not more) enjoyable foods you CAN eat than ones you should limit. Sometimes it is just a matter of learning to prepare foods differently, rather than eliminating them completely. If you like to cook, this is your opportunity to become creative, learning new recipes or finding ways to change old ones. There are many good cookbooks on the market today to help you make this process more enjoyable. Some of these tips were outlined on pages 217-223 of this chapter, and more can be found in the references listed at the end of the chapter.

"I eat too fast or I finish eating before everyone and find myself reaching for seconds."

Eating too fast happens for a couple of reasons. One may be that you are limiting yourself to only two or three meals a day, and not eating or drinking between meals. This can leave you so hungry at mealtime that you practically inhale your food. Another reason may be that you have not had a chance to slow down and relax before eating. Slowing down your eating can help you decrease the amount of food you eat. If you find you are too hungry, feeling stressed out, or in a hurry, try one or more of the following:

- **Try not to skip meals.** In this way you are less likely to overeat at the next meal.

- **Allow yourself to snack on healthy foods between meals.** In fact, plan your snacks for mid-morning and afternoon. Keep a banana, some raw vegetables, or a few crackers with you for those "snack attacks."

- **Eat more frequent, smaller meals.** This may also be easier on your digestive system, which won't be overwhelmed by a large meal eaten in a hurry.

- **Chew your food well.** Food is an enjoyable necessity! Chewing your food well also eases the burden on your digestive system.

- **Drink plenty of water!** Six to eight glasses of water per day is recommended. This helps you to eat less and helps prevent medication side effects, aids elimination, and keeps the kidneys functioning properly.

- **Try a relaxation method about a half hour before you eat.** Several methods are discussed in Chapter 5.

"I can't do it on my own."

Losing weight isn't easy, but it can be done. Sometimes you just need some outside support. For help, you can contact any of the following resources:

- **A registered dietitian** through your provincial regulatory body, or listed on the Dietitians of Canada website (www.dietitians.ca).

- **A support group** in your community where you can meet other people who are trying to lose weight or maintain a healthy weight. Many community and recreation centres offer these programmes.

- **A weight reduction course** offered by your local health department or hospital, the community school, or even your employer.

Another motivation for losing weight is remembering that losing some of those extra kilograms can help to relieve some of your symptoms, such as joint pain and shortness of breath, as well as to help control your blood glucose, cholesterol, and blood pressure. In these cases, losing is winning, and that can be your new positive thinking and self-talk to help you carry on when it starts to get difficult to stick with the changes you are making.

COMMON PROBLEMS WITH GAINING WEIGHT

"I don't know how to add kilograms."

Here are some ways to increase the amount of calories and/or nutrients you eat. Unfortunately, these may also add some fat to your eating plan. Check with your doctor or a registered dietitian to see which of the following tips are appropriate for you.

- Eat smaller meals more often during the day.

- Don't skip meals.

- Eat high-calorie foods first at each meal, saving the vegetables, fruits, and beverages for later.

- Snack on calorie-rich foods such as avocados, nuts, seeds, nut butter, or dried fruits.

- Drink high-calorie beverages such as shakes, malts, fruit nectars, fruit whips, and eggnogs.

- Use low-fat or whole milk to prepare creamed dishes with meat, fish, or poultry.

- Top salads, soups, and casseroles with nuts or seeds.

- Add milk or milk powder to sauces, gravies, cereals, soups, and casseroles.

- Use melted cheese on vegetables and other dishes.

- Add butter, margarine, oils, and creams to dishes (1–3 tablespoons [15–45 mL] per day).

"Food doesn't taste as good as before."

If you have had a tracheostomy, are receiving oxygen through a nasal cannula, or are taking certain medications, you may have noticed a decrease in your taste sensations. To compensate, you may have also noticed that you've been increasing the amount of salt you add to your foods. Be careful of this because a high sodium intake can cause water retention or "bloating," which can result in increased blood pressure. To avoid this, try enhancing the flavors of foods by:

- Experimenting with herbs, spices, lemon juice, and other seasonings. Start with just about ¼ teaspoon (5 mL) in a dish for four people.

- Modifying recipes to include a wide variety of ingredients to make the food look and taste more appealing.

- Chewing your food well. This will allow the food to remain in your mouth longer and provide more stimulation to your taste buds.

If the decline in taste is keeping you from eating enough and, therefore, getting essential nutrients, you may need to adjust the calorie content of the foods you can manage to eat. Tips for doing this are mentioned above.

"It takes so long to prepare meals. By the time I'm done, I'm too tired to eat."

If this is a problem for you, then it's time to develop a plan, because you need to eat to maintain your energy level. Here are some hints to help:

- Plan your meals for the week.

- Go to the grocery store and buy everything you will need.

- Break your food preparation into steps, resting in between.

- Cook enough for two, three, or even more servings, especially if it's something you really like.

- Freeze the extra portions in single-serving sizes. On the days when you are really tired, thaw and reheat one of these pre-cooked, frozen meals.

- Ask for help, especially for those big meals or at family gatherings.

"Sometimes eating causes discomfort." Or "I'm afraid I'll become short of breath while I'm eating." Or "I really have no appetite."

People who experience shortness of breath or who find it difficult and physically uncomfortable to eat meals tend to eat less. For some, eating a large meal causes indigestion, discomfort, or nausea. Indigestion, along with a full stomach, reduces the space your breathing muscles have to expand and contract. This can aggravate breathing problems. If this is a problem for you:

- Try eating four to six smaller meals a day, rather than the usual three larger meals. This reduces the amount of energy you need to chew and digest each meal.

- Avoid foods that produce gas or make you feel bloated. You can determine which foods affect you this way by trying different foods and observing the results. Often these foods include vegetables such as cabbage, broccoli, brussels sprouts, varieties of onions, beans, and fruits like raw apples, melons, and avocados, especially if eaten in large quantities.

- Eat slowly, taking small bites and chewing your food well. You should also pause occasionally during a meal. Eating quickly to avoid an episode of shortness of breath can actually bring one on. Slowing down and breathing evenly reduces the amount of air you swallow while eating.

- Practise a relaxation exercise about half an hour before mealtime, or take time out for a few deep breaths during the meal.

- Eat some easy fast food like yogurt or drink fruit nectar when you wake up in the middle of the night.

"I can't eat much in one sitting."

There is no real need to eat only three meals a day. In fact, for many it is recommended that four to six smaller meals be eaten. If you choose to do this, include "no fuss," high-calorie snacks like shakes, muffins and other baked products, and protein bars as part of these extra meals. If you still can't finish a whole meal, be sure to eat the portion of your meal that is highest in calories first. Save the vegetables, fruits, and beverages for last.

COMMON PROBLEMS WITH MAINTAINING WEIGHT

"I've been on a LOT of diets before and lost a lot of weight. But I've always gained it back, and then some. It's so frustrating, and I just don't understand WHY this happens!!!"

Many of us have probably experienced this problem, which occurs because the diet was short-term and calorie-restricted; it did not emphasize changes in eating habits. In fact, this is the problem with many "diets." They involve such drastic changes in both what we eat and the way we eat and they cannot be tolerated or sustained for long. Because your body does not know when more food will be available again, it reacts physiologically to this deprivation, slowing its metabolism to adapt to the lower number of calories consumed. Then, when you've had enough of the diet, or have lost the weight and returned to your old eating habits, you gain the weight back. Sometimes you even gain back more weight than you lost. Again, the body is responding physiologically, replenishing its stores, usually in the form of fat. This fat serves as a concentrated energy source to be called upon again when calories are restricted. This causes the weight to go up and down in cycles, which, as mentioned before, is unhealthy and very discouraging.

This situation is further complicated by feelings of deprivation, as you probably had to give up your favourite foods. Therefore, when you reach your goal weight, you begin to eat all of those foods again freely and most likely in larger quantities.

The key to maintaining a healthy weight is developing healthy eating habits that you enjoy and that fit into your lifestyle. We have already discussed many of these tips earlier in this chapter. Here are a few more:

- **Set a small weight-range goal that you consider to be healthy for you.** Weights fluctuate naturally. By setting a range, you will allow yourself some flexibility.

- **Monitor your activity level.** Once you have lost some weight, exercise three to five times a week to improve your chances of keeping the weight off. If possible, gradually increase your activity level.

"I do okay maintaining my weight for a short time. Then something happens beyond my control, and my concerns about what I eat become insignificant. Before I know it I've slipped back into my old eating habits."

If you had only a little slip, don't worry about it. Just continue as if nothing happened. If the slip is longer, try to evaluate why: Is there a situation or circumstance requiring a lot of attention now? If so, weight management may be taking a back seat for a while. This is okay. The sooner you realize this, the better; just try to set a date when you will start your weight management program again. You may even want to join a support group and stay with it for at least four to six months. If so, look for one that:

- Emphasizes good nutrition and the use of a wide variety of foods.

- Emphasizes changes in eating habits and patterns.

- Gives support in the form of ongoing meetings or long-term follow-up.

- Does not make miraculous claims or guarantees. (If it sounds too good to be true, then it probably is!)

- Does not rely on special meals or supplements.

Eating well does not mean that you can never eat certain foods. It means learning to eat a variety of foods in the right quantities to maintain your health and/or better manage your disease symptoms. This involves changing your eating patterns and emphasizing foods that are lower in fat, sugar, and sodium. These changes are also important for effective weight management. If you choose to make some of the changes suggested in this chapter, remember that you should not feel like you are punishing yourself, or that this is a life sentence to boring, bland food. As a self-manager, it's up to you to find the changes that are best for you. And if you experience setbacks, identify the problems and work at resolving them. Remember, if you really want to, you can do it!

Community Resources

Nutrition Information

Health Canada – Food and Nutrition: www.hc-sc.gc/fn-an/index_e.html

Eating Well With Canada's Food Guide: www.healthcanada.gc.ca/foodguide or publications@hc-sc.gc.ca. Telephone: 1-866-225-0709.

Dial-A-Dietitian

B.C.: 1-800-667-3438 or 604-732-9191 / www.dialadietitian.org/

Ontario: 1-877-510-5102

In all other provinces, use the Dieticians Canada website for a professional near you. www.dietitians.ca

Provincial and Territory Health Ministries

B.C. Ministry of Health: 1-800-465-4911 or 250-952-1742

Alberta Health and Wellness: 310-0000 toll free, then 780-427-7164

Saskatchewan Health: 1-800-667-7766

Manitoba Health: 1-800-392-1207

Ontario Ministry of Health and Long-Term Care: 1-800-267-8097 or 416-326-1234

Quebec Ministry of Health and Social Services: 418-643-5321

Newfoundland and Labrador Health and Community Services: 709-729-4984

North West Territories Health and Social Programs: 867-920-8877

Yukon Health and Social Services: 1-800-661-0408, local 3673; or 867-667-3673

Nunavut Health and Social Services: 867-975-5700

New Brunswick Health: 506-457-4800

Nova Scotia Department of Health: 1-800-387-6665 or 902-424-5818

Prince Edward Island Ministry of Health: 902-368-6130

(continued on next page)

Community Resources

Heart and Stroke Foundation of Canada: 1-888-HSF-INFO, www.heartandstroke.ca
Provincial Offices
B.C: 1-800-473-4636 or in Vancouver: 604-736-4404
Alberta, NWT and Nunavut: 403-264-5549
Saskatchewan North: 306-244-2124
Saskatchewan South: 780-451-4545
Manitoba: 204-949-2000
Ontario: 416-489-7111
Quebec: 1-800-567-1551 or 514-871-1551
Newfoundland and Labrador: 709-753-8521
Nova Scotia: 1-800-423-4432 or 902-423-7530
Prince Edward Island: 902-892-7441

Canadian Cancer Society: 416-961-7223, www.cancer.ca
BC and Yukon Division: 604-872-4400
Alberta and NWT Division: 1-800-661-2262 or 403-228-4487
Saskatchewan Division: 1-877-977-HOPE or 306-790-5822
Manitoba Division: 1-888-532-6982 or 204-774-7483
Ontario Division: 1-800-268-8874 or 416-488-5400
Quebec Division: 514-255-5151
Nunavut Division: 416-961-7223
Newfoundland and Labrador Division: 1-888-753-6520 or 709-753-6520
New Brunswick Division: 1-800-455-9090 or 506-634-6272
Nova Scotia Division: 1-800-639-0222 or 902-423-6183
Prince Edward Island Division: 1-866-566-4007 or 902-566-4007

Community Resources

National Cancer Information Service: 1-888-939-3333

B.C. Cancer Information Line: 1-888-939-3333 or 604-879-2323

Canadian Diabetes Association: 1-800-268-4656, www.diabetes.ca
B.C. Diabetes Information and Support Centre: 1-800-268-4656 or 604-732-4636
Northern Alberta and NWT Regional Leadership Centre: 1-800-563-0032 or 780-423-1232

Southern Alberta Regional Leadership Centre: 403-266-0620

Saskatchewan Diabetes Information and Support Centre: 1-800-782-0715

Saskatchewan North Regional Leadership Centre: 306-933-1238

Saskatchewan South Regional Leadership Centre: 306-584-8445

Manitoba and Nunavut Area Winnipeg Regional Leadership Centre):
         1-800-226-8464 or 204-925-3800

South East Ontario Regional Leadership Centre: 613-384-9374

Newfoundland and Labrador Regional Office: 709-754-0953

Nova Scotia Halifax or Sydney Diabetes Resource Centres): 1-800-326-7712 or
         902-453-4232

New Brunswick Regional Office: 1-800-884-4232 or 506-452-9009
         Prince Edward Island Regional Office: 902-894-3005

Canadian Diabetes Association: 1-800-268-4656, www.diabetes.ca
Diabetes Quebec: 1-800-361-3504 or 514-259-3422 or call Info Diabetes at
         1-800-361-3504 (ext. 233)-or 514-259-3422 (ext. 233)

Public Library

Local Health Library

Suggested Further Reading

General

Adams, Shelley. Whitewater Cooks. Nelson, B.C.: Whitecap Books, 2009.

Canadian Diabetes Association. *Beyond the Basics: Meal Planning for Healthy Eating, Diabetes Prevention and Management, 2007*. A series of binder inserts that can be ordered online at www.diabetes.ca/literature

Canadian Diabetes Association. *The Glycemic Index, 2007*. Handout and Binder Insert. Can be ordered at www.diabetes.ca/literature

Dietitians of Canada. *Simply Great Food: 250 Quick, Easy and Delicious Recipes.* Toronto: Robert Rose Inc., 2007.

Ferguson, Carol and McMillan, Murray. T*he New Canadian Basics Cookbook.* Toronto: Penguin Books Canada, 2005.

Josephson, Ramona. *HeartSmart Nutrition: Shopping on the Run.* Toronto: Douglas & McIntyre, 2003.

Lindsay, Anne. *The New Lighthearted Cookbook.* Toronto: Key Porter, 2005.

Olson, Anna and Olson, Michael. *Cook at Home.* Vancouver, Toronto, New York: Whitecap Books, 2005.

Stern, Bonnie. *The Best of HeartSmart Cooking*, Toronto: Random House Canada, 2006.

Where People Feast, An Indigenous Cookbook. Dolly Watts and Annie Watts. Vancouver: Arsenal Pulp Press, 2007.

http://www.diabetes.ca/section-about/nutritionindex.asp. The nutrition section of the Canadian Diabetes Association with up-to-date nutrition information specific to people with diabetes.

http://www.dietitians.ca. Website of the Dietitians of Canada with current nutrition information and easy-to-use interactive features, including a menu planner; targeting consumers; as well as information for educators and nutrition professionals.

http://www.hc-sc.gc.ca/fn-an/food-guide-aliment/index_e.html. Part of Health Canada's website, this section features a guided tour of Canada's Food Guide and an interactive tool (My Food Guide) for personalizing information in the food guide.

http://www.worldshealthiestfoods.org/. A non-profit, free consumer website featuring unbiased scientific information about foods that can promote health and energy. Includes recipes and tips of the week, as well as the latest research and breaking nutrition news.

Vegetarian Eating

Brooks Brown, Celia. *Entertaining Vegetarians.* Vancouver, Toronto, New York: Whitecap Books, 2005.

Jones, Bill. *Sublime Vegetarian.* Scarborough, Ont: Harper Collins Canada, 2003.

Jones, Bill. *Chef's Salad.* Vancouver, Toronto, New York: Whitecap Books, 2003.

Katzen, Mollie. *The New Enchanted Broccoli Forest.* Berkeley, CA: Ten-Speed Press, 2000.

Audrey Alsterberg, Wanda Urbanowicz, *Rebar Modern Food Cookbook.* Vancouver: Big Ideas Publishing, 2001.

Weight Control

Katzen, Mollie and Willet, Walter. *Eat, Drink and Weigh Less: A Flexible and Delicious Way to Shrink Your Waist Without Going Hungry.* Berkeley, CA: Ten-Speed Press, 2007.

Lindsay, Anne. Light Kitchen: *Easy and Delicious Meals for a Healthy Weight.* Mississauga, Ont.: John Wiley and Sons Canada, 2002.

Weight Watchers. *Make it in Minutes: Easy Recipes in 15, 20 and 30 Minutes.* Mississauga, Ont.: John Wiley and Sons Canada, 2001.

Podleski, Janet and Greta Podleski, *Eat, Shrink & Be Merry.* Waterloo, Ont.: Granet Publishing Inc., 2005.

MANAGING YOUR MEDICINES

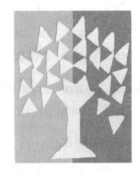

14

HAVING A CHRONIC ILLNESS USUALLY MEANS TAKING ONE OR MORE MEDICATIONS. Thus a very important management task is to understand your medications and to use them appropriately. This chapter will help you do just that.

A FEW GENERAL WORDS ABOUT MEDICATIONS

We see many advertisements for medications in magazines and through satellite television. If we have e-mail, we get daily plugs for medications online. These ads are aimed at convincing us that if we just use this pill or get this prescription, our symptoms will disappear. We will be cured. In Canada, direct advertising of prescription medication is not allowed, outside of trade media. Many of us, though, visit the U.S. regularly, and see the ads in newspapers, magazines and on television. At the same time, we have been taught to avoid excessive medications, and have all heard about or experienced some of the ill effects of medications. What confusion!

Your body is its own healer and, given time , most common symptoms and disorders will improve. The prescriptions filled by the body's internal pharmacy are frequently the safest and most effective treatment. So patience, careful self-observation, and monitoring are excellent therapeutic choices.

It is also true that medications can be a very important part of managing a chronic illness. These medications do not cure the disease. They generally have one or more of the following purposes:

1. **They relieve symptoms through their chemical actions.** For example, an inhaler delivers medications that help expand the bronchial tubes and make it easier to breathe, or a nitroglycerin tablet expands the blood vessels, allowing more blood to reach the heart, thus quieting angina.

2. **Other medications are aimed at preventing further problems.** For example, medications that thin the blood help prevent blood clots, which cause strokes and heart problems.

3. **A third type of medication helps to improve the disease or slow the disease process.** For example, nonsteroidal anti-inflammatory drugs can help arthritis by quieting the inflammatory process. Likewise, antihypertensive medications can lower blood pressure.

4. **Finally, there are medications to replace substances that the body is no longer producing adequately.** This is how insulin is used by someone who is diabetic.

In all cases, the purpose of medication is to lessen the consequences of disease or to slow its course. You may not be aware that the medications are doing anything. For example, if a drug is slowing the course of the disease, you may not feel anything, and this may lead you to believe that the drug isn't doing anything. It is important to continue taking your medications, even if you cannot see how they are helping. If this concerns you, ask your doctor.

We pay a price for having such powerful tools. Besides being helpful, all medications have undesirable side effects. Some are predictable and minor, and some are unexpected and life-threatening. From 5% to 10% of all hospital admissions are due to drug reactions.

EXPECT THE BEST

Any medication sets off two reactions in your body. The first is determined by the chemical nature of the medication. The second is triggered by your beliefs and expectations for the medication. Any time you take medications, your beliefs and confidence can change your body chemistry and your symptoms. This reaction is called the "placebo effect."

Thousands of scientific studies have now demonstrated the power of the placebo—the power of our mind. When people take a plain sugar pill, about one-third of them improve. Placebos relieve headaches, ulcers, asthma, arthritis, hay fever, colds, warts, constipation, angina, insomnia, and pain after surgery. Cholesterol levels, blood pressure, blood counts, gastric acidity, and even immune function have been altered by taking a placebo.

The placebo effect clearly demonstrates that our positive beliefs and expectations turn on our self-healing mechanisms. You can learn to take advantage of your powerful internal pharmacy. Every time you take a medication, you are swallowing your expectations and beliefs as well as the pill. So try to expect the best!

- **Examine the beliefs you have about the treatment.** If you tell yourself, "I'm not a pill taker," or, "Medications always give me bad side effects," how do you think your body is likely to respond? If you don't think the prescribed treatment is likely to help your symptoms or condition, your negative beliefs will undermine the therapeutic effect. You can counteract those negative images and change them to more positive ones.

- **Many people find it easier to associate healthful images with vitamins than with medications.** Each vitamin pill affirms that the person taking it is doing something positive to prevent disease and promote health. If you regard all medications as health-restoring and health-promoting, like vitamins, more powerful mental benefits might be realized.

- **Imagine how the medicine is helping you.** Develop a mental image of how the medication is helping your body. For example, if you are taking thyroid hormone replacement medication, tell yourself it is filling a missing link in your body's chemical chains, and helping to balance and regulate your metabolism. For some, forming a vivid mental image is helpful. An antibiotic, for example, might be seen as a strong broom sweeping germs out of the body. Don't worry if your image of what's happening chemically inside of you is not 100% physiologically correct. It's your belief in a clear, positive image that counts.

- **Keep in mind why you are taking the medication.** "Because my doctor told me to" is not nearly as effective as understanding how the medication is helping you. Suppose you are given chemotherapy for cancer. You've been told that it is highly toxic and that it's likely to cause your hair to fall out and nauseate you. How do you think you will feel? You could revise the expectation. Think of chemotherapy as a very powerful medication designed to kill rapidly producing cells like cancer cells. Other rapidly growing cells in your body may also be affected, such as the cells that line your hair follicles and your stomach. But fortunately, your healthy cells can recover and reproduce themselves, while the weak, poorly formed cancer cells are killed off. So if you have nausea or hair loss, remember that it's temporary, and that the primary effect of chemotherapy is to destroy the cancer cells.

WHAT IS A SIDE EFFECT?

A side effect is any effect other than the one you want. Usually, it is an undesirable effect. Some side effects are stomach problems, constipation or diarrhea, sleepiness, and dizziness. It is important to know the common side effects for the medications you take. Sometimes people say they can't or won't take a drug because of possible side effects. This is a reasonable response. However, before making a decision to stop taking a drug or refusing to take it, there are some questions you should ask yourself and your doctor.

Are the benefits from this medication more important than the side effects?
The use of chemotherapy for people with cancer is a good example. While these drugs have side effects, many people still choose the drugs because of their life-saving qualities. To take or not to take a drug is your decision. However, it should always be looked upon as "will I be better off with the drug despite its side effects?"

Are there some ways of avoiding the side effects or making them less severe?
Many times the way you take the drug—for example, with food or without food—can make a difference. Ask your doctor or pharmacist for advice on this question.

Are there other medications with the same benefits but fewer side effects?
Often there are several drugs that do the same thing but react differently in different people. Unfortunately, no one knows how a drug will react in you until you have taken it. Therefore, your doctor may have to try several medications before hitting on the one that is best for you. For this reason, when getting a new medication, it is always best to ask for a prescription for only a week or two, with a refill for a month. In this way, if the drug does not work out, you will not have had to pay for what you do not use.

TAKING MULTIPLE MEDICATIONS

It is not uncommon for patients with multiple problems to be taking multiple medications: a medication to lower blood pressure, anti-inflammatory drugs for arthritis, a pill for angina, a bronchodilator for asthma, antacids for heartburn, a tranquillizer for anxiety, plus a handful of over-the-counter remedies and herbs. Remember, the more medications you are taking, the greater the risk of adverse reactions. Fortunately, it is often possible to reduce the number of medications and the associated risks. It requires forging an effective partnership with your doctor. This involves participation in determining the need for the medication, selecting the medication, properly using the medication, and reporting back to your doctor the effect of the medication.

An individual's response to a particular medication varies depending on age, metabolism, activity level, and the waxing and waning of symptoms characteristic of most chronic diseases. Many medications are prescribed on an as-needed ("PRN") basis so that you need to know when to begin and end treatment and how much medication to take. You need to work out a plan with your doctor to suit your individual needs.

For most medications, your doctor depends on you to report what effect, if any, the drug has on your symptoms and what side effects you may be experiencing. Based on that critical information your medications may be continued, increased, discontinued, or otherwise changed. In a good doctor–patient partnership, there is a continuing flow of information. There are important things you need to let your doctor know and critical information you need to receive.

Unfortunately, this vital interchange is too often shortchanged. Studies indicate that fewer than 5% of patients receiving new prescriptions asked any questions of their physicians or pharmacists. Doctors tend to interpret patient silence as understanding and satisfaction with the information received. Mishaps often occur because patients do not receive adequate information about medications and don't understand how to take them or fail to follow instructions given to them. Safe, effective drug use depends on your understanding of the proper use, the risks, and the necessary precautions associated with each medication you take. You must ask questions.

Many patients are reluctant to ask their doctor questions, fearing to appear ignorant or to be challenging the doctor's authority. But asking questions is a necessary part of a healthy doctor–patient relationship.

The goal of treatment is to maximize the benefit and minimize the risks. This means taking the fewest medications, in the lowest effective doses, for the shortest period of time. Whether the medications you take are helpful or harmful often depends on how much you know about your medications and how well you communicate with your doctor.

WHAT YOU NEED TO TELL YOUR DOCTOR

Even if your doctor doesn't ask, there is certain vital information you should mention to her or him.

Are you taking any medications?

Report to your physician and dentist all the prescription and nonprescription medications you are taking, including birth control pills, vitamins, aspirin, antacids, laxatives, and herbal remedies. This is especially important if you are seeing more than one physician. Each one may not know what the others have prescribed. Knowing all the medications and herbs you are taking is essential to correct diagnosis and treatment. For example, if you have symptoms like nausea or diarrhea, sleeplessness or drowsiness, dizziness or memory loss, impotence or fatigue, they may be due to a drug side effect rather than a disease. It is critical for your doctor to know what medications you are taking to help avoid problems from drug interactions. It is helpful to carry an up-to-date list with you or at least know the names and dosages of all the medications you are taking. Saying that you are taking "the little green pills" usually doesn't help identify the medication. Sometimes it is beneficial to bring in all your medications (including over-the-counter medications) in a bag so that your doctor can review them, advising you on which to continue and which to stop or discard. You can also write a list of all the medications you are taking and their dosages. In this way your doctor doesn't have to spend valuable minutes looking through your medical chart.

Have you had allergic or unusual reactions to any medications?

Describe any symptoms or unusual reactions you have had to any medications taken in the past. Be specific: Which medication and exactly what type of reaction. A rash, fever, or wheezing that develops after taking a medication is often a true allergic reaction. If any of these develop, call your doctor at once. Nausea, ringing in the ears, light-headedness, agitation, and so on are likely to be side effects rather than true drug allergies.

Do you have any major chronic diseases or other medical conditions?

Many diseases can interfere with the action of a drug or increase the risk of using certain medications. Diseases involving the kidneys or liver are especially important to mention since these diseases can slow the metabolism of many drugs and increase toxic effects. Your doctor may also avoid certain medications if you now or in the past have had such diseases as hypertension, peptic ulcer disease, asthma, heart disease, diabetes, or prostate problems. Also be sure to let your doctor know if you are possibly pregnant or are breast-feeding since many drugs cannot be safely used in those situations.

What medications were tried in the past to treat your disease?

If you have a chronic disease, it is a good idea to keep your own written record of what medications were tried in the past to manage the condition and what the effects were. Knowing your past responses to various medications will help guide the doctor's recommendation of any new medications. However, just because a medication did not work successfully in the past does not necessarily mean that it can't be tried again. Diseases change and may become more responsive to treatment.

WHAT YOU NEED TO ASK YOUR DOCTOR (OR PHARMACIST)

Do I really need this medication?

Some physicians decide to prescribe medications not because they are really necessary, but because they think patients want and expect drugs. Physicians often feel pressure to do something for the patient, so they reach for the prescription pad. Don't pressure your physician for medications. Many new medications are heavily advertised and promoted by pharmaceutical companies before the full range of side-effects and hazards are known. Some medications, such as Vioxx, are found to be dangerous and are withdrawn from use after heavy marketing. Be cautious about requesting the newest medications. If your doctor doesn't prescribe a medication, consider that good news rather than a sign of rejection or disinterest. Ask about herbs and other nondrug alternatives. Many conditions can be treated in a variety of ways, and your physician can explain alternative choices. In some cases lifestyle changes such as exercise, diet, and stress management should be considered before making a choice. When any treatment is recommended, also ask what the likely consequences are if you postpone treatment. Sometimes the best medicine is none at all.

What is the name of the medication?

If a medication is prescribed, it is important that you know its name. Write down both the brand name and the generic (or chemical) name. If the medication you get from the pharmacy doesn't have the same name as the one your doctor prescribed, ask the pharmacist to explain the difference.

What is the medication supposed to do?

Your doctor should tell you why the medication is being prescribed and how it might be expected to help you. Is the medication intended to prolong your life, completely or partially relieve your symptoms, or improve your ability to function? For example, if you are given a diuretic for high blood pressure, the medication is given primarily to prevent later complications (i.e., stroke or heart disease) rather than to stop your headache. On the other hand, if you are given a pain reliever like ibuprofen (Motrin), the purpose is to help ease the headache. You should also know how soon you should expect results from the medication. Drugs that treat infections or inflammation may take several days to a week to show improvement, while antidepressant medications and some arthritis drugs typically take several weeks to begin working.

How and when do I take the medication, and for how long?

Understanding how much of the medication to take and how often to take it is critical to the safe, effective use of medications. Does "every six hours" mean "every six hours while awake"? Should the medication be taken before meals, with meals, or between meals? What should you do if you accidentally miss a dose? Should you skip it, take a double dose next time, or take it as soon as you remember? Should you continue taking the medication until the symptoms subside or until the medication is depleted?

The answers to such questions are very important. For example, if you are taking a non-steroidal anti-inflammatory drug for arthritis, you may feel better within a few days, but you should still take the medication as prescribed to maintain the anti-inflammatory effect. Or, if you abruptly stop taking steroid medications used for severe asthma as soon as the wheezing improves, you are likely to relapse. If you are using an inhaled medication for treatment of asthma, the way you use the inhaler critically determines how much of the medication actually gets into your lungs. Taking the medication properly is vital. Yet when patients are surveyed, nearly 40% report that they were not told by their physicians how to take the medication or how much to take. If you are not sure about your prescription, call your doctor.

What foods, drinks, other medications, or activities should I avoid while taking this medication?

The presence of food in the stomach may help protect the stomach from some medications while it may render other drugs ineffective. For example, milk products or antacids block the absorption of the antibiotic tetracycline, so this drug is best taken on an empty stomach. Some medications may make you more sensitive to the sun, putting you at increased risk for sunburn. Ask whether the medication prescribed will interfere with driving safely. Other drugs you may be taking, even over-the-counter drugs and alcohol, can either amplify or inhibit the effects of the prescribed medication. Taking aspirin along with an anticoagulant medication can result in enhanced blood thinning and possible bleeding. The more medications you are taking, the greater the chance of an undesirable drug interaction. So ask about possible drug-drug and drug-food interactions.

What are the most common side effects, and what should I do if they occur?

All medications have side effects. You need to know what symptoms to be on the look-out for and what action to take if they develop. Should you seek immediate medical care, discontinue the medication, or call your doctor? While the doctor cannot be expected to tell you every possible adverse reaction, the more common and important ones should be discussed. Unfortunately, a recent survey showed that 70% of patients starting a new medication did not recall being told by their physicians or pharmacists about precautions and possible side effects. So it may be up to you to ask.

Are there any tests necessary to monitor the use of this medication?

Most medications are monitored by the improvement or worsening of symptoms. However, some medications can disrupt body chemistry before any telltale symptoms develop. Sometimes these adverse reactions can be detected by laboratory tests such as blood counts or liver function tests. In addition, the levels of some medications in the blood need to be measured periodically to make sure you are getting the right amounts. Ask your doctor if the medication being prescribed has any of these special requirements.

Can an alternative or generic medication that is less expensive be prescribed?

Every drug has at least two names, a generic name and a brand name. The generic name is the name used to refer to the medication in the scientific literature. The brand name is the company's unique name for the drug. When a drug company develops a new drug in Canada, it is granted exclusive rights to produce that drug for 20 years. After this 20-year period has expired, other companies many market chemical equivalents of that drug. These generic medications are generally considered as safe and effective as the original brand-name drug, but often cost half as much. In some cases, your physician may have a good reason for preferring a particular brand. Even so, if cost is a concern, ask your doctor if there is a less expensive, but equally effective, medication available.

Is there any written information about the medication?

Realistically, your doctor may not have time to answer all of your questions in great detail. Even if your physician carefully answers the questions, it is difficult for anyone to remember all of this information.

Fortunately, there are many other valuable sources of information you can turn to: pharmacists, nurses, package inserts, pamphlets, and books. Several particularly useful books and online resources to consult are listed at the end of this chapter.

HOW TO READ THE PRESCRIPTION LABEL

There is a lot of information on every prescription label. The following picture will help you learn how to read the labels on your prescriptions.

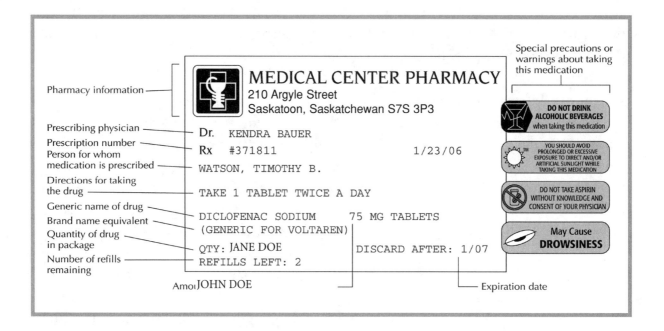

A SPECIAL WORD ABOUT PHARMACISTS

Pharmacists are an underutilized resource. They have gone to school for many years to learn about medications, how they act in your body, and how they interact with each other. Your pharmacist is an expert on medications. You can often call him or her on the phone. In addition, many hospitals, medical schools, and schools of pharmacy have medication information services where you can call and ask your questions. As a self-manager, don't forget pharmacists. They are important and helpful consultants.

REMEMBERING TO TAKE YOUR MEDICINE

No matter what medication is prescribed, it won't do you any good if you don't take it. Nearly half of all medicines are not taken regularly as prescribed. There are many reasons why this occurs: forgetfulness, lack of clear instructions, complicated dosing schedules, bothersome side effects, cost of the medications, and so on. Whatever the reason, if you are having trouble taking your medications as prescribed, discuss this with your doctor. Often, simple adjustments can make it easier. For example, if you are taking five different medications, sometimes one or more can be eliminated. If you are taking one medication three times a day and another four times a day, your doctor may be able to simplify the regimen, perhaps even prescribing medications that you need to take only once or twice a day. Understanding more about your medications, including how they can help you, may also help motivate you to take them regularly.

If you are having trouble taking your medications, ask yourself the following questions and discuss the answers with your doctor.

- Do you tend to be forgetful?

- Are you confused about the instructions for how and when to use the medications?

- Is the schedule for taking your medications too complicated?

- Do your medications have bothersome side effects?

- Is your medicine too expensive for you to afford?

- Do you feel your disease is not serious or bothersome enough to need regular medications? (Some diseases such as high blood pressure, high cholesterol, or early diabetes may not have any symptoms.)

- Do you feel that the treatment is unlikely to help?

- Are you denying that you have a disease that needs treatment?

- Have you had a bad experience with the medicine you are supposed to be taking, or another medication?

- Do you know someone who had a bad experience with the medication, and are you afraid that something similar will happen with you?

- Are you afraid of becoming addicted to the medication?

- Are you embarrassed about taking the medication, view it as a sign of weakness or failure, or fear you'll be judged negatively if people know about it?

If forgetting to take your medications is a major problem, then here are some suggestions:

- **Place the medication or a reminder next to your toothbrush, on the meal table, in your lunch box, or in some other place where you're likely to "stumble over" it.** (But be careful where you put the medication if children are around.) Or you might put a reminder note on the bathroom mirror, the refrigerator door, the coffee maker, the television, or some other conspicuous place. If you link taking the medication with some well-established habit like meal times or watching your favorite television program, you'll be more likely to remember.

- **Make a medication chart listing each medication you are taking and when you take it; or check off each medication on a calendar as you take it.** You might also buy a "medication organizer" at the drugstore. This container separates pills according to the time of day they should be taken. You can fill the organizer once a week so that all of your pills are ready to take at the proper time. A quick glance at the organizer lets you know if you have missed any doses and prevents double dosing.

- **Get a watch that can be set to beep at pill-taking time.** There are also "high-tech" medication containers available that beep at a pre-programmed time to remind you to take your medication.

- **Ask other family or household members to help remind you to take your medications.**

- **Don't let yourself run out of your medicines.** When you get a new prescription, mark on your calendar the date a week before your medications will run out. This will serve as a reminder to get your next refill. Don't wait until the last pill.

If you plan to travel, put a note on your luggage reminding you to pack your pills. Also, take along an extra prescription in your carry-on luggage in case you lose your pills or your luggage.

SELF-MEDICATION

In addition to medications prescribed by your doctor, you, like most people, may take non-prescription or over-the-counter (OTC) medications and herbs. In fact, within every two-week period nearly 70% of people will self-medicate with one or more drugs. Many OTC drugs are highly effective and may even be recommended by your doctor. But if you self-medicate, you should know what you are taking, why you are taking it, how it works, and how to use medications wisely.

In Canada, there are more than 15,000 distinct nonprescription drug products available, although some 500 products generate approximately 90% of sales. Overall, these products represent about 500 active ingredients. There are also in excess of 40,000 natural health products currently available in Canada. This amounts to approximately $3.6 billion spent on self-medication products. Increased research, testing, and regulation could bring more products to the Canadian market soon. Unfortunately, the majority of the public receives its education on OTC products and supplements solely from TV, radio, newspaper, and magazine advertising where many of their claims are either not true or subtly misleading.

You need to be aware of the barrage of drug advertising aimed at you. The implicit message of such advertising is that for every symptom, every ache and pain, every problem, there is a product solution. While many of the OTC products are effective, many are simply a waste of your money and a diversion of your attention from better ways of managing your illness.

If you self-medicate, here are some suggestions:

- **Always read drug labels and follow directions carefully.** The label must by law include names and quantities of the active ingredients, precautions, and adequate directions for safe use. Careful reading of the label, including review of the individual ingredients, may help prevent you from ingesting medications that have caused problems for you in the past. If you don't understand the information on the label, ask a pharmacist or doctor before buying it.

- **Do not exceed the recommended dosage or length of treatment unless discussed with your doctor.**

- **Use caution if you are taking other medications.** Over-the-counter and prescription drugs can interact, either canceling or exaggerating the effects of the medications. If you have questions about drug interactions, ask your doctor or pharmacist before mixing medicines.

- **Try to select medications with single active ingredients rather than the combination ("all-in-one") products.** In using a product with multiple ingredients, you are likely to be getting drugs for symptoms you don't even have, so why risk the side effects of medications you don't need? Single-ingredient products also allow you to adjust the dosage of each medication separately for optimal symptom relief with minimal side effects.

- **When choosing medications, learn the ingredient names and try to buy generic products.** Generics contain the same active ingredient as the brand-name product, usually at a lower cost.

- **Never take or give a drug from an unlabeled container or a container whose label you cannot read.** Keep your medications in their original labeled containers or transfer them to a labeled medication organizer or pill dispenser. Do not make the mistake of mixing different medications in the same bottle.

- **Do not take medications left over from a previous illness or that were prescribed for someone else, even if you have similar symptoms.** Always check out medications with your doctor.

- Pills can sometimes get stuck in the esophagus, the "feeding tube." To help prevent this, be sure to **drink at least a half glass of liquid with your pills and remain standing or sitting upright for a few minutes after swallowing.**

- **If you are pregnant or nursing, have a chronic disease, or are already taking multiple medications, consult your doctor before self-medicating.**

- **Store your medications in a safe place away from the reach of any children.** Poisoning from medications is a common and preventable problem. The bathroom medicine chest is not automatically a particularly secure or dry place to store medications. Consider a lockable tool chest or fishing box.

- Many medications have an expiration date of about two to three years. **Dispose of all expired medications.**

Medications can help or harm. What often makes the difference is the care you exercise and the partnership you develop with your doctor.

Suggested Further Reading

Canadian Pharmacists Association. *Patient Self-care.* 2002.

Silverman, Harold. *The Pill Book,* 11th ed. New York: Bantam Doubleday, 2004.

Useful Websites to Learn About Medications

www.pharmacists.ca

www.pharmacists.ca/patientguide

Saskatchewan Lung Association
www.sk.lung.ca
An excellent resource naming both generic and brand name medications. Click on lung disease, then respiratory drugs explained. This site is very detailed and up-to-date.

Canadian Arthritis Society
www.arhtritis.ca
Consumer's Guide to Arthritis Medications
Another superb resource, with both generic and brand name medications. Click on Programs and Resources, and then click on Printed Publications in the General section.

MAKING TREATMENT DECISIONS

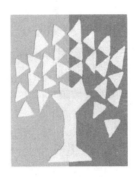

15

W E HEAR ABOUT NEW TREATMENTS, NEW DRUGS, NUTRITIONAL SUPPLEMENTS, AND ALTERNATIVE TREATMENTS ALL THE TIME. Hardly a week goes by without a new treatment of some kind being reported in the news. Drug companies and nutritional supplement companies run commercials during the television news and place large ads in newspapers and magazines. Our e-mail boxes are filled with promises of new treatment or cures from spammers. We are bombarded in the market or pharmacy with signs and packaging for over-the-counter alternative treatments.

What can we believe? How can we decide what might be worth a try?

An important part of managing our own care is being able to evaluate these claims so that we can make an informed decision about trying something new. Dr. William Feldman explains how Canadian patients and family members can find and evaluate the evidence necessary to make decisions about their health care in his new book *Take Control of Your Health: The Essential Roadmap to Making the Right Health Care Decisions.*There are some important questions that should be asked in the process of making a decision about any mainstream medical treatment, as well as complementary and alternative treatments.

1. Where did you learn about this?

Was it reported in a scientific journal, supermarket tabloid, print or TV ad, or a flyer you picked up somewhere? Did your doctor suggest it?

The source of the information is important. Results that are reported in a respected scientific journal are more believable than those you might see in the supermarket tabloid or on an advertising flyer. Results reported in scientific journals, such as the *Canadian Medical*

Association Journal, the *New England Journal of Medicine, Lancet,* or *Science,* are usually from research studies. These studies are carefully reviewed for scientific integrity by other scientists, who are very careful about what they approve for publication. Many alternative treatments and nutritional supplements, however, have not been studied scientifically, so they are not as well represented in the scientific literature as medical treatments are. If this is the case, you need to be extra careful and critical about analyzing what you read.

2. Were the people who got better like you?

In the past, many studies were done with easy-to-get people, so older studies were often done on college students, nurses, or white men. This has changed, but it is still important to find out if the people that got better were like you. Were they from the same age group? Did they have a similar lifestyle? Did they have the same health problems as you do? Were they the same sex and race? If the people aren't like you, the results may not be the same for you.

3. Could anything else have caused these positive changes?

We talked to a woman who had just returned from a two-week stay at a spa in the tropics, and reported that her arthritis improved dramatically because of the special diet and supplements she had received. But it's hard to attribute her improvement totally to the treatment, when the warm weather, relaxation, and pampering may have had a lot to do with her improvement!

It is important to look at everything that has changed since starting the treatment. It is common to take up a generally healthier lifestyle when starting a new treatment—could that be playing a part in the improvement? Have you started another medication or treatment at the same time? Has the weather improved? Are you under less stress than before you started the treatment? Can you think of anything else that could have affected your health?

4. Does treatment suggest stopping other medications or treatments?

Does it require that you stop taking another basic medication because of dangerous interactions? If the other medication is important, this will require a discussion with your health care provider before making a change.

5. Does treatment suggest not eating a well-balanced diet?

Does it eliminate any important nutrients or stress only a few nutrients that could be harmful to you? Maintaining a balanced diet is important for your overall health. Make sure that you're not sacrificing important vitamins or that you're getting them from another source if you change your eating habits. Also make sure that you're not putting excessive stress on your organs by concentrating on only a few nutrients.

6. Can I think of any possible dangers/harm?

Some treatments take a toll on your body. All treatments have side effects and possible risks. Make sure that you and your health care provider have a thorough discussion about what these may be. Only you can decide if the potential problems are worth the possible benefit, but you must have all the information in order to make that decision.

Many people think that if something is natural, it must be good for you. This may not be true. "Natural" isn't necessarily better just because it comes from a plant or animal. In the case of the powerful heart medication digitalis, which comes from the foxglove plant, it is "natural" but the dosage must be exact or it could be dangerous. Hemlock comes from a plant, but it is a deadly poison. Some treatments may be safe in small doses but dangerous in larger doses. Be careful.

There is no regulatory agency that is responsible for determining if what is listed on the label of a nutritional supplement is actually what's in the bottle, except in Germany. Supplements don't have the same safeguards as medications. Do some research about the company selling the product before you try it.

7. Can I afford it?

Do you have the money to give this treatment the time it needs to produce an improvement? Is your health strong enough to maintain this new regimen? Will you be able to handle it emotionally? Will this put a strain on your relationships at home and work?

8. Am I willing to go to the trouble/expense?

Do you have the necessary support in place?

If you ask yourself all of these questions and decide to try a new treatment, it is very important to inform your health care professional about it if this is something you are doing on your own. After all, you are partners, and you will need to keep him or her informed on your progress during the time you are taking the treatment.

The Internet can respond to new treatments very quickly, and is therefore a place to go for up-to-date information about these treatments. If you use the Internet as a source of information about medications or other treatments, it is important to be cautious. Not everything found on the Internet is correct, or even safe. Therefore, to find the more reliable sources look at the author or sponsor of the site and the URL address. Addresses ending in .edu, .org, and .gov are generally more objective and reliable; they originate from universities, nonprofit organizations, and governmental agencies. Some .com sites can also be good, but because they come from commercial or for-profit organizations, their information might be biased, as they may be trying to promote or sell their own products. One good source for information about questionable treatments is Quackwatch, a nonprofit corporation whose purpose is to combat health-related frauds, myths, fads, and fallacies (www.quackwatch.org). They also have other sites that are accessible from Quackwatch. Another website that exposes various hoaxes, especially in regard to chain e-mails, is Snopes (www.snopes.com/). For more information on finding resources on the Internet and elsewhere, see Chapter 3.

Suggested Further Reading

Dector, Michael. *Navigating Canada's Health Care*. Toronto: Penguin Canada, 2006.

Feldman, William. *Take Control of Your Health: The Essential Roadmap to Making the Right Health Care Decisions*. Toronto: Key Porter Books, 2007.

MANAGING CHRONIC LUNG DISEASE

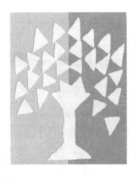

16

SHORTNESS OF BREATH, TIGHTNESS IN THE CHEST, WHEEZING, PERSISTENT COUGHING, AND THICK MUCUS. If you have chronic lung disease, these symptoms may be all too familiar. While there are many types of lung disease, the most common are asthma, chronic bronchitis, and emphysema. In each of these diseases there is an obstruction of the airflow in and out of the lungs. Chronic bronchitis and emphysema are often referred to as chronic obstructive pulmonary disease (COPD) or chronic obstructive lung disease (COLD). Although asthma, chronic bronchitis, and emphysema can be described separately, in truth, many patients have a mixture of these diseases and the treatment and self-management approaches often overlap.

UNDERSTANDING ASTHMA

Our understanding of asthma is changing. Until recently, the focus of attention was on *bronchospasm*, tightening of the muscles of the airways (bronchioles) (see Figure 16.1). In asthma, the airways are very sensitive and when exposed to irritants such as smoke, pollens, dusts, or cold air the muscle contracts, the membrane shrinks, and the airway narrows (see Figure 16.2). As the airway narrows, the flow of air is obstructed or blocked, producing an "asthma attack" or flare with shortness of breath, coughing, chest tightness, and wheezing (a high-pitched whistling sound as air pushes through narrowed airways). Treatment is aimed at relaxing the temporarily tightened airway muscles.

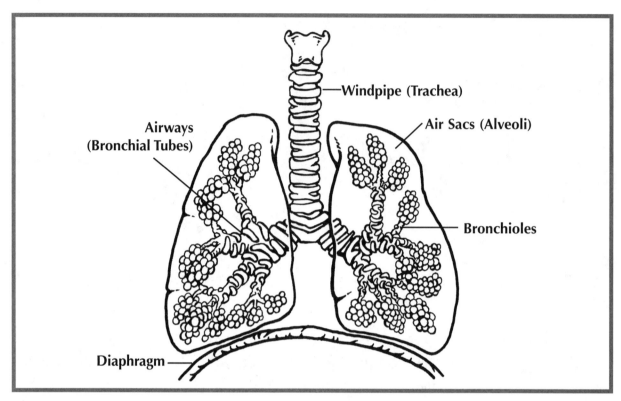

Figure 16.1 **Normal Lungs**

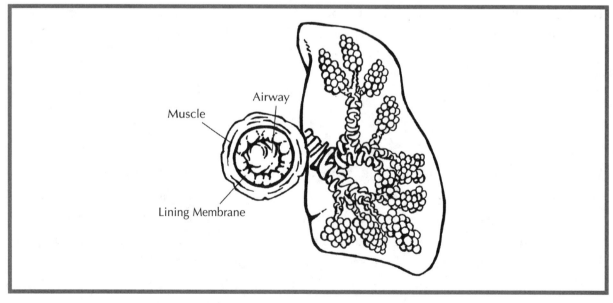

Figure 16.2 **The Bronchiole or Small Airway**

However, research has shown that tightening of the airways (bronchospasm) is not the whole picture in asthma. The irritants or triggers also cause *inflammation* of the membrane, with swelling of the airways and excessive mucus production. Chemicals are released from the surface lining of the airways that cause the inflamed airways to become even more sensitive to irritants. A vicious circle is set up, leading to more bronchospasm and more inflammation.

Therefore, it is often not enough to treat the acute flare of bronchospasm with bronchodilator medications that relax the muscles in the airways. Effective treatment involves *avoiding irritants* in the environment and the use of anti-inflammatory medications such as corticosteroids or cromolyn to reduce the swelling, inflammation, and excessive reactivity of the airways. Environmental control strategies and anti-inflammatory medications must be used even when you are not feeling any symptoms in order to help *prevent* acute attacks. Avoiding smoking and secondhand smoke is especially important for people with asthma.

Asthma varies dramatically from person to person. Symptoms may consist of mild wheezing or shortness of breath at night (asthma symptoms tend to be worse during sleep). The attacks may be mild and infrequent. The acute episodes may be severe and life-threatening. For most people, asthma can be effectively managed. But your involvement as an active partner in care is essential. You can learn to avoid triggers that make symptoms worse, monitor lung function, and take action to prevent symptoms and acute attacks. You can develop a plan with your doctor to recognize and effectively treat symptoms. You can also learn how to breathe effectively and exercise properly. While these measures cannot completely cure or reverse the disease, they can help you reduce symptoms and live a full, active life. By taking an active role in self-management, you should be able to participate fully in work and leisure activities, sleep through the night without coughing or wheezing, and avoid emergency visits to the doctor and hospitalizations for asthma.

UNDERSTANDING CHRONIC BRONCHITIS

Chronic bronchitis is a chronic *inflammation and thickening of the lining of the airways* (bronchial tubes). The inflammation narrows the opening of the airways and interferes with the flow of air. The inflammation also causes the glands that line the airways to produce excessive amounts of thick mucus, further obstructing breathing. The result is often a chronic cough that produces mucus (sputum) and shortness of breath. For diagnosis of chronic bronchitis, the cough must be present for at least three months each year during two consecutive years. At first, the sputum and cough tend to occur just in the winter months, but soon may occur year round. As the disease progresses, shortness of breath may become more severe.

Chronic bronchitis is primarily caused by smoking. Air pollutants, dusts, and toxic fumes can also contribute. These irritants keep the airways continually inflamed and swollen. The key to management is to stop smoking and avoid other irritants. If this is done, especially early in the disease, the condition can often be prevented from getting worse. If you have chronic bronchitis, you should get a *yearly influenza (flu) vaccine and a once-in-a-lifetime pneumococcal pneumonia vaccine.* If you have a respiratory condition or are above age 65 you may need a second vaccination. Also, avoid exposure to anyone with a cold or influenza; these infections can greatly aggravate the symptoms of bronchitis. Your doctor may also recommend the use of medications to *thin and liquefy mucus* as well as occasional treatment with *antibiotics* if symptoms get worse (increased cough with yellow-brown sputum, increased shortness of breath, and/or fever). Some of the medications that might be prescribed are discussed in more detail later in this chapter.

UNDERSTANDING EMPHYSEMA

In emphysema, the tiny air sacs *(alveoli)* at the very ends of the airways are damaged (see Figure 16.1). The air sacs lose their natural elasticity, become overstretched, and often break. The damaged air sacs are less able to transmit fresh oxygen into the bloodstream and to get rid of carbon dioxide wastes. The tiniest airways also narrow, lose their elasticity, and tend to collapse during exhalation. The stale air gets trapped in the air sacs and fresh air cannot be brought in.

A large amount of lung tissue can be destroyed before symptoms appear. This is because most of us have more lung capacity than we need. However, at a certain point, the lung capacity is diminished to the point where you begin to notice shortness of breath with exertion and physical activity. As the disease progresses, the shortness of breath becomes worse with less exertion and eventually may be present even at rest. A cough producing mucus may also occur.

Smoking is the major cause of emphysema. While cigarette smoking is the most common and dangerous cause, cigar and pipe smoking are also damaging. Even if you do not smoke, daily exposure to passive, or "secondhand," smoke is almost as bad. It is important that your home, car, and workplace be smoke-free. There is also a rare hereditary type of emphysema caused by the deficiency of an enzyme that normally protects the elastic tissue in the lungs.

Emphysema tends to get progressively worse, especially if smoking continues. The key to prevention and treatment is avoiding all smoking. Although quitting smoking sooner rather than later is better, quitting at any stage of the disease can help preserve remaining lung function. People with emphysema can learn a variety of self-management strategies, from proper breathing to efficient exercise, in order to maximize the ability to lead an active life. Medications and oxygen can sometimes be helpful in emphysema, as described below.

Asthma, chronic bronchitis, and emphysema most often overlap, so you may have one or more of them. While the treatment varies somewhat depending on the specific symptoms and disease, some of the principles and strategies of management are similar (see Table 16.1, "Chronic Lung Disease at a Glance"). In addition to the self-management strategies described throughout this book, let's take a closer look at some of the management approaches specific to chronic lung disease.

AVOIDING IRRITANTS AND TRIGGERS

The best way to manage chronic lung disease is to avoid the things that make it worse. Several types of irritants can trigger the symptoms of asthma and worsen the symptoms of other types of chronic lung disease. Fortunately, you can learn to eliminate or avoid many of the irritants and, when that isn't possible, at least gain control over others.

Smoking

Whether you smoke yourself or are around people who smoke, smoking irritates and damages the lungs. The hot smoke dries, inflames, and narrows the airways. The poisonous gases paralyze the cilia, the tiny hairlike sweepers in your airways that help clean out dirt and mucus. The carbon monoxide in cigarette smoke robs your blood of oxygen and makes you feel tired and short of breath. The irritation from smoking makes infections more likely and can irreversibly destroy the air sacs deep in the lungs. *Smoking is the principal cause of chronic bronchitis and emphysema and a major trigger of asthma.* The good news is that most of these harmful effects can be eliminated by quitting smoking and by avoiding secondhand smoke.

Table 16-1. **Chronic Lung Disease at a Glance**

	ASTHMA	CHRONIC BRONCHITIS	EMPHYSEMA
FEATURES			
Sensitivity to triggers	common	sometimes	no
Spasm of airways	common	sometimes	sometimes
Inflammation (*swelling*) of airways	common	common	rare
Excess mucus	sometimes	common	sometimes
Damaged air sacs	no	no	common
SYMPTOMS			
Cough	common	common	sometimes
Shortness of breath	sometimes	sometimes	common
Wheezing	common	sometimes	sometimes
Mucus	sometimes	sometimes	common
PROGNOSIS (OUTLOOK)			
	symptoms almost always controllable with treatment	treatment and removal of triggers may slow early disease	damage is permanent, but progression may be slowed
PREVENTION			
Avoid triggers	important, especially smoking	important, especially smoking	important, especially smoking
Immunizations	influenza (annual)	influenza (annual)	influenza (annual)
	pneumonia	pneumonia	pneumonia
TREATMENT			
Bronchodilators:			
Adrenaline-like	common	sometimes	sometimes
Theophylline	sometimes	sometimes	sometimes
Ipratropium	sometimes	common	common
Anti-inflammatory:			
Steroids	common	sometimes	sometimes
Cromolyn sodium	common	never	never
Expectorants/mucolytics	rare	sometimes	sometimes
Antibiotics	rare	common	sometimes
Oxygen	rare	sometimes	common
Breathing exercises	sometimes	common	common

Air Pollution

Dirt and fumes added to the air, whether from automobile exhaust, industrial wastes, household products, aerosol sprays, or wood smoke from fireplaces, can irritate sensitive airways. On particularly smoggy days, check your radio and TV for air pollution alerts and try to stay indoors as much as possible.

Cold Weather/Steam

For some people, very cold air can irritate the airways. If you can't avoid the cold air, try breathing through a cold-weather mask (available at most drugstores) or a scarf. For some people steam, such as from showers, can also be a trigger.

Allergens

An allergen is anything that triggers an allergic reaction. If you have asthma, an attack may be triggered by both outdoor and indoor allergens. Avoiding allergens completely can become a full-time job. Still, a few sensible measures significantly reduce exposure. When pollen and mold spore counts are high, an air-conditioned environment is best.

For some people, however, the major allergic triggers are found indoors in the form of house-dust mites, animal dander, and molds. Often pet dogs, cats, and birds have to be banished from the house or at least from bedrooms if a person reacts to pet allergens. Bathe dogs and cats weekly to reduce allergens. House-dust mites tend to live in mattresses, pillows, carpets, upholstered furniture, and clothing. A severely allergic person should cover the mattress and pillows with airtight covers after having them vacuumed, wash bedding weekly in hot water, avoid sleeping or lying on upholstered furniture, remove carpets from the bedroom, and, if possible, avoid dusting and vacuuming. Damp mopping is recommended rather than dusting or vacuuming, which can scatter allergens in the air. Also, change heating and air-conditioning filters each month. Avoid air cleaners that produce ozone; these can make asthma worse. It may take some time and repeated cleaning to rid the environment of harmful levels of pet, mite, or dust allergens.

Household products like perfumes, room deodorizers, fresh paint, and certain cleaning products can also trigger asthma symptoms in susceptible people. For some people, indoor air cleaners can be helpful in reducing allergens in the air. For some people with asthma, allergy testing can help identify specific allergic triggers, and "allergy shots" (immunotherapy) may help desensitize a person to certain allergens. Certain foods (e.g., peanuts, beans, nuts, eggs, shellfish, and milk products) and food additives (e.g., sulfites in wine and dried apricots) can also trigger asthma symptoms in some people.

Sometimes people with asthma or other respiratory conditions also have gastric reflux in which acid from the stomach can back up and irritate the esophagus and airways. This may or may not cause heartburn symptoms. The irritation of the airways may cause trouble breathing. Treatment of reflux includes keeping your head and chest elevated when sleeping; avoiding smoking, caffeine, and foods that irritate the stomach; and, when necessary, taking antacids and acid-blocking medications.

Medications

Certain medications can cause wheezing, shortness of breath, and coughing in some people. These include anti-inflammatory medications like aspirin, ibuprofen, and naproxen, as well as beta-blockers (such as propranolol) used to treat high blood pressure, heart disease, and migraine headaches.

Infections

Colds, influenza, sinus infections, and infections of the airways and lungs can make breathing more difficult for those with chronic lung problems. While you can't prevent all infections, you can reduce your risks. Make sure to get an influenza immunization (flu shot) each year in the early fall and a one-time vaccine for pneumococcal pneumonia. Try to avoid people with colds. To cut down on the spread of viruses, wash your hands frequently and don't rub your nose and eyes. Also, discuss with your doctor how to adjust your medications if you get an infection. Early treatment can often prevent serious illness and hospitalization.

Exercise

Exercise can be a problem or a benefit for people with chronic lung disease. On one hand, physical activity can improve strength and enhance the capacity of the heart and lungs. On the other hand, vigorous physical exercise can trigger asthma symptoms and cause uncomfortable shortness of breath in people with chronic lung disease. There are ways to choose exercise routines (see Chapters 6 through 9) and adjust your medications before exercising to prevent exercise-induced asthma. If being able to exercise comfortably is a problem, discuss this with your physician.

Emotional Stress

Emotional stress does not cause chronic lung disease. However, it can make the symptoms worse by causing the airways to tighten and breathing to become rapid and shallow. Many of the breathing and relaxation exercises in this book can help prevent the worsening of symptoms. Also, learning how to manage your disease helps you feel more in control and less stressed in general.

The effect of triggers can be additive. For example, your cat alone may not trigger an acute attack, but if you add a cold, cleaning chemicals, or stress, then an attack may occur.

A Note About Medications

Some medications change rapidly, others remain the same for many years. This next section explains common medications currently in use. The meds you are using may differ. An excellent resource for all drugs commonly in use in Canada for lung disease is the Saskatchewan Lung Association website (www.sk.lung.ca). The site has current information about both generic and brand name medications and side effects of these medications.

MONITORING LUNG DISEASE

Lung disease does not stay the same all the time. Sometimes it will be in better control than at other times. By monitoring your symptoms, you can often predict when a flare-up is coming and do something about it before it gets worse.

There are two ways to monitor lung disease. It is important to use at least one of them. For best results, use both symptom monitoring (for asthma, COPD, bronchitis, and emphysema) and peak flow monitoring (for asthma).

1. Symptom Monitoring (for Asthma, COPD, Bronchitis, Emphysema)

This method requires that you pay attention to symptoms and how you are feeling. You can tell that a flare-up is coming when:

- Symptoms (coughing, wheezing, shortness of breath, increased or thickened sputum, new fever, increased fatigue) occur more often than usual, or there are a greater number of symptoms than usual;

- More puffs than usual are needed of quick-relief medicine, or the medicine is required more often that two times a week (other than for physical activity);

- Symptoms are causing you to wake up at night more frequently.

If you are having such symptoms, discuss them with your doctor or health professional. Unfortunately, symptoms are not always good indicators of the severity of the disease, response to treatment, or future problems.

2. Peak Flow Monitoring (for Asthma)

This method uses a tool called a peak flow meter to measure if the breathing tubes are opened enough for normal breathing. Peak flow measurements can let you know when a flare-up is starting (even before symptoms increase) and can help you to figure out how bad the flare-up is.

If you have moderate or severe asthma, the peak flow meter can become a best friend. It can be a very helpful tool by alerting you to problems before they become severe. It can help you and your doctor know when medications need to be increased and when they can be safely tapered. It can help you distinguish between worsening asthma and breathlessness caused by anxiety or hyperventilation. Most of all, it can help you manage your asthma better.

- When the peak flow reading is closer to the personal best (see below), the breathing tubes are more open. The asthma is in better control.

- When the peak flow reading is farther away from the personal best, the breathing tubes are more closed than they should be. Even if you feel okay, a lower peak flow reading can be a sign that a flare-up is starting and you need to take action and adjust your medications (see Action Plan on pages 281–282).

Note: Different peak flow meters may give different readings, so always use the same peak flow meter.

How To Use A Peak Flow Meter

1. Put the indicator at the bottom of the scale.

2. Stand up straight.

3. Breathe in as much air as your lungs will hold.

4. Place the mouthpiece of the flow meter in your mouth and close your lips around the mouthpiece.
   - Be sure the mouthpiece is on top of your tongue.
   - Be sure no holes are covered by your hands or fingers.

5. Blow out as *hard and fast* as you can into the meter.

6. Write down the peak flow reading.

7. Repeat these steps three times. The highest of the three readings is your peak flow reading. Do not average the readings.

These are general instructions. Please follow the specific instructions that come with your meter and have your doctor, nurse, or respiratory therapist observe your technique to get accurate results.

Figuring Out the "Personal Best" Peak Flow

At a time when you are feeling well, measure and write down the peak flow two times a day for one to two weeks. The "personal best" peak flow reading is the highest peak flow reading you get at least three separate times. After you figure out your "personal best" peak flow, write it down.

When To Measure the Peak Flow

- After you have figured out the "personal best" peak flow, the peak flow should ideally be checked every morning before you take the asthma medicine or at least twice a week.

- If you are having asthma symptoms (or if you have a cold or the flu), it's important to check the peak flow at least twice a day.

Using An Asthma Diary

You can keep track of symptoms and peak flow measurements by writing them in an asthma diary. (Your medical professional can give you one, or you can make your own.) Keeping an asthma diary can help you figure out:

- What triggers the asthma

- Whether the medicines are working

- When flare-ups are starting

Asthma Self-Management Plan

Work out a plan with your doctor about what specific actions you should take based on your peak flow measurements (see sample Asthma Self-Management Plan). For example, if your peak flow reading drops to 50–70% of your personal best or predicted measurements, your doctor may instruct you to increase your inhaled bronchodilator medications or perhaps start a steroid medication. You'll need to work out an individual plan of action with your doctor. If you wait until your symptoms get worse, they will be more difficult to treat. Early action and adjustment of your medications can make a critical difference.

Asthma Self-Management Plan

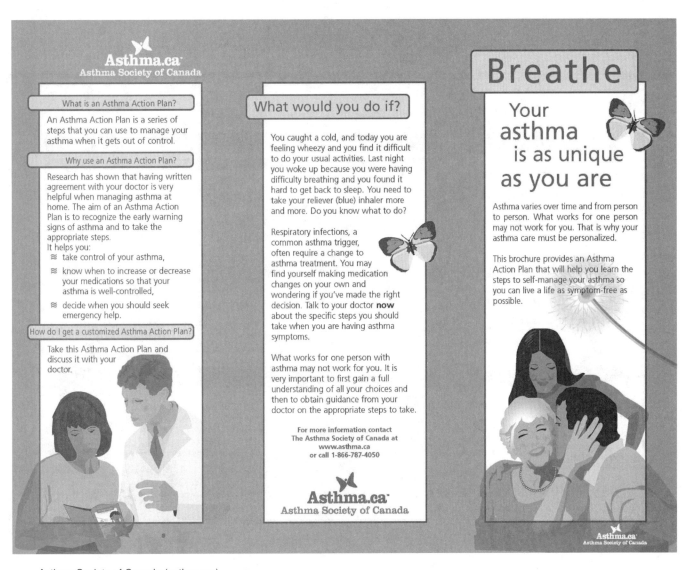

Asthma Society of Canada (asthma.ca)

Asthma Self-Management Plan

Asthma Action Plan (Sample)

Name: _____

Doctor's Name: _____

Date: _____

Hospital/Emergency Room Phone Number: _____

Doctor's Phone Number: _____

This Action Plan is a guide only. Always see a doctor if you are unsure what to do.

Green Zone – I have symptom-free asthma

I have no symptoms:
- I have no cough, wheeze, chest tightness or shortness of breath
- I do not cough or wheeze when I exercise or sleep
- I can do all my usual activities
- I do not need to take days off work

To remain symptom-free, I need to take these controller medications every day

Medication	How much to take	When to take it

Yellow Zone – I have asthma symptoms

- I cough, wheeze, have chest tightness or shortness of breath during the day, when I exercise, or sleep
- I feel like I am getting a cold or the flu
- I need to use my reliever inhaler more than three times a week for my asthma symptom

I need to either increase my controller medication, or add on a different controller

First ■ Take _____ 2 puffs, every _____ hours, as needed.
(Reliever)

Second ■ Increase _____ to _____ day, for _____ days, or until you are back in the green zone.
(Controller)
If no improvement in _____ hours, call or visit your Doctor.

Red Zone – I am in danger and need help

Any of the following:
- I have been in the Yellow Zone for 24 hours
- My asthma symptoms are getting worse
- My reliever does not seem to be helping
- I can not do any type of activity
- I am having trouble walking or talking
- I feel faint or dizzy
- I have blue lips or fingernails
- I am frightened
- This attack came on suddenly

Go directly to the nearest Emergency Room of your local hospital

First This is an emergency. Dial 911.

Second While waiting for the ambulance, take

■ 2 puffs of _____ every 10 minutes.
(Reliever inhaler)

Asthma Society of Canada (asthma.ca)

Medications

Effective management of chronic lung disease often involves a combination of medications.* Bronchodilator medications are designed to relax the muscles surrounding the airways and open the airways wider. Most inhaled bronchodilators can be used frequently and work within minutes to relieve the wheezing and shortness of breath. The exception is salmeterol (Serevent)), which should be used no more often than every 12 hours. Anti-inflammatory medications may also be prescribed to reduce the inflammation, swelling, and reactivity of the airways. For those with chronic bronchitis or emphysema, medications to loosen mucus (mucolytics and expectorants) as well as antibiotics may be used.

Some of the medications may be used to relieve symptoms such as wheezing, while others may be used to prevent symptoms. Some medications may be used to both treat and prevent. When the medications are being used to prevent symptoms, they must be taken regularly, *even when symptoms are not present.* Too often people stop their medications because they feel better. Discuss with your doctor which medications to continue and which may be stopped as symptoms improve.

Some people worry that they will become addicted to the medications or that they may become "immune" and no longer respond to the medication. *None of the medications used to treat lung disease are addictive. Nor do patients become "immune" to the medications.* If your medications are not working well to control your symptoms, discuss this with your doctor so that adjustments can be made.

Bronchodilator Medications

Adrenaline-like Medications (Beta-Adrenergic Agonists)

Examples: albuterol (Proventil, Ventolin), pirbuterol (Maxair), metaproterenol (Alupent, Metaprel), terbutaline (Brethine, Bricanyl). Salmeterol (Serevent) and formaterol (Foradil) should not be used more frequently than every 12 hours and should always be taken along with an inhaled corticosteroid. Advair (fluticasone/salmeterol) is a combination of salmeterol (Serevent) and an inhaled corticosteroid, fluticasone (Flovent).

How They Work: These medications are similar to adrenaline (epinephrine), a substance produced in the body. They stimulate tiny nerve receptors in the smooth muscles that surround the airways and cause the muscles to relax, rapidly reversing the bron-

---

* Because research about medications is changing rapidly, we suggest that you consult your physician, pharmacist, and/or a recent drug reference book for the latest information.

chospasm, opening the airways, and making breathing easier. These medications are most often inhaled, but some can also be taken orally (pills or liquids). In the emergency room or hospital, they may be given by injection.

Possible Side Effects: Shakiness, tremor, nervousness, restlessness, irregular or increased heart rate, insomnia, nausea, headache. The side effects tend to be less with inhaled medications than with the oral form of the medications.

Comments: The inhaled form takes only a minute or two to begin working while the oral form may require more than 30 minutes to start relieving symptoms (see "How To Use An Inhaler" on page 289). These medications may be used regularly to help prevent asthma symptoms or on an "as needed" basis to treat suddenly worsening symptoms. It is usually easier and takes less medication to prevent symptoms or to stop an episode in its early phase than later. Always carry an inhaled bronchodilator with you so that it is available at the first sign of increasing symptoms. Inhaled bronchodilators can also be used 5 to 15 minutes before exercising by people who tend to develop wheezing during or after exercise. While the bronchodilator medications can help quickly relieve the muscle tightness and associated narrowing of the airways, they do not treat the underlying inflammation. Therefore, if you are having to use the inhaled brochodilator often (twice a week or more), discuss this with your doctor. You may need an additional anti-inflammatory medication.

Theophylline

Example: aminophylline (Slophyllin, Somophyllin, Slobid, Theo-Dur, Resbid, Theolair-SR, etc.)

How It Works: This medication relaxes the muscles surrounding the airways to reduce wheezing and shortness of breath. It can be used to treat an asthma attack or on a regular basis to prevent airway constriction. The medication can be given intravenously (I.V.) in the hospital or taken orally as a pill or liquid. The oral forms of the medication take 45 minutes or more to begin working.

Possible Side Effects: Stomach upset (heartburn and nausea), diarrhea, irritability, headache, dizziness, shakiness, insomnia, nervousness, frequent urination, difficulty urinating (especially in men with prostate gland enlargement), rapid or irregular heartbeat, and, rarely, seizures. Taking the medication with meals can help reduce the stomach irritation.

Comments: Monitoring theophylline is often important. Your doctor may order blood tests to measure the levels of theophylline in your blood. If it is too low, it may not be effective. If it is too high, it may be toxic. The usual therapeutic range is 5–20 mcg/mL. Theophylline is prescribed somewhat less frequently today because of the more widespread use of the beta-adrenergic bronchodilators and corticosteroid medications. Theophylline may be used in combination with these other medications. The long-acting forms of theophylline are convenient (taken only twice a day) and can be useful in controlling nighttime wheezing in some people.

Ipratropium Bromide

Example: Atrovent

How It Works: This newer medication blocks constriction of the airways and inhibits mucus secretion. It is used more commonly to treat emphysema and chronic bronchitis than to treat asthma. It is available in inhaled form.

Possible Side Effects: Dry mouth and throat, cough, headache, nausea, and blurred vision.

Comments: This medication, unlike the adrenaline-like bronchodilators described above that work within minutes, takes longer to open the airways and needs to be used regularly to be maximally effective.

Anti-Inflammatory Medications (Symptom "Preventers/Controllers")

Cromolyn Sodium

Example: Intal

How It Works: This inhaled medication prevents asthma attacks by inhibiting the release of chemicals in the airways that cause inflammation, allergic reactions, and narrowing of the airways. Since it has an anti-inflammatory effect and is used to prevent asthma attacks, it should be used regularly, not just when symptoms worsen. It can also be used to prevent symptoms that occur from exercise or allergens (such as pets or pollens), if it is used 5 to 60 minutes before contact.

Possible Side Effects: Cough

Comments: It is difficult to predict which people will benefit from cromolyn. You may need to use the medication for a full 4 to 6 weeks before you know how well it will work for you. If you are taking an inhaled bronchodilator as well as inhaled cromolyn, use the bronchodilator first and wait 5 minutes before using the cromolyn. This increases the amount of cromolyn reaching the smaller airways.

Inhaled Corticosteroids

Examples: beclomethasone (QVAR, Vanceril), triamcinolone (Azmacort), flunisolide (Aerobid), fluticasone propionate (Flovent)

How They Work: These medications gradually decrease inflammation, swelling, and spasm of the airways and prevent overreaction of airways to asthma triggers like allergens. You may have to take the inhaled steroid medication for 1 to 4 weeks to see its full benefit. The inhaled steroids are now being recommended for use more often in patients with recurrent or moderately severe symptoms. Since inhaled steroids are not rapid acting, they are not helpful in the immediate treatment of a severe asthma attack.

Possible Side Effects: Coughing, hoarseness, and yeast (candida) infections in the mouth. The risk of irritation and infection can be greatly reduced by using a spacer or holding chamber (see page 279) and by rinsing excess medication out of your mouth after inhaling (we call this "swish and spit"). Because only small amounts of inhaled steroids reach the bloodstream, they tend to have fewer and less serious side effects than does long-term use of oral steroids (see below). (Note: The corticosteroid medications used to treat asthma are completely different from the anabolic steroids sometimes taken illegally by athletes.)

Comments: If you are taking an inhaled bronchodilator as well as an inhaled steroid, use the bronchodilator first and wait 5 minutes before using the inhaled steroid medication. This increases the amount of steroid medication reaching the smaller airways.

Systemic Corticosteroids ("Burst" Medicines)

Examples: prednisone, dexamethasone (Decadron), methylprednisolone (Medrol), triamcinolone (Aristocort)

How They Work: The corticosteroids or steroid medications work gradually to both prevent and reduce inflammation, swelling and spasm of the airways, and overreaction of the airways to asthma triggers like allergens. They can be taken orally or given intravenously (I.V.). It usually takes several hours for the steroid medications to begin reducing airway inflammation. They are often prescribed as a "burst" medicine during a severe asthma attack.

Possible Side Effects: With short-term treatment (less than 2 weeks), there appear to be no serious long-term effects, but you may experience slight weight gain, increased appetite, mood swings, fluid retention, and stomach upset. However, long-term steroid treatment with doses above 10 mg per day can result in more serious side effects including stomach ulcers, menstrual irregularities, muscle cramps, acne, thinning of bones (osteoporosis), cataracts, thinning and bruising of the skin, and disruption of adrenal gland function. Stomach upset can be reduced by taking the oral steroid medication along with food. Inhaled steroid medications (see above) have fewer side effects. (The types of corticosteroid medications used to treat asthma are not like the anabolic steroids taken illegally by some athletes, which can have devastating effects on the liver, heart, and muscles.)

Comments: If you are taking oral steroid medications, **do not** suddenly stop taking them. They need to be slowly tapered over days to weeks on a schedule worked out with your doctor.

Leukotriene Inhibitors

Examples: montelukast (Singulair), zarfirlukast (Accolate)

How They Work: This medication blocks substances in the body called leukotrienes and can help control chronic ashtma. This medication is used daily to prevent asthma and should not be used to relieve an acute asthma attack.

Possible Side Effects: Unusual weakness, stomach upset, diarrhea, dizziness, cough, headache, trouble sleeping, or mouth pain.

Expectorants and Mucolytics

Examples: water, guaifenesin, potassium iodide, acetylcysteine, iodinated glycerol (Organidin)

How They Work: These agents may help make mucus thinner and easier to cough up. Make sure to drink an adequate amount of water to liquefy and thin mucus (6–8 glasses a day).

Possible Side Effects: Varies with the product.

Antibiotics

Examples: ampicillin, amoxicillin, azithromycin, penicillin, erythromycin, tetracycline, sulfa antibiotics (Septra, Bactrim), cephalosporins, quinolones

How They Work: Antibiotics help the body fight bacterial infections. People with chronic lung disease are prone to develop bacterial infections of the airways (bronchitis) or the lungs (pneumonia).

Possible Side Effects: These vary with the specific antibiotic but sometimes include nausea, vomiting, and diarrhea. Rashes, increased difficulty breathing, or fever may indicate a more serious allergic reaction, and the antibiotic should be stopped until a doctor is consulted.

Comments: Always take your antibiotic for the full time prescribed (usually 5–10 days or longer) even though you feel better. If you stop too soon, the infection may recur. Follow the instructions with each antibiotic. For example, tetracycline should not be taken with any milk products or antacids, since they interfere with the absorption of the drug and reduce its effectiveness.

Inhalation Treatments

Metered-Dose Inhaler (MDI)

Some lung medications such as bronchodilators, corticosteroids, and cromolyn can be taken by inhalation. They come in a special canister called a metered-dose inhaler (MDI). When used properly, inhalers can be a highly effective way of quickly delivering medication to your lungs. By breathing medicine directly into the lungs instead of swallowing it in a pill form, you absorb less medication into the bloodstream, causing fewer side effects while allowing higher concentrations of medicine to reach the lungs.

However, learning to use an inhaler properly is more difficult than swallowing a pill. It takes proper instruction and some practice. The instructions given below are good as background information, but *it is essential to have a health professional knowledgeable about inhaler use observe you periodically to check your technique. Improper use of inhalers is one of the most important reasons for failure to control symptoms. So, if you are prescribed an inhaler, make sure to get help in using it properly.*

Using the Medications: With medications, use the quick-acting symptom-relieving (bronchodilator) medication first. Wait several minutes for it to open up the breathing tubes so that the preventive (inhaled anti-inflammatory) medication can get into your lungs better.

Spacers or Holding Chambers: To make using an inhaler easier, safer, and more effective, we strongly recommend using a spacer device or holding chamber. This is a chamber (usually a specially designed tube or bag) into which you spray the medication from the inhaler. You then inhale the medication from the spacer. The spacer makes it more likely that you can inhale the smaller, lighter droplets of medication farther into your airways. The spacer also collects on its walls some of the larger, heavier droplets of medication that would otherwise settle in your mouth or throat. This can reduce side effects such as yeast infections in the case of inhaled steroids. Some spacer devices have a whistle that sounds if you are inhaling too rapidly. This also reminds you not to take a fast breath. A fast breath deposits more of the medication in your mouth and less in your lungs.

Spacers are easier to use than metered-dose inhalers alone. You don't have to worry about pointing the spray in the right direction, and your inhalation doesn't have to be as carefully timed and coordinated with the spray. Since more of the medication reaches your lungs and less is left in your mouth with a spacer, the medication tends to be safer and more effective. This is especially important if you are using a steroid inhaler.

How To Use An Inhaler: Using a spacer with a metered-dose inhaler (MDI) is the most efficient way to get the most medication to your lungs. Here is the correct way to use an MDI **with a spacer**:

1. Shake the inhaler, remove the inhaler cap, and place the mouthpiece of the inhaler into the spacer.

2. Remove the cap from the spacer.

3. Hold the inhaler upright with the mouthpiece at the bottom.

4. Tilt your head back slightly and breathe out slowly and completely.

5. Place the spacer's mouthpiece in your mouth.

6. Press down on the inhaler to spray one puff of medication into the spacer and then start breathing in slowly (press then inhale). Hold your breath for 10 seconds. This will let the medication settle in your lungs.

7. If you need to take a second dose, wait 30 seconds to allow the inhaler valve to refill.

Although using an MDI with a spacer is usually recommended, here are ways to use an MID **without a spacer:**

1.　Shake the inhaler as directed and remove the cap.

2.　Hold the inhaler upright with the mouthpiece at the bottom.

3.　Tilt your head back slightly, and breathe out slowly and completely.

4.　Position the inhaler in one of two ways:

   - Place the inhaler 1 inch (2.5 centimeters) to 2 inches (5.1 centimeters) in front of your open mouth, without closing your lips over it. Some studies indicate this method is slightly better at delivering the medication to your lungs, but some people may find this method difficult.

   - Place the inhaler in your mouth. This method is easier for most people and reduces the risk that any of the medication will get into your eyes.

5.　Start breathing in slowly, evenly, and deeply, and press down on the inhaler one time (inhale, then press).

6.　Hold your breath for 10 seconds. This will let the medication settle in your lungs.

7.　If you need to take a second dose, wait 30 seconds to allow the inhaler valve to refill.

If you are using a corticosteroid inhaler, rinse your mouth out with water after use. Do not swallow the water. Swallowing the water will increase the chance that the medication will get into your bloodstream. This may increase the side effects of the medication. Some powder may build up on the inhaler, but it is not necessary to clean the inhaler every day. Occasionally rinse the spacer or mouthpiece, cap, and case.

Common Errors to Avoid When Using An Inhaler

- Forgetting to shake the canister
- Holding the inhaler upside down
- Breathing through your nose
- Failing to hold your breath
- Inhaling too fast

How Many Puffs Are Left in the Metered-Dose Inhaler? An inhaler may still seem to release puffs of medicine, even when there is no medicine left. The best way to tell how many puffs of medicine are left is to keep track of how many puffs have been used already. There are two ways you can do this:

1. Read the label on a new canister to find out how many puffs it contains. Write down one number for each puff on a sheet of paper. For example, if your caniser has 100 puffs in it, you would write each number from 1 to 100 on a sheet of paper. Each time you take a puff of the medicine, cross off a number. When all the numbers are crossed off, the canister doesn't have any more medicine in it.

2. Divide the number of puffs of medicine in the inhaler by the number of puffs you or your child uses each day. This gives you the number of days the medicine will last and lets you know when you will need to start using a new canister. For example, if the inhaler has 100 puffs and you take 2 puffs a day, the inhaler will last 50 days (100 puffs divided by 2 puffs a day = 50 days).

Count off the days on a calendar and mark the day when the inhaler will be empty. Ask your medical professional for a refill before you run out of medicine.

Note: If you cannot find the number of puffs on the label of the inhaler, ask your medical professional or your pharmacist for help.

Caution: In the past, some people tried to float their MDI canister in water to figure out how many puffs were left. *This method does not work.* We recommend that you use one of the two methods described above.

Dry Powder Inhalers

Dry powder inhalers (DPIs) deliver the medicine as a powder. They are used without a spacer. To use a dry powder inhaler, you need to be able to breathe air in quickly and deeply.

Nebulizers

Nebulizers are machines that deliver quick-relief medicine as a fine mist. They are often used in the clinic or the emergency room to give a 5- to 10-minute "breathing treatment," or at home for people who cannot use an inhaler with a spacer correctly. Nebulizers are bulky and are less convenient than using an inhaler. Taking four to six puffs of quick-relief medicine from an inhaler with a spacer, when done correctly, works just as well as a breathing treatment with a nebulizer.

Oxygen Therapy

For some people with chronic lung disease, their lungs cannot supply the body with enough oxygen from ordinary air. If you are tired and short of breath because there is too little oxygen in your blood, your doctor may order oxygen equipment for you to use at home. Oxygen is a medicine. It is not addicting. Yet some people try not to use it for fear of becoming dependent on it. Supplemental oxygen, however, can provide just the extra boost your body needs to remain comfortable or to perform daily activities without extreme shortness of breath. Most importantly it may well slow down your disease and make your brain function better. Some people may require continuous use of oxygen, while others may need oxygen only to help them with certain activities such as exercise.

Oxygen comes in large tanks of compressed gas or small portable tanks of either gas or liquid oxygen. If you are using oxygen, be sure to know the proper dose (flow rates and when to use it and for how long), how to use the equipment, and how to know when to order more. Although your oxygen tank will not explode or burn, oxygen can help other things burn faster. So keep the tank at least 10 feet away from any open flame, including cigarettes.

HOW TO BREATHE MORE EFFECTIVELY

Breathing Exercise

It is not surprising that breathing is a central concern of people with lung disease. Yet many people find it surprising that proper, effective breathing is a skill that has to be learned. It is not necessarily something that every adult does well naturally. This is especially important for people with lung disease. You can learn some ways to breathe that will enhance the functioning of your respiratory system.

Diaphragmatic or abdominal breathing helps strengthen respiratory muscles (especially the diaphragm) and helps rid the lungs of stale, trapped air. One of the primary reasons people with lung disease feel short of breath and can't seem to get enough air in, is because they don't get the old air out. Fresh air can't come in if the lungs are already filled with stale air. These breathing exercises can help you more fully empty your lungs and take advantage of your full lung capacity. (See pages 52–55 for instructions on how to do the breathing exercises.)

Posture

If you are slouched over and constricted, it may be very difficult to breathe in and out. Certain body postures make it easier to exhale and inhale fully. For example, if you are sitting, try leaning forward from the hips with a straight back. You can then rest your forearms on your thighs or rest your head, shoulders, and arms on a pillow placed on a table. Or use several pillows at night to make breathing easier. See page 55.

Clearing Your Lungs

Sometimes excess mucus blocks the airways, making it difficult to breathe. Your doctor or respiratory therapist may recommend certain specific positions for "postural drainage." For example, by lying on your left side on a slant with your feet higher than your head, you may be able to help the mucus from certain areas of the lung drain more effectively. Ask your doctor, nurse, or respiratory therapist which, if any, postures would be helpful for you. Also, remember that drinking at least 6 glasses of water a day (unless you have ankle swelling) may help liquefy and loosen the mucus. See page 54.

Controlled Coughing

A well-executed cough, producing a strong jet of air, is an effective way of clearing mucus from the airways. On the other hand, a weak, hacking, tickle-in-the-throat type of cough can be exhausting, irritating, and frustrating. You can learn to cough from deep in your lungs and put air power into a cough to clear the mucus. Start by sitting in a chair or on the edge of the bed with your feet firmly on the floor. Grasp a pillow firmly against your abdomen with your forearms. Take in several slow, deep belly breaths through your nose and as you exhale fully with pursed lips, bend forward slightly and press the pillow into your stomach. On the fourth or fifth breath, slowly bend forward while producing two or three strong coughs without taking any quick breaths between coughs. Repeat the whole sequence several times to clear the mucus. See page 54.

Exercise Training

Among the simplest and most effective ways to improve your ability to live a full life with chronic lung disease is to exercise. Physical activity strengthens the muscles, improves mood, increases energy level, and enhances the efficiency of the heart and lungs. Although exercise does not reverse the damage to the lungs, it can improve your ability to function within whatever limits you have due to your lung disease. (See Chapter 9 for discussion of physical fitness and exercise for people with chronic lung disease.)

Exercise is good for the heart and lungs. However, some people with asthma may cough or wheeze when they exercise. If you do, you may wish to discuss with your doctor using 2 puffs of albuterol (Ventolin, Proventil) or cromolyn (Intal) 15 to 30 minutes before starting exercise. Wearing a scarf or a mask over your face in cold weather may help prevent the cold air from triggering asthma. Swimming usually does not trigger asthma.

Asthma, chronic bronchitis, and emphysema are by definition not curable. But you can, in partnership with your doctor, work to reduce the symptoms and improve your ability to live a rich, rewarding life.

A special thanks to Cheryl Owen, RN, and Karen Freimark for help with this chapter.

Community Resources

Canadian Allergy, Asthma, and Immunology Foundation
774 Echo Drive, Ottawa Ont., K1S 5N8
Tel.: (613)-730-6272

Asthma Society of Canada
4950 Yonge Street, Suite 2306, Toronto, Ontario, M2N 6K1
Toll Free: 1-866-787-4050

Allergy/Asthma Information Association
Vaughan, Ont., L4H 3H9
Toll Free: 1-800-611-7011
B.C.
Toll Free :1-877-500-2242

Prairies/NWT/Nunavut)
Toll Free: 1-866-456-6651

Ontario
Toll Free: 1-888-250-2298

Quebec
Toll Free: 1-866-694-0679

Atlantic
Toll Free: 1-866-761-6600

The Lung Association, National Office
1750 Courtwood Crescent, Suite 300, Ottawa, Ont. K2C 2B5
Toll-Free: 1-888-566-LUNG (5864)

British Columbia Lung Association
Toll-Free: 1-800-665-LUNG (5864)

Lung Association of Alberta & NWT
Toll Free: 1-888-566-LUNG (5864)

(continued on next page)

Community Resources

Lung Association of Saskatchewan
Toll-Free: 1-888-566-LUNG (5864)

Manitoba Lung Association
Telephone: (204) 774-5501

Ontario Lung Association
Toll Free: 1-800-972-2636

The Quebec Lung Association/ l'Association pulmonaire du Québec
Toll-Free: 1-800-295-8111

New Brunswick Lung Association
Toll Free: 1-800-565-LUNG (5864)

Lung Association of Nova Scotia
Telephone: (902) 443-8141

Prince Edward Island Lung Association
Toll-Free: 1-888-566-LUNG (5864)

Newfoundland & Labrador Lung Association
Toll Free: 1-888-566-LUNG (5864)

Community Asthma Care Centre
(There are 50 CACCs across Canada, as well as many other asthma centres. Below is a
website that lists their locations, as well as a sample of asthma centres in all the provinces.)
http://www.asthma.ca/adults/community/locator.php

Alberta
Northeast Community Health Centre
Edmonton
Telephone: 780-472-5000

British Columbia
Kelowna General Hospital
Kelowna
Telephone: 250-862-4222

(continued on next page)

Community Resources

Manitoba
Seven Oaks Hospital
Winnipeg
Telephone: 204-661-7255

Ontario
Lakeridge Health Port Perry
Port Perry
Telephone: 613-737-2344

New Brunswick
North East Health Network Regional Hospital Centre
Bathurst
Telephone: 506-544-2447

Newfoundland
Western Health Care Corporation
Corner Brook
Telephone: 709-637-5298

Nova Scotia
Fishermen's Memorial Hospital
Lunenberg
Telephone: 902-634-8801

Prince Edward Island
Asthma Education Centre, Prince Edward County Hospital
Telephone: 902-438-4252
Charlottetown

Saskatchewan
S.E. Health District
Telephone: 306-634-0410
Estevan

Suggested Further Reading

American Lung Association of Western Pennsylvania. *Self-Help: Your Strategy for Living With COPD,* 3rd ed. Palo, Alto, Calif.: Bull Publishing, 1997.

Hodder, Rick and Susan Lightstone. *Every Breath I Take: A Guide to Living with COPD.* Toronto: Stoddart, 2001.

Marcus, Bess, Jeffrey S. Hampl, and Edwin B. Fisher. *How To Quit Smoking Without Gaining Weight.* New York: Pocket Books, 2004.

Plaut, Thomas F., and Teresa B. Jones. *Asthma Guide for People of All Ages.* Amherst, Mass.: Pedipress, 1999.

Shimberg, Elaine Fantle. *Coping With COPD.* New York: St. Martin's Press, 2003.

MANAGING HEART DISEASE AND HIGH BLOOD PRESSURE

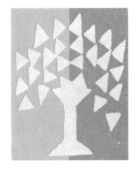

17

THE MODERN MANAGEMENT OF HEART DISEASE AND HIGH BLOOD PRESSURE SAVES LIVES, KEEPS PEOPLE OUT OF THE HOSPITAL, AND DRAMATICALLY REDUCES THE RISKS OF HEART ATTACKS AND STROKES. The success in treatment comes from a combination of lifestyle changes, medications, and, if necessary, procedures to improve the function of the heart. The result is that many heart attacks and strokes are prevented, and that many people with heart disease can look forward to long, healthy, and enjoyable lives.

There are many forms of heart disease. The arteries that supply the heart muscle can be blocked, as in atherosclerosis. The valves inside the heart that control the flow of blood can be damaged, as in valvular heart disease. The electrical system that controls the beating of the heart can be disrupted resulting in irregular heart rhythms (arrhythmias). The heart muscle can be damaged and unable to effectively push the blood to the lungs and the rest of the body, as occurs in heart failure.

The most common form of heart disease is coronary artery disease and is the one that leads to most heart attacks and heart failure. Coronary arteries are "pipelines" or blood vessels that wrap around the heart. The coronary arteries deliver the oxygen and nutrients the heart needs to perform its job. Healthy arteries are elastic, flexible, and strong. The inside lining of a healthy artery is smooth, so blood flows easily. Arteries narrow as they become clogged with cholesterol and other substances. This is called atherosclerosis, also known as coronary artery disease (CAD), and the blocked area is called a stenosis.

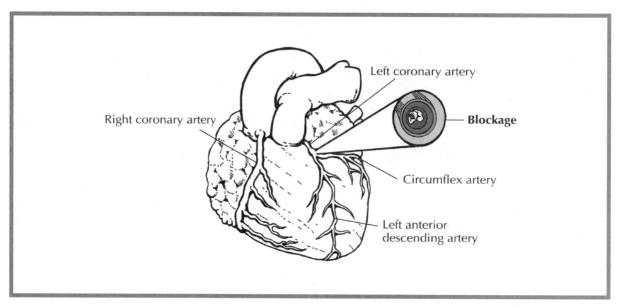

Figure 16.1 **The Heart's Arteries**

Atherosclerosis is a gradual process that occurs over many years. The first step is damage to the wall of the artery. This damage is caused by a number of factors, including: high cholesterol and/or triglycerides, diabetes, smoking, and high blood pressure. The initial damage allows the low-density lipoprotein cholesterol (LDL cholesterol, the "bad" cholesterol) to enter the artery wall. The next step is an inflammatory response. White blood cells gobble up the LDL-cholesterol particles. This results in the formation of large, fatty cells called foam cells. The foam cells form fatty streaks, which are the earliest sign of atherosclerosis. The beginning of these fatty deposits can appear as early as the teenage years.

Over time, more cholesterol is deposited and the fatty areas grow larger and larger. These fatty areas are called plaques, which can completely block off blood flow in an artery, or may crack open, causing a blood clot to form at the injured site. In both cases, blood flow to the heart is blocked and one may experience angina (temporary chest pain) or a heart attack. A heart attack is also known as a myocardial infarction (MI) and, if not treated immediately, can cause permanent damage to the heart muscle. When a part of the heart muscle has been damaged, that part can no longer help the heart pump blood. The pain of angina or a heart attack may be on the left side of the chest over the heart but may also radiate to the shoulders, arms, neck, and jaw. Some people with angina or a heart attack may also experience nausea, sweating, shortness of breath, and fatigue.

Finally, people with heart disease may notice irregular heartbeats. This is caused by irregularities in the conduction system or electrical wiring of the heart. Damage to this system can result in irregular heartbeats, palpitations, skipped beats, or racing beats. Physicians refer to these as arrhythmias or dysrhythmias.

Most irregular heartbeats are minor and not dangerous. However, some forms of arrhythmias can cause problems. Dangerous arrhythmias are often accompanied by episodes of fainting or prolonged irregular heartbeats. Such arrhythmias may be more dangerous for people with severely weakened hearts and those with heart failure. If you notice occasional irregular heartbeats, take note of how frequently they occur, how long they last, how fast your heart is beating (check your pulse), and how you feel during the episode. That information will help your doctor decide whether or not your arrhythmias are dangerous. Remember that infrequent, short bouts of irregular beats are common among many people, both with and without heart disease. They are generally not cause for concern and should not require activity restrictions or treatment with drugs.

Most people with coronary artery disease have at least one of the above symptoms. However, the presence of one of these symptoms does not automatically mean you have heart disease.

Seek Emergency Care Immediately

If you are having symptoms that might mean a heart attack or stroke, you must seek medical care immediately. New treatments are available that can dissolve blood clots in the blood vessels of the heart and brain and restore blood flow. However, these treatments must be given within hours of the heart attack or stroke—the sooner, the better. In Canada, call 9-1-1 or emergency health services if you experience:

Heart Attack Warning Signs
- Severe, crushing, or squeezing chest pain (like someone is sitting on your chest)
- Pain that spreads to the jaw, arms, neck, and/or back
- Pain not relieved by rest or heart medications (nitroglycerin)
- Chest pain occurring with any of the following: rapid and/or irregular heartbeat, sweating, nausea or vomiting, shortness of breath, or light-headedness
- Chest pain that lasts longer than 15 minutes when there is no obvious cause

Stroke Warning Signs
- Weakness, numbness, or paralysis of the face, arm, or leg, especially on only one side of the body, that does not go away in a few minutes
- Blurred or decreased vision in one or both eyes that does not clear with blinking
- Newly developed difficulty speaking or understanding simple statements

In addition, people with heart disease can develop symptoms under varying conditions. For example, one person may develop angina and shortness of breath at the end of a brisk 5-mile walk. Another person may notice those same symptoms at rest. Although both people experience angina and shortness of breath, the significance of their symptoms is probably not the same. For example, the first person would be able to safely exercise at an intensity below the level that causes his or her angina. The second person, on the other hand, is severely limited by the symptoms and is at high risk for a heart attack.

The same symptoms can represent different levels of concern for different people. The following section will help you identify dangerous symptoms and understand their implications for your future outlook. Remember, if you are ever in doubt about the severity of a symptom you are experiencing, contact your doctor. He or she is your best resource for discussing these issues.

WHAT DOES HEART DISEASE DO?

When ischemia occurs, the blood supply is less than the heart muscle requires. The cells of the heart muscle usually weaken and may even die. Your body may let you know that the heart is not getting enough oxygen by giving you the sensation of a squeezing pain or pressure in your chest, commonly known as angina or angina pectoris. In some people with coronary artery disease, this sensation can radiate from the chest to other parts of the body, including the shoulders, arms, neck, and jaw. The reason angina radiates to other parts of the body is uncertain. It is probably due to the referral of pain along nerve fibers that run close to the heart and go to other parts of the body.

Some people with heart disease experience sweating and nausea. These are usually associated with angina and are probably caused by certain chemicals released by the body in response to stressful events (such as angina). These chemicals may stimulate nerve endings that control sweating and the sensation of nausea.

Other symptoms of coronary artery disease include unusual shortness of breath and fatigue. Shortness of breath and fatigue are probably caused by temporary weakening of the heart during an episode of angina, and result from the lack of proper blood supply to the heart muscle itself. As a result of the shortage of blood, the heart is unable to pump out all the blood it receives. This creates two problems:

- Blood may back up into the lungs, causing shortness of breath.

- The rest of the body will not receive the blood supply it needs, leading to fatigue and further shortness of breath.

When this weakening of the heart is severe and persistent, it is called heart failure. Fortunately, not everyone with heart disease experiences heart failure. For those who have episodes of heart failure, treatments are available to improve their symptoms and future outlook (see page 307 for treatment information).

WHAT IS THE OUTLOOK FOR PEOPLE WITH HEART DISEASE?

With lifestyle changes, use of medications, and, if necessary, cardiac procedures, most people with heart disease do very well, even those who have had a heart attack. Some people with coronary heart disease do not have any symptoms. For others, physical exertion or an emotional upset will sometimes bring on predictable pain.

Predictable episodes of angina are relatively safe. They can teach you to avoid the levels of exercise or emotional upset that cause angina. If the angina does occur, you can use medicines to relieve the angina and prevent the heart from being overworked.

Unpredictable episodes, on the other hand, may occur at any time for no apparent reason. Because of their unpredictable nature, these episodes are considered to be more dangerous. The underlying cause for all angina is the same: the heart's cells are not getting enough oxygen.

Angina and other symptoms of coronary artery disease are worrisome because they can be associated with one of the most serious outcomes of coronary artery disease—a myocardial infarction, or heart attack. A heart attack results when the blood supply to an area of the heart is suddenly and completely blocked, leading to heart muscle damage or even death.

For those who survive a heart attack, the severity of heart muscle damage varies from person to person. Generally speaking, the more severe the heart attack, the more heart muscle damage. People with mildly damaged hearts generally do quite well. Some people may have no evidence of ongoing ischemia (the lack of blood supply and oxygen to the heart). Their outlook is very good. Less than 1% of such people have another heart attack the following year.

People with mildly damaged hearts who have episodes of ischemia after their heart attack are at a slightly higher risk of having a future heart attack. Still, only a small number of such people will develop a heart attack during the year following the initial heart attack.

People with severely damaged hearts, on the other hand, are generally at higher risk for subsequent heart attacks. Approximately 10–15% of such people have a heart attack during the subsequent year. In addition, they may develop episodes of heart failure and be physically limited in what they can do. Treatments, including surgical and medical therapies, have been shown to improve the symptoms of heart disease. In many cases, they also improve the long-term outlook, or prognosis, of the disease. (See treatment section on page 300.)

The level of impairment is also somewhat variable, even among people with the same severity of disease. Some people with relatively normal hearts after a heart attack will live relatively normal lives. Others may be limited by the emotional or psychological burdens they feel from having an imperfect heart. They may experience anxiety or depression. They may develop a fear of sexual intimacy. While each person will respond differently, it is important to remember that it is common for people to have worries, anxiety, and even depression. It's also important to remember that these feelings can be helped with improved understanding and control of their disease.

With time, a person with heart disease may experience a worsening of symptoms, such as angina (chest discomfort), shortness of breath, or fatigue. Sometimes symptoms will worsen temporarily due to a simple, underlying cause, such as the resumption of cigarette smoking, a change in medications, or suffering an emotionally upsetting experience. At other times, a worsening of symptoms represents a worsening of the coronary artery disease, potentially necessitating more vigorous medical or even surgical therapy.

How can one tell the difference? Call your physician whenever you are concerned about a new symptom. Dangerous symptoms include the development of:

- any new chest discomfort,

- unusual shortness of breath,

- dizziness or fainting,

- prolonged irregular heartbeats,

- sudden weight gain*, or

- ankle swelling.*

DIAGNOSING HEART DISEASE

Sometimes the symptoms of heart disease are clear and "classic," such as chest pain with physical activity or exertion. Fortunately, there are now many tests available to determine if heart disease is present and how severe it is. The following are the more common tests and treatments you might have to determine the health of your heart.

---

* Sudden increased weight or ankle swelling may indicate worsening heart failure.

Blood Tests

Blood tests to measure fatty-like substances (cholesterol and triglycerides) in the blood may be done to estimate your risk of heart disease or the effect of cholesterol-lowering medications. If you are having chest pains, your physician may order special blood tests of cardiac enzymes to confirm the diagnosis of a heart attack.

Electrocardiogram (EKG)

An EKG measures your heart's electrical activity. It can show a lack of oxygen to the heart, a heart attack, heart enlargement, and irregular heart rhythm. It is a "snapshot" of your heart's activity. Sometimes EKGs need to be repeated to see if a heart attack is occurring. An EKG cannot predict your risk for a future heart attack.

Echocardiogram

Painless ultrasound waves are bounced off the heart. This produces detailed images of the heart. A computer converts echoes and displays them on a TV screen. The pictures are recorded on videotape or paper. It can show heart size, heart motion, valve function, and certain types of heart damage. This test may also be done with exercise (stress testing) to assess the response of the heart to stress.

Stress Test

Sometimes problems only appear when the heart is under some type of increased stress. This test is done while exercising on a treadmill or stationary bicycle. An EKG is attached to the chest to get continuous information about the heart during exercise or stress. The EKG, blood pressure, and symptoms are monitored during the test and a few minutes after the test. A stress test is done to:

• Evaluate stress-related symptoms.

• Confirm suspicion of heart disease.

• Evaluate treatment.

- Assess progress after a heart attack.

- Determine irregularities in heart rhythm.

A "positive" test result suggests the presence of coronary artery disease.

Nuclear Scans

A weak radioactive substance such as thallium, sestamibi, or technetium is injected into a vein. A scanner or special camera is used to take two sets of pictures, with and without stress (induced by exercise or medication), which are compared. This test shows blood distribution to the heart muscle and how well the heart is pumping.

Cardiac Catheterization and Coronary Angiography

A long plastic tube called a catheter is inserted through a major blood vessel (usually in the groin area) and gently guided into the heart. A dye is then injected into the catheter. This allows the coronary arteries to show up on X-rays. This test helps your physician decide the best treatment to follow if the arteries are clogged. It can also give information about the function of the heart muscle and the valves.

HIGH BLOOD PRESSURE

High blood pressure, known as hypertension, increases the risk of heart disease, stroke, and kidney and eye damage. Blood pressure is a measurement of the amount of pressure in an artery. The systolic pressure is the pressure in the artery when the heart contracts and pushes out a wave of blood. The diastolic pressure is the pressure when the heart relaxes between pumps.

The pressures are recorded as millimeters of mercury (mm Hg). When the blood pressure is written down, the systolic pressure is always written first, followed by a slash (/) and then the diastolic pressure. So a blood pressure of 120/80 ("120 over 80") means that the systolic pressure is 120 mm Hg and the diastolic pressure is 80 mm Hg. Both numbers are important since both high systolic and high diastolic pressures can cause damage.

Hypertension, or "high blood pressure," is often referred to as a "silent" disease. This is because most people with hypertension have no symptoms and cannot really tell or feel if their blood pressure is high without measuring it. If your blood pressure is high and you feel perfectly well, it may be hard to believe that anything is wrong or needs to be treated. High blood pressure (unless it is extremely high) does not usually cause headaches, dizziness, nervousness, or pounding of the heart. However, hypertension may not stay silent. Over a period of years, untreated high blood pressure can damage blood vessels throughout the body. In some people, this damage to blood vessels can eventually cause strokes, heart attacks, heart failure, or damage to the eyes or kidneys. The reason for treating high blood pressure is to prevent these serious complications. That's why it is extremely important to control your blood pressure even if you do not have any symptoms and feel perfectly well.

Why do you have hypertension? Over 90% of hypertension is called "primary" or "essential," which really means that the cause is not known.

What is normal blood pressure? The standards have been changing. A healthy or optimal blood pressure is below 120 systolic and 80 diastolic. "Prehypertension" is below 140 systolic and 90 diastolic. High blood pressure, or hypertension, is considered at or above 140 systolic and 90 diastolic. For most people lower blood pressure usually means less risk of complications. Both the systolic and diastolic pressures are important measures of the health of the cardiovascular system.

Your blood pressure, however, varies minute to minute. Hypertension is diagnosed when blood pressure measurements are high on two or more separate occasions. Except in severe cases, the diagnosis is never based on a single measurement. That's one reason it is important to have repeated measurements of your blood pressure.

Some people's blood pressure tends to go up only in the doctor's office. This is a stress reaction called "white-coat hypertension." This is one reason it is very helpful in both diagnosing hypertension and monitoring the effects of treatment to have additional blood pressure measurements taken outside the clinic or hospital. Being able to measure your blood pressure at home (self-monitoring) or at a pharmacy, may allow you to collect better information about what your blood pressure is throughout the day, not just in the doctor's office. This may help monitor how your blood pressure responds to lifestyle changes (diet, exercise, relaxation) and ensure you are on safe and effective dosages of antihypertensive medications. It's important to take your blood pressure the right way, though. See the Heart and Stroke Foundation website for tips on self-monitoring (see Resources for further information).

HEART FAILURE

"Heart failure" does not mean that your heart has stopped working or is going to stop. It means that your heart's pumping ability is weaker than normal; your heart still beats, but with less force.

Heart failure is a group of symptoms. Heart failure can be treated and its symptoms managed, even when the heart cannot be returned to normal. What are the signs and symptoms of heart failure? You may have one or more of the following:

Excessive tiredness, fatigue, and weakness

When your heart is not pumping with enough force, your muscles do not get enough oxygen to meet their needs. You may be more tired than usual and not have enough energy for normal activities.

Shortness of breath

Sometimes breathing becomes more difficult. You may experience difficulty catching your breath, frequent/hacking cough, difficulty breathing when lying flat, or waking up at night due to difficulty breathing.

Weight gain

A common sign of heart failure is weight gain due to fluid retention. When your body is holding on to extra fluid, your weight will go up. Sometimes this weight gain happens rapidly. In other cases, slow, progressive weight gain occurs. You may feel a swelling sensation in feet and ankles, shoes and socks too tight, rings on fingers too tight, bloated stomach, tightness at waistline, or shortness of breath.

Changes in the frequency of urination

Your kidneys help your body get rid of extra fluid when you urinate. More blood may be pumped to your kidneys at night because your brain and muscles are resting and need less blood. Additional blood to your kidneys allows them to "catch up" during the night while you are at rest. You may experience more frequent urination at night or decreased urination at all times.

Although heart failure is a serious condition, steps to manage the symptoms and lead a full, productive life include checking your weight each day and reducing the amount of sodium in your diet.

Weigh yourself daily and keep records of your weight. Why? Sudden or steady weight gain can be a warning sign that your body is holding on to fluid. This fluid can lead to symptoms such as shortness of breath and swelling of feet, ankles, and abdomen.

How to Weigh Yourself

- Weigh at about the same time every day. We suggest weighing every morning, just after waking up (after urinating and before eating).

- Weigh with the same amount of clothing on, or without clothing.

- Use the same scale.

- Check to be sure the scale is set to zero before weighing yourself.

- Make sure the scale is on a hard surface.

- Write your weight on the daily weight log or other record.

- Repeat weighing if you have doubts about the scale or your weight.

- Bring your daily weight log to all your medical appointments.

Call your physician or health care professional if you have:

- weight gain of one kilogram (or more) in a day

- weight gain of 2 kilograms in 5 days

- shortness of breath

Eat Healthy, Low-Sodium Foods

Sodium is an important mineral that helps regulate fluid levels in your body. Too much sodium makes your body hold on to too much fluid. People with heart failure need to eat less sodium to avoid retaining excess fluid. We only need about 500 milligrams of sodium per day. However, most people eat 4,000 to 6,000 milligrams of sodium per day. Sodium is a naturally occurring mineral and is present in most foods in various amounts. Most of the sodium we eat comes from processed foods like luncheon meats, condiments, and canned, jarred, or packaged foods (including frozen foods). Ordinary table salt is made up of sodium and chloride. A teaspoon of table salt has about 2,000 milligrams of sodium. Cutting down on processed foods and table salt is a good way to reduce the sodium we get from food. Cutting down on sodium takes time to get used to, but eventually you will enjoy the natural flavours of food. Reducing sodium in the diet may also help some people with hypertension reduce their blood pressure.

Ways to keep sodium levels below 2,000 mg per day:

- Eat mainly fresh foods.

- Read food labels for sodium content.

- Choose foods that have 140 mg of sodium per serving or less (refer to food label on package for serving size).

- Choose low-sodium foods when eating in restaurants.

- Choose restaurants that offer low-sodium foods and preparation methods.

UNDERSTANDING THE RISKS

Below are listed some of the more important risk factors that contribute to the development of heart disease and may also increase the risk of stroke. The good news is that nearly all of these risk factors can be changed and your risk of heart disease dramatically lowered.

Smoking

Smoking damages the inner lining of the blood vessels and raises blood pressure. Quitting is the best thing you can do for your health. The successful quitters do so on their own. Fortunately, there are now a variety of behavioral support programs (from telephone counseling to group programs) and medications (from nicotine gum and patches to calming medications) that can significantly improve the chances of quitting.

High cholesterol

Cholesterol is a fat-like substance in the blood. It can cause fatty deposits called plaque to build up and narrow your blood vessels. The higher your cholesterol level, the greater your risk for heart disease. Lowering the amount of saturated fat and eating a generally healthy diet may help lower cholesterol levels. Aggressively lowering LDL cholesterol with diet and medications can considerably reduce the risk of heart attacks and strokes.

Diabetes

If you have diabetes, your risk for heart disease more than doubles because high blood sugar damages the blood vessels. By controlling your diabetes and taking certain heart-protective medications you can greatly lower the risk of heart attack and stroke.

High blood pressure

High blood pressure occurs when blood presses too hard against the walls of the blood vessels. This damages the lining of the vessels. Controlling your blood pressure lowers the risk of heart disease and stroke.

Lack of exercise

Exercise strengthens your heart. It can also lower your cholesterol and blood pressure and help you control your weight. Inactive people double their risk for heart disease. Even small amounts of daily physical activity can lower your risk of heart disease and help you feel better and have more energy (see Chapters 6, 8, and 9).

Stress

Stress increases your blood pressure and heart rate, which can damage the lining of the blood vessels and lead to heart disease. (See Chapter 5.)

Excess weight

Being overweight makes your heart work harder and can raise your LDL ("bad") cholesterol and blood pressure, and increase your chances of developing diabetes. Excess weight around the midsection increases your risk the most. Regular exercise and a healthy diet are the most important steps to help prevent weight gain, maintain weight, or lose weight.

Alcohol

While low levels of alcohol intake (1 drink per day) may reduce the risk of heart disease, higher alcohol use can increase the risk of both heart disease and hypertension. So, if you do use alcohol, limit the use.

Age and gender

Blood vessels slowly narrow and harden with age. The older you are, the greater your risk for heart disease. Men older than 45 and women older than 55 are at increased risk. Note that heart disease is the leading cause of death in both men and women. It is not just a "man's disease."

Family history

Your risk for heart disease may be higher if you:

- Have a father or brother who has had heart disease before age 55.

- Have a mother or sister who has had heart disease before age 65.

PREVENTION AND TREATMENT OF HEART DISEASE AND HIGH BLOOD PRESSURE

There are three general approaches to help prevent and treat heart disease:

1. Lifestyle changes

2. Medications

3. Procedures and surgery

Most people will benefit from one or more of these approaches.

What Is the Role of Lifestyle Changes and Non-Drug Treatments?

The build-up of fatty deposits that block the coronary arteries can often be prevented. The key lifestyle changes (described above) include:

• Not smoking

• Exercising

• Eating a healthy, low-fat diet

• Maintaining a healthy weight

• Managing stress

• Limiting alcohol intake

Medications

A variety of medications are available to treat heart disease and high blood pressure. In addition, some of these medications are very useful in preventing future complications such as heart attacks, stroke, and kidney damage.* It used to be thought that medications were only to be used if lifestyle changes such as diet and exercise failed to make the needed improvements. Newer research suggests that along with lifestyle changes, certain medications may be helpful for nearly everyone with heart disease to reduce the risk of heart attacks, death, and strokes.

---

* Because research about medications is changing rapidly, we suggest that you consult your physician, pharmacist, and/or a recent drug reference book for the latest information.

Below we briefly discuss some of the most common and effective medications. If you have heart disease, diabetes, stroke, peripheral vascular disease, chronic kidney disease, or an abdominal aortic aneurysm, be sure to consult your doctor to find out if some or all of these heart-protective medications are right for you.

Aspirin

Example: enteric coated "baby" aspirin (81 mg)

How It Works: Aspirin works by reducing the stickiness of the blood platelets, which is what helps the blood clot. Aspirin prevents the platelets from clumping together and sticking to the walls of the arteries and blocking them. Aspirin is sometimes referred to as a blood thinner.

Possible Side Effects: Aspirin can cause stomach irritation (gastritis) and may even cause small ulcers and bleeding. Usually, taking the low-dose (81 mg) aspirin with a special coating ("enteric coated") and taking the aspirin with food can protect the stomach. While aspirin can reduce the overall risk of strokes caused by blood clots, it can slightly increase the risk of having a certain type of stroke from bleeding (hemorrhagic).

Comments: Most people think aspirin is just for aches and pains, but it is also a very helpful medicine for your heart and blood vessels. If you are at risk for developing heart disease—or even if you have already had a heart attack—taking an aspirin every day can help prevent heart attacks or dying from a heart attack or stroke. Sometimes a newer medication called clopidogrel (Plavix) is used to help prevent blood clots.

Cholesterol-Lowering Statins (HMG-CoA Reductase Inhibitors)

Examples: cholestyramine, colestipol, niacin, lovastatin, pravastatin, simvastatin, gemfibrozil, and probucol. (We have listed generic names, as formulations differ. Ask your doctor to recommend which is best for you.)

How They Work: Statins work to lower your LDL (bad) cholesterol, which clogs arteries by blocking the production of cholesterol in the liver. They also increase your HDL (good) cholesterol, reduce your triglycerides, and may help to prevent blood clots and inflammation inside your arteries. The latest evidence suggests that even if your cholesterol levels are within the desirable range, if you have heart disease or diabetes, taking a statin medication can further lower your risk.

Possible Side Effects: Most people who take these medications have few or no side effects. Some people experience mild muscle aching, upset stomach, gas, constipation, abdominal pain, or cramps. Liver damage and severe muscle pain (or rhabdomyolysis) is a rare side effect that occurs in very few people who use statins. If you experience severe muscle pain, severe weakness, or brown urine, contact your health care professional immediately.

Comments: Statins may help reduce the risk of a heart attack or stroke for people who take them daily. If you have heart disease or diabetes, taking a statin medication may be helpful even if your cholesterol levels are normal for people who do not have these diseases. Other medications may also be used to lower cholesterol and reduce triglycerides.

Beta-Blocking Agents

Examples: metoprolol, atenolol, propranolol, acebutolol, nadolol.

How They Work: Beta-blockers reduce the workload of the heart by relaxing the heart muscle and slowing down the heart rate. This allows your heart to pump blood more easily. Beta-blockers are used to treat high blood pressure, heart failure, irregular heart beats, blocked arteries, and angina (chest pain). This medication reduces sudden death (without symptoms or warning) from heart attack in people with coronary heart disease.

Possible Side Effects: Most people who take this medication have few or no side effects. Some people report a tired feeling. Some people develop a very slow heart rate or low blood pressure, which can make you feel light-headed. People with well-controlled asthma can usually take a beta-blocker without any problem. In rare cases, the asthma can worsen. If you have uncontrolled asthma, you should not take beta-blockers because they may make your asthma worse. People with diabetes can usually take beta-blockers without any problem, although they may reduce the ability to feel the symptoms of a very low blood sugar level (hypoglycemia).

Comments: Beta-blockers are used to treat high blood pressure, heart failure, irregular heartbeat, blocked arteries, and angina (chest pain). It can take two to three months to get used to a beta-blocker. It helps to remember that:

- Early side effects usually go away over time.

- You may need to take a beta-blocker for two to three months before it makes you feel better.

- Even when a beta-blocker does not make you feel better, it can still help protect your heart from getting weaker. This medication significantly reduces sudden death (without symptoms or warning) from heart attack in people with coronary heart disease or a previous history of a heart attack.

- Since beta-blockers slow your heart rate, it may change your "target heart rate range" and "maximal heart rate" if you use these to monitor the intensity of your exercise.

Angiotensin-Converting Enzyme (ACE) Inhibitors

Examples: lisinipril (Prinivil, Zestril), captopril (Capoten), enalopril (Vasotec)

How They Work: ACE inhibitors act by blocking the formation of angiotensin II, an enzyme in the body that causes constriction of blood vessels. This causes the blood vessels to relax and widen, increases the flow of oxygen-rich blood to the heart, and lowers blood pressure.

Possible Side Effects: Most people who take this medication have few or no side effects. Some people get a mild cough or tickle in the back of the throat. The cough is usually not very bothersome, and it is not always necessary to stop the ACE inhibitor medication. Very rarely, some people who take ACE inhibitors have swelling of the face, eyes, lips, tongue, or throat or difficulty breathing, and should seek immediate care. Some people experience headaches or dizziness.

Comments: Most people think ACE inhibitors are just for lowering blood pressure, but they are also a very helpful medicine for your heart and blood vessels. They can help reduce symptoms and improve survival in heart failure. They are also used to treat and prevent kidney problems, especially in people who also have diabetes.

Calcium-Channel Blockers

Examples: : nifedipine, diltiazem, verapamil, amlodipine

How They Work: They manage angina by dilating the blood vessels, leading to an increased blood supply to the heart muscle itself and reduced blood pressure.

Possible Side Effects: Headache, ankle swelling, dizziness, flushing, and constipation are experienced by 10–20 per cent of people on calcium-channel blockers.

Comments: Calcium blockers are an effective treatment for heart disease and high blood pressure, but speak to your doctor to ensure you get the most appropriate medication for your particular situation.

Diuretics

Examples: : hydrochlorothiazide, furosemide, chlorthalidone, indapamide, and triamterene/hydrochlorothiazide. (We have listed generic names for this category, as formulations differ. Ask your doctor to recommend which is best for you.)

How They Work: Diuretics or "water pills" help by reducing the amount of fluid in the body. Your body gets rid of this excess fluid when you urinate. Getting rid of this excess fluid decreases the amount of work your heart needs to do. This can reduce blood pressure, swelling, and excess fluids. Some diuretics also help the blood vessels relax and widen to reduce blood pressure.

Possible Side Effects: Diuretics can cause frequent urination, weakness and fatigue, and sometimes leg cramps. They may lead to low potassium levels in the blood. They may also interfere with control of blood glucose in diabetes or control of uric acid levels in gout. Blood tests can be done to monitor the safe use of diuretics.

Comments: Certain diuretics not only reduce blood pressure but have been shown to reduce the risk of heart attacks and stroke. They are also used to reduce the build-up of fluid in the lungs, which can occur in heart failure. Take your last dose of diuretic medication no later than 6:00 p.m. so that you will not need to get up as often at night to urinate.

There are many other medications used to treat heart disease, heart failure, high blood pressure, and irregular heart rhythms. If one medication is not working for you or is causing side effects, discuss this with your doctor. Usually an alternative medication can be found that will work well for you. (See Chapter 4.)

PROCEDURES AND SURGERY

Coronary or "Balloon" Angioplasty

Coronary angioplasty relieves the symptoms of coronary artery disease by improving blood flow to the heart by opening the blockages. A catheter with a balloon at the tip is inserted into the artery to widen a narrow passage in the vessel. Your physician may choose to insert a tiny mesh tube called a stent to help keep the narrowed vessel open. Many stents contain medications ("drug-eluting stents") that can help prevent the artery from clogging up again.

Coronary Artery Bypass Surgery

Bypass surgery creates a new route for blood flow to your heart. A blood vessel from your leg or chest wall is used to create a detour around the blockage in the coronary artery. One or more blocked arteries may be bypassed. The surgery usually requires several days in the hospital, and the recovery time can be several months.

THE OUTLOOK

The outlook for preventing heart disease and for helping people with heart disease lead longer, fuller lives has never been better. The combination of healthy lifestyle practices and selective use of medications, coupled with cardiac procedures when needed, has dramatically lowered the risk of heart attacks, strokes, and early deaths. Much can be done by patients to self-manage heart disease (from eating well and exercising to managing stress and regularly taking medications as prescribed) and work with their health care team to help improve both the quality and quantity of life.

Resources for Further Information

Heart and Stroke Foundation of Canada
222 Queen Street, Suite 1402
Ottawa, ON K1P 5V9
Telephone: 613-569-4361
www.heartandstroke.ca

Heart and Stroke Foundation of Manitoba
The Heart and Stroke Building
6 Donald Street
Winnipeg, Manitoba R3L 0K6
Telephone: 204-949-2000

Heart and Stroke Foundation of New Brunswick
133 Prince William Street, Suite 606
Saint John, New Brunswick E2L 2B5
Telephone: 506-634-1620 or 1-800-663-3600

Heart and Stroke Foundation of Newfoundland & Labrador
1037 Topsail Road
Mount Pearl, Newfoundland A1N 5E9
Telephone: 709-753-8521

Heart and Stroke Foundation of Nova Scotia
5161 George St. 7th Floor
Halifax, Nova Scotia B3J 1M7
Toll Free: 1-800-423-4432

Heart and Stroke Foundation of Ontario
2300 Yonge Street, Suite 1300
PO Box 2414
Toronto, Ontario M4P 1E4
Telephone: 416-489-7111

Heart and Stroke Foundation of Prince Edward Island
180 Kent Street P.O. Box 279
Charlottetown, Prince Edward Island C1A 7K4
Telephone: 902-892-7441

Heart and Stroke Foundation of Quebec
1434 Sainte-Catherine Street West, Suite 500
Montreal, Quebec H3G 1R4
Telephone: 1-800-567-8563

Heart and Stroke Foundation of Saskatchewan
Saskatchewan North Saskatoon)
279 - 3rd Ave N.
Saskatoon, Saskatchewan S7K 2H8
Telephone: 306-244-2124

Saskatchewan South Regina)
2360-2nd Ave.,
Regina, Saskatchewan S4R 1A6
Telephone: 306-569-8433

Health Canada
www.hc-sc.gc.ca

Suggested Further Reading

Baker, Dr. Brian and Dorien, Dr. Paul. *A Change of Heart: Recovering from Heart Disease in Body and Mind.* Toronto, ON. Random House of Canada, 1998.

Gretzky, Walter. *On Family, Hockey and Healing.* Toronto: Random House Canada, 2002.

Heart and Stroke Foundation of Canada. *Managing Congestive Heart Failure, 2003*

Heart and Stroke Foundation of Canada. *Recovery Road.* 2000.

Kavanagh, Dr. Terence. *Take Heart.* Toronto: Key Porter Books, 1998.

MANAGING ARTHRITIS

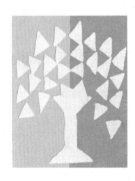

18

What is arthritis? The word "arthritis" means inflammation of a joint. However, as the word has come to be used, arthritis commonly means virtually any kind of damage to a joint. The most common form of arthritis is osteoarthritis. It is the arthritis that generally affects us as we age, causing knobby fingers, swollen knees, or back pain.

Osteoarthritis is not caused by inflammation, although sometimes it may result in inflammation of a joint. The cause of osteoarthritis is not precisely known but involves degeneration or a wearing away of the cartilaginous ends of bone. Because of the degeneration, the bone surfaces become rough and don't move smoothly on one another. Also, the bone ends grow out in the form of spurs (called osteophytes) that create, for instance, the knobs on fingers and heel spurs. Because of these rough surfaces, the lining of the joint is sometimes irritated and makes more than the normal amount of joint fluid. The extra fluid results in swelling.

There are many kinds of arthritis due to inflammation. The most common forms are those caused by rheumatic diseases such as rheumatoid arthritis, metabolic diseases such as gout, and psoriasis. With these diseases, the lining of the joint becomes inflamed and swollen, and also secretes extra fluid. As a result, the joint becomes swollen, warm, red, and tender. If present for a time, inflammatory arthritis also results in destruction of cartilage and bone. Such destruction can ultimately lead to deformity. The cause of the inflammation associated with these diseases is not precisely known, but with respect to gout it is clearly related to the formation of uric acid crystals in the joint fluid, and in the case of rheumatic diseases it is thought to be due to a form of autoimmunity (an immune or allergic reaction of the body against itself).

Most arthritic diseases do not affect only the joints. Joints are crossed by tendons from nearby muscles that move the joints and by ligaments that stabilize the joints. When the joint lining is inflamed, or the joint is swollen or deformed, those tendons, ligaments, and muscles can be affected. They may become inflamed, swollen, stretched, displaced, thinned out, or even broken. Also, in many places where tendons or muscles move over each other or over bones, there are lubricated surfaces to make the movement easy. These surfaces are called bursae; with arthritis, they too may become inflamed or swollen, causing bursitis. Thus, arthritis of any kind does not simply affect the joint. It can affect all of the structures in the region of the joint.

WHAT DOES ARTHRITIS DO?

From the foregoing discussion, you can see what arthritis does. As a result of irritation, inflammation, swelling, or joint deformity, it causes pain. The pain may be present all the time or only sometimes, as when moving the joint. Of all the symptoms of arthritis, pain is the most common.

Arthritis can also limit motion. The limitation may be due to pain, to swelling that prevents normal bending, to deformity of the joint or tendons, or to weakness in nearby muscles.

In addition, arthritis can cause problems in areas distant from the arthritis. For example, if the joints of a leg have arthritis, that leg may be favoured during walking or other motion. When favouring occurs, posture is often altered and an extra burden is placed on other muscles and joints. Abnormal posture or extra burdens can create pain in the affected areas.

One dramatic result of arthritis is stiffness. Stiffness of joints and muscles is particularly apparent after periods of rest such as sleeping and sitting. The stiffness makes it difficult to move. However, if you are able to get going, or if you can get heat to the affected joint and muscles (hot pad or hot shower), the stiffness lessens or disappears. For most people, the stiffness lasts only a short while; for an unlucky few, it can last all day. The cause of this stiffness is not clearly known.

Another common consequence of arthritis is fatigue. Here, again, the precise cause is not known. Inflammation itself causes fatigue. So does chronic pain, and so does the effort of movement when joints and muscles don't work right. In addition, fatigue is caused by the worries and fears that often accompany arthritis. Whatever its cause, or combination of causes, fatigue is an issue confronting most arthritis patients.

Fibromyalgia is a condition that is not inflammatory but creates muscle and joint pain similar to that of many patients with chronic inflammatory arthritis. Its cause is not yet known. It usually exists alone but sometimes accompanies a rheumatic disease. Anti-inflammatory treatment does not help. However, much of the self-management therapy used by patients with chronic arthritis is beneficial.

A final consequence of arthritis and fibromyalgia is depression. People with these conditions often have trouble doing what they need or want to do. This can make them feel helpless, angry, and withdrawn, which may lead to depression. Depression can make other symptoms such as pain, fatigue, and disability seem worse. It can reduce an individual's work or social functioning. It can damage family relationships, as well as the capacity for independent living. Usually the depression is the situational type, meaning that it comes from the difficulties caused by the arthritis and is not a mental illness. Often it improves when the arthritis improves, but it can also be helped through self-management and by the use of antidepressant medication.

Obviously, arthritis can have very damaging effects. In a sense, one might assume that the outlook for a person with chronic arthritis would be bleak. Actually, it is not. Much can be done to offset or eliminate the harmful effects of chronic arthritis. This and related books have been written to describe how that may be achieved. The remainder of this chapter will describe elements of appropriate management, some of which are developed in much greater detail elsewhere in this book.

PROGNOSIS, OR WHAT DOES THE FUTURE HOLD?

Most arthritic diseases, if left untreated, would have different outcomes for different people. Some people would progress more or less steadily to deformity. Others would experience disease that waxed and waned over many years, possibly getting slowly worse but maybe not. A lucky few would have the disease disappear spontaneously. With modern treatment, most patients fall in the last two categories, with far fewer patients proceeding to severe deformity than did years ago.

However, as people live longer without deformity, they also live longer with the various symptoms and problems created by arthritis. That is, they live a life that has been changed in some way by arthritis and, possibly, by the undesirable effects of treatment.

There is no real cure for any of the forms of chronic arthritis. With luck, the arthritis will subside partially or completely on its own. Medical treatment can usually suppress the symptoms and the inflammation, but often must be continued indefinitely. Proper self-management can add greatly to improvement and to the prevention of disability. This depends largely on the participation of the person with arthritis and the family. Therefore, prognosis, or what the future holds, cannot be predicted accurately for any individual. It depends partly on medical treatment and on the management program, partly on good fortune, and partly on the individual's own self-management efforts.

HOW IS CHRONIC ARTHRITIS TREATED?

Drug Treatment

Since there is no cure for most chronic arthritis, medical treatment is aimed at preventing or controlling inflammation and pain, and improving physical function. The drugs commonly used either help pain or reduce inflammation, or do both. When inflammation is reduced, pain usually declines and function increases.

Most types of chronic arthritis fluctuate in severity. That is, they get better and worse by themselves. The drugs can speed improvement but they do not cure. Therefore, they must usually be used for long periods of time. The commonly used drugs fall into four categories:

1. **Nonsteroidal anti-inflammatory drugs (NSAIDs).** These drugs have both pain-reduction and anti-inflammatory effects. Of all anti-inflammatory drugs, these are the weakest. They are usually the first drugs used to treat arthritis because they are often helpful and tend to have the least severe side effects. Representatives of this group include aspirin, Motrin, Indocin, Clinoril, Naprosyn, and Voltaren. In a way, acetaminophen (Tylenol) also falls in this group; it reduces pain but has no anti-inflammatory effect. When there is no inflammation involved in the arthritis, as is commonly the case with osteoarthritis, the anti-inflammatory activity of the drug is of no known importance; the benefit is derived from the pain-reducing effect, and therefore aspirin or Tylenol may be as effective as the other NSAIDs.

   Three new NSAIDs have been made available: Celebrex, Vioxx, and Bextra. In the pharmacy field, they fall in the COX-2 inhibitor category. This means that the drugs are designed to have anti-arthritic abilities similar to other NSAIDs but to be less damaging to the stomach and intestines. In practice, the "less damaging" property may be true, but the anti-arthritic effect is no better than that of other NSAIDs and may be less. Also, the drugs are expensive. They have recently been withdrawn from sale or restricted in use because, over time, they can cause heart and blood vessel disease. Potential damage to stomach and intestines by any NSAID can be greatly reduced simply by taking the drug in the middle of meals.

2. **Second-line or "disease-modifying" drugs.** The drugs in this category are all anti-inflammatory drugs, which are more powerful than the NSAIDs but are also potentially more toxic. The term "disease-modifying" is intended to imply healing of inflammatory arthritis, but healing from these drugs has not been proved. Members of this group of drugs are gold, penicillamine, methotrexate, Azulfidine, Plaquenil, and a new drug, leflunomide (Arava). They are usually used in inflammatory arthritis if NSAIDs fail. They are not used for osteoarthritis.

   In recent years, evidence has emerged indicating that earlier use of second-line agents slows the progression of the disease. Because the NSAIDs do not achieve such slowing, many patients with rheumatoid arthritis are receiving treatment with second-line agents early in the course of their disease. Such an early benefit from second-line agents has not yet been shown for other forms of chronic inflammatory arthritis.

3. **Corticosteroids.** Corticosteroids are powerful anti-inflammatory drugs that also suppress immune function. Both effects are helpful with inflammatory arthritis, especially for rheumatic diseases in which autoimmune abnormalities appear to play a role in causing the arthritis. Most corticosteroids in use are synthetic versions of a normal human hormone, cortisol, which is present in everybody and exerts a mild masculinizing effect in women. Corticosteroids are the most rapid-acting and effective of the anti-arthritic drugs, but may cause serious adverse effects when used for long periods of time. Prednisone is the most commonly used corticosteroid. One last note: Corticosteroids should not be stopped suddenly. Talk with your physician if you are thinking about stopping your use of steroids. This is important.

4. **Cytotoxic drugs.** These drugs, developed to treat cancer, also have anti-inflammatory and immunosuppressive effects. Examples include Cytoxan, Imuran, Leukeran, cyclosporine, CellCept, and Rituxan. These drugs can be quite toxic and only sometimes have clear advantages over other anti-arthritic drugs. They are usually used only after other drugs have failed to control the problem. They are never used for osteoarthritis.

5. **New biological agents.** Recent evidence has shown that a biological material called "tumor necrosis factor" (TNF) plays an important role in the inflammation of rheumatoid arthritis. TNF is a product of some of the cells involved in the inflammatory and immune responses and is a member of the cytokine family. Two methods of counteracting TNF have been developed, both of which neutralize TNF. One treatment uses an antibody to TNF called infliximab (Remicade) or adalimumab (Humira). The other treatment method uses a soluble receptor that is obtained from cells to neutralize the TNF. This material is called etanercept or Enbrel. Remicade is given intravenously, whereas Humira and Enbrel are injected subcutaneously (under the skin). These drugs are very expensive.

For osteoarthritis, two other therapies have been introduced. Both are intended to improve damaged cartilage or substitute for it. One is glucosamine, taken orally. The other is hyaluronan, injected into the joint. Studies suggest that glucosamine diminishes symptoms from osteoarthritis in the short term with a potency similar to low doses of NSAIDs. However, the studies are not definitive and long-term outcomes have not been established. Fortunately, glucosamine appears to have no significant adverse effects. Use of hyaluronan is more complicated because it requires injections, studies have not demonstrated real benefit to people with arthritis, and the treatment is expensive. Both methods of treatment appear not to be of decisive benefit to people with osteoarthritis; they have no theoretical or practical value in other forms of arthritis.

At times, other drugs are used. An example is colchicine, which, along with many of the above-mentioned drugs, is effective in treating gout. Antibiotics are used when the arthritis is due to infection.

Only occasionally do the drugs used to treat arthritis provide an immediate benefit. Usually many days or even weeks are necessary before the full effects of the drug are felt. Corticosteroids and colchicine are the exceptions; they can often produce benefit in a matter of hours.

It is almost impossible to predict beforehand whether any of the drugs will be helpful. Therefore, the treatment of chronic arthritis with drugs is a trial-and-error process, in which the physician usually starts with the mildest medications and proceeds to more powerful drugs if the milder forms fail to benefit the patient.

Most drugs for arthritis are taken by mouth. However, some (corticosteroids, methotrexate, gold, colchicine, Remicade, Humira, and Enbrel) can be or are given by injection into skin, muscles, or veins. Injection of corticosteroids directly into inflamed joints can sometimes be very beneficial.

Problems can be caused by the toxic effects of the drugs. All drugs can cause harm as well as benefit. Sometimes a particular drug can be very helpful but also cause so much harm that it cannot be used. Again, it is impossible to predict which drugs will be harmful. With some of the drugs, toxic effects cannot be recognized by the individual and, therefore, the individual must be monitored with blood counts, liver function studies, and/or analyses of urine. People starting on any drug treatment for chronic arthritis should make sure they understand the signs and symptoms of potential harm such as rash, upset stomach, or unusual thoughts, and notify the physician if such symptoms appear.

Sometimes, despite drug treatment, joints are damaged to the point where they cannot be effectively used. Fortunately, today, surgical techniques allow for the replacement of many types of joints, and some of the replacement joints function almost as well as natural joints.

Some years ago, each type of inflammatory arthritis was treated with a particular group of drugs. Today, almost all of the above drugs are used for any type of inflammatory arthritis. The choice of drugs depends on the person's condition and needs; commonly, milder drugs are used first and more powerful ones are used when milder ones fail. However, as mentioned earlier, stronger drugs are now often used earlier in rheumatoid arthritis in an effort to prevent joint destruction.

Drug treatment is usually helpful. However, it is by no means the only form of treatment. Other forms fall under the general heading of management methods and involve the active participation of the person with arthritis.

MANAGEMENT OF CHRONIC ARTHRITIS

In addition to treatment with drugs or surgery, there are many other ways to achieve good management of chronic arthritis. Certainly as much as for any disease, proper management of arthritis follows the principles outlined in the first two chapters of this book. To understand a complete arthritis management program, it is useful to recall the many consequences of arthritis previously mentioned.

The goal of proper management is not just to avoid pain and reduce inflammation; it is to maintain the maximum possible use of affected joints and the best possible function. This involves maintaining the fullest motion of the joint and the greatest strength in muscles, tendons, and ligaments surrounding the joint. *The key to this goal is exercise.* Exercise, discussed in detail in Chapters 6 through 9, is an essential part of any good management program. The exercise should be regular, consistent, and as vigorous as possible. The Arthritis Society has developed two exercise programs, Joint Works™, which is land-based, and Water Works™, which is done in warmer water swimming pools. While exercise may increase pain temporarily, it will not make the arthritis worse. In fact, failing to exercise can make arthritis symptoms worse because of physical deconditioning. The rule of thumb is that you should not have more pain after you exercise than before you start.

Heat is a helpful part of arthritis management. It reduces stiffness and makes movement easier. Many people find that heating joints just before exercise makes the exercise easier. Heat associated with rest can be very soothing. Occasionally, people find cooling of the joint with ice to be comforting. Cooling, however, does not increase mobility.

Control of fatigue is important. Rest periods between activities and restful sleep at night are essential for control. When pain disturbs sleep at night, different types of beds (foam beds, water beds) and the use of mild sedation can be of significant help. For some people with arthritis, low doses of anti-depression medication at bedtime will effectively control night pain.

Sometimes, when joint function remains limited, use of assistive devices can be of benefit. Many types of devices are available and are described in the books listed at the end of this chapter.

Altering your eating plan has little value with most types of chronic arthritis, particularly osteoarthritis and rheumatoid arthritis. (What you eat, however, is important for gout, where use of alcohol and eating certain meats can provoke attacks. People with gout should discuss this with their physicians.) In rare cases, food allergies can cause attacks of arthritis. There is some evidence that eating oils from cold-water fish can help people with rheumatoid arthritis; however, the benefit is small. Of course, it is not wise to be overweight, because that places an extra burden on joints. Most people with chronic arthritis should eat balanced, pleasurable meals and maintain a normal weight. Ways to do this are discussed in Chapter 13.

It is not surprising that sometimes in the struggle against arthritis, an individual becomes depressed. *It is important to recognize the depression and to seek advice from health professionals.* There are many ways to combat depression; the important thing is to know it is present and take steps to control it.

Most people with chronic arthritis are able to lead productive and satisfying, independent lives. The most important step in achieving this is to take an active part in managing your own arthritis. All of the components of management mentioned here either are the responsibility of the individual or are best done with the individual's participation. The rest of this book is devoted to making your participation most effective.

Community Resources

The Arthritis Society
www.arthritis.ca
e-mail: info@arthritis.ca

The Arthritis Society has Regional Offices in every province and territory. Books, brochures, information on local events, and current information on medication and treatment are available. The website features exercise tips, research information, and online shopping. Call the 1-800 number for referrals to telephone counselling service, and programs and resources in your community.

Suggested Further Reading

Arthritis Foundation Staff. *Living Better with Fibromyalgia*. Atlanta, Ga.: Arthritis Foundation, 1996.

Backstrom, Gayle, and Bernard Rubin. *When Muscle Pain Won't Go Away: The Relief Handbook for Fibromyalgia and Chronic Muscle Pain*, 3rd ed. Dallas, Tex.: Taylor Publishing, 1998.

Change Your Life! Simple Strategies to Lose Weight, Get Fit, and Improve Your Outlook. Atlanta, Ga.: Arthritis Foundation, 2002.

Davidson, Paul. *Chronic Muscle Pain Syndrome: The 7-Step Plan to Recognize and Treat It—and Feel Better All Over*, Berkley trade ed. New York: Berkley Books, 2001.

Fries, James F. *Arthritis: A Comprehensive Guide to Understanding Your Arthritis*, 5th ed. Reading, Mass.: Perseus, 2000.

Horstman, Judith. *The Arthritis Foundation's Guide to Alternative Therapies*. Atlanta, Ga.: Arthritis Foundation, 1999.

Koehn, Cheryl. Taysha Palmer and John Esdaile. *Rheumatoid Arthritis: Plan to Win.* Don Mills, Ont.: Oxford University Press, 2001.

Lorig, Kate, and James Fries. *The Arthritis Helpbook*, 6th ed. Reading, Mass.: Perseus, 2006.

Mosher, Dianne, Howard Stein, and Gunnar Kraag. *Living Well with Arthritis: A Sourcebook for Understanding and Managing Your Arthritis.* Toronto: Penguin Canada, 2006.

Millar, A. Lynne. *Action Plan for Arthritis: Your Guide to Pain-Free Movement.* Windsor, Ont.: Human Kinetics, 2003.

Sayce, Valerie, and Ian Fraser. *Exercise Beats Arthritis: An Easy-to-Follow Program of Exercise,* 3rd ed. Palo Also, Calif.: Bull Publishing, 1998.

Other Resources

The Arthritis Society. *Arthritis Answers Newsletter.* Available online or through Regional Development Offices.

MANAGING DIABETES

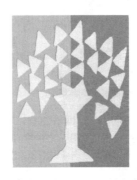

19

WHILE DIABETES IS A SERIOUS DISEASE, YOU CAN LIVE A LONG AND HEALTHY LIFE AND PREVENT COMPLICATIONS. Living well with diabetes requires both good medical care and effective self-management. Although there is much that health care providers can do, you must take responsibility for learning about diabetes and managing the daily decisions and actions necessary to deal with the disease. Before looking at all the options for self-management, however, let's talk about diabetes and its causes.

WHAT IS DIABETES?

Diabetes is a disorder of the body's endocrine system. It is a disease of the pancreas but also involves other organs and systems of the body, including the liver and digestive system. Diabetes causes the body to have difficulty using food to fuel the body and provide energy. To understand diabetes, it is helpful to know a little about the digestion process, the function of the pancreas and insulin in the body, and how these relate to diabetes. (See Figure 19.1.)

Some of the food we eat (carbohydrates and sugars) is broken down in the digestion process into a simple sugar called glucose. The glucose is absorbed into the bloodstream from your stomach, which makes your blood glucose levels rise. In order for the cells of your body to use the glucose from your blood as fuel, it needs the help of insulin. Insulin is a hormone produced by the pancreas, a small gland located below and behind your stomach. Insulin acts as a bridge that helps the blood glucose get from the bloodstream into the cells. Once inside the cells, the glucose is used to regenerate body tissue and provide energy.

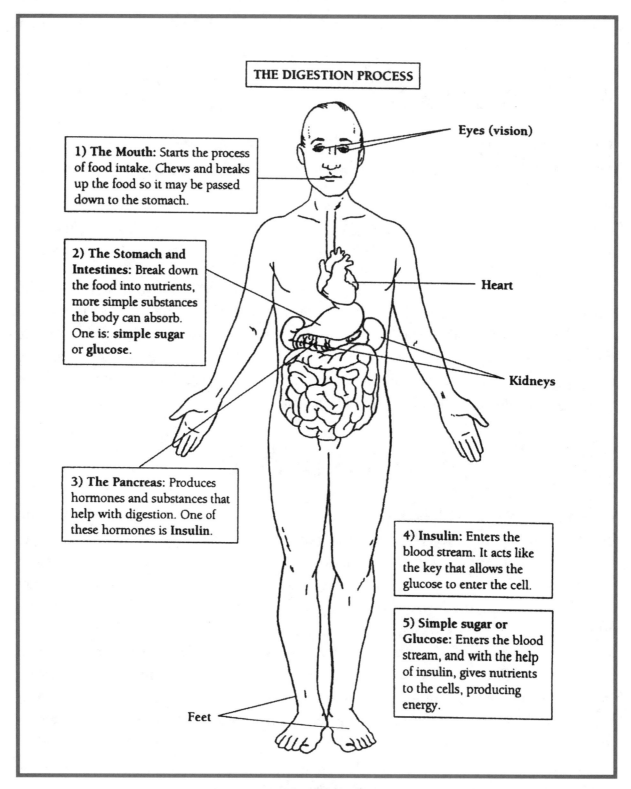

Figure 19.1 **The Digestion Process**

Glucose in the body can be compared to the gasoline in a car; they are each a fuel and a source of energy. Gasoline alone, however, is not enough to make the car move. We also need a key to start the motor, which allows the gasoline to be converted into energy. Like the car, our bodies also need a key that enables us to use glucose as energy. Insulin is this key; it carries the glucose from the bloodstream into the cells, where it produces energy for the body. Insulin is required for all life functions. Without it, we die.

In diabetes, insulin is not able to carry out its function properly because either the pancreas does not produce sufficient insulin, or the insulin that is produced cannot be used efficiently by the body. As a result, glucose rises to high levels in the blood. When the kidneys filter the blood, excess glucose spills out in the urine. This causes one of the symptoms of diabetes, which is frequent urination and large amounts of glucose in the urine. This is how diabetes got its name, diabetes mellitus. The Greek word *diabetes* means "to pass through," and the Latin word *mellitus* means "sugar" or "honey."

The cells of your body require a continual source of energy in order to survive. If glucose is not available from the blood due to a lack of insulin, body fat is broken down to be used for energy. When excess fat is broken down in the liver, acids called ketones are produced. Large amounts of ketones in the body can lead to a serious condition called diabetic ketoacidosis.

High blood glucose levels over time can damage blood vessels and nerves in vital organs throughout the body. This can cause heart disease, heart attacks and strokes; nerve damage causing tingling and numbness in hands and feet; kidney damage; eye damage causing vision problems; more frequent and serious infections and, possibly, loss of a limb due to poor circulation and nerve damage. By learning to manage your diabetes and controlling blood glucose levels, these complications can be prevented or delayed.

There are many different types of diabetes with many different causes. Despite ongoing studies in diabetes research, the exact cause of diabetes is still not known. Table 19.1 compares the two most common types, Type 1 and Type 2 diabetes. There is one thing common to all types of diabetes: The body does not produce enough insulin, or it cannot use the insulin that is produced.

Type 1 Diabetes

Type 1 diabetes usually starts in childhood, but it may also be diagnosed in adults. It appears to be more common in white Northern European populations. It is the type of diabetes that is primarily the result of the insulin-producing cells of the pancreas being destroyed. This form includes cases due to an autoimmune process, where the body's own immune system destroys the insulin-producing cells of the pancreas. In other cases of Type 1 diabetes, the causes of destruction of the insulin-producing cells are unknown. Destruction of the insulin-producing cells may be triggered by environmental factors in genetically predisposed people according to recent research published by the Canadian Diabetes Association. All people with Type 1 diabetes require insulin every day.

Type 2 Diabetes

Type 2 diabetes usually starts in adulthood, but it may also be diagnosed in children. It is the type of diabetes where the body can be resistant to insulin produced by the pancreas, or else the pancreas does not produce sufficient insulin. Insulin resistance means that the body is not effective in moving glucose from the blood into the cells. As a result, the glucose builds up in the blood because the body cannot use it efficiently.

Type 2 diabetes tends to run in families and appears to be more common in ethnic minority groups such as Aboriginal, Hispanic, Asian and Canadian First Nations populations, according to current information from the Canadian Diabetes Association. This form of diabetes also involves other body systems and organs such as the digestive system, the liver, muscles and body fat. The onset may be associated with other factors such as being overweight, an inactive lifestyle, eating habits, stress or some other illness.

Some people with Type 2 diabetes may be able to control their condition through a prescribed eating plan, exercising regularly and managing their weight. Others will require oral medications or insulin in order to control their blood glucose levels.

An important difference between Type 1 and Type 2 diabetes is that people with Type 1 diabetes require insulin every day in order to survive. People with Type 2 diabetes may or may not require insulin to manage their condition. Some similarities in symptoms can appear in both Type 1 and Type 2 diabetes. These include fatigue, increased appetite, blurry vision, frequent urination, excessive thirst, changes in mood, infections, and unexplained weight loss.

SELF-MANAGEMENT

No matter what kind of diabetes you have, there are two major self-management tasks to keep in mind. The first is to achieve and maintain a target blood glucose level. This means

Table 19.1 **Overview of Type 1 and Type 2 Diabetes**

Characteristics	Type 1 Diabetes (insulin dependent)	Type 2 Diabetes (may or may not need insulin and may need oral medications)
Age	Usually begins before age 20, but can occur in adults	Usually begins after age 40, but can occur in young adults and children
Insulin	Little or no insulin is produced by the pancreas	The pancreas produces insulin, but it may not be enough or it cannot be used by the body
Onset	Sudden	Slow
Sex	Males and females equally affected	More females are affected
Heredity	Some hereditary tendency	Strong hereditary tendency
Weight	Majority experience weight loss and are thin	Majority are overweight
Ketones	Ketones found in the urine	Usually there are no ketones in the urine
Treatment	Insulin, healthy eating, exercise, self-management	Healthy eating, exercise, self-management, and when necessary, oral medication and/or insulin

balancing all treatment methods, which includes healthy eating, exercise, managing stress and emotions, taking insulin or oral medications, and monitoring your blood glucose levels. The second task is to detect early any problems or complications caused by diabetes. Of course these two are very closely linked because high blood glucose levels cause many of these problems and complications. Diabetes care depends upon our daily commitment to self-management practices. Self-management comes more easily when we have the knowledge and skills required to manage diabetes on a day-to-day basis. We can ask for education and support from diabetes health care specialists. Some of the management tasks are discussed in more detail in the next section.

Maintaining Target Blood Glucose Levels

We know that the body gets nutrients and glucose through the digestive process. The blood carries this glucose to the body's cells, where it is converted into energy. Therefore, it is important to have a certain amount of glucose in your blood all the time, for your body to use for energy throughout the day. The goal of diabetes management is to maintain a blood glucose level appropriate for your condition. Target blood glucose levels for people with diabetes should fall within the following ranges

- Fasting, or before meals: 4.0 - 7.0 mmol/L
- 2 hours after a meal: 5.0 - 10.0 mmol/L
- 2 hours after a meal if the A1c target is not being met: 5.0 - 8.0 mmol/L
- A1c (3 month average):   7 % or less

The A1c is a test ordered by your doctor and is usually done every 3 months. It reflects the average of a person's blood glucose level over a 3 -month period.

Because blood glucose levels are recorded in mmol/L, and A1c levels are recorded as percentages, an A1c of 7 % does not mean that the average blood glucose level over 3 months was 7 mmol/L. Here are examples of what the A1c reflects.

Average blood glucose level, mmol/L	A1c %
7.5	6
9.5	7
11.5	8

Even if your A1c is 7 %, your average blood glucose over the past 3 months has been 9.5 mmol/L.

It is important to know what blood glucose level to aim for and maintain. The problems occur when the blood glucose level is either too high, called hyperglycemia, or too low, hypoglycemia. It is helpful to understand the causes and symptoms of high and low blood glucose (see Table 19.2) as well as what to do if your blood glucose level is too high or low.

Your job as a self-manager is to keep your blood glucose level as close as possible to your target level and to avoid too high or too low values. This is achieved by maintaining a balance between healthy eating, activity and exercise, and oral medications and/or insulin. In addition, strong emotions and illness can also affect blood glucose levels; therefore, knowing how to manage these effectively can help in controlling your diabetes.

Note: The blood glucose targets and A1c levels quoted above are from the 2008 Canadian Diabetes Association Clinical Practice Guidelines. Throughout Canada and the Territories, A1c is measured in mmol/L and percentages. You may notice that in handouts or articles on diabetes from the United States, blood glucose levels are measured in mgm/dL. A conversion chart might be helpful if you are reading articles from the United States or on the Internet.

HOME BLOOD GLUCOSE MONITORING

One of the most important self-management tasks is learning how to monitor your blood glucose level. This helps you to know what your blood glucose level is, and to maintain your target blood glucose level. As we said at the beginning, keeping your blood glucose level under control is a balancing act. Of course, there are tests that your doctor can do to monitor your condition, including the blood glucose tests (fasting or nonfasting) and the A1c. However, the most important tests are the ones you do at home on a daily basis.

Monitoring your blood glucose helps you know if the strategies you are using to control your diabetes are working. Only through monitoring and recording the results can you judge the success of your program and make appropriate adjustments. It is important to monitor your blood glucose regularly. How often you test is generally determined by the type of diabetes you have, how stable your blood glucose levels are, what medications or insulin you are taking and how you feel. The Canadian Diabetes Association Clinical Practice Guidelines recommend that people with Type 1 diabetes should monitor their blood glucose at least 3 times a day and more frequently if on intensive insulin manage-

Table 19.2 Causes and Symptoms of Hyperglycemia and Hypoglycemia In People With Diabetes (Mild, Moderate, to Severe)

HYPERGLYCEMIA (blood glucose level too high)	HYPOGLYCEMIA (blood glucose level too low)
CAUSES: Too little, or poorly timed insulin or oral medication Too much food or wrong types of food, especially foods high in carbohydrates; poorly timed or irregular meals Less exercise, etc. Using old or poor quality insulin; overuse of insulin sites Emotional stress Illness, such as fever, colds, flu or surgery	**CAUSES:** Too much, or poorly timed insulin; some types of oral medications. Not enough food; not eating regularly; late or missed meals; eating less carbohydrate without adjusting insulin More exercise without adjusting food or insulin Drinking alcohol on empty stomach Emotional stress Illness, such as stomach flu, vomiting
SIGNS AND SYMPTOMS: Slow onset in type 2; rapid onset in type 1 if insulin omitted Unusual, excessive thirst Frequent urination Fatigue, extreme tiredness Blurry vision Headaches Frequent or persistent infections Unexplained weight loss Nausea and vomiting Deep, rapid breathing Fruity-smelling breath High levels of ketones in the urine	**SIGNS AND SYMPTOMS:** Sudden, rapid onset. Cold, clammy skin or sweating Hard, fast heartbeat Hunger Numbness or tingling (in fingers and toes) Shaking, confusion, nervousness or irritability Slurred speech Headache Convulsions Night sweats Restless sleep Unconsciousness

ment. People with Type 2 diabetes on once-a-day insulin plus oral medications should test at least once daily at different times of the day. For all individuals with diabetes, more frequent blood monitoring before and after meals should be undertaken if more information is required to achieve desired blood glucose levels. You can work out an appropriate plan with your doctor and diabetes educator. Below we discuss the different ways that people with diabetes monitor their blood glucose level, as well as the advantages and disadvantages of each method.

Observing Symptoms

While it is important to recognize and know how you feel when your blood glucose is very low or high, this is not the best method for controlling your diabetes for two reasons. First, many people do not experience any symptoms until their blood glucose levels are already too high or too low. This makes it very difficult to stay within their appropriate blood glucose range. Second, many of the symptoms that someone might experience can be similar for both conditions: high and low blood glucose. Without knowing what the actual blood glucose level is, it is difficult to determine what steps to take to treat it.

Blood Glucose Monitoring

The main method of self-monitoring is testing your blood. This is a simple test that can be done at home or anywhere. To do the test, you need a small device called a blood glucose monitor or meter and test strips. There are several different types of meters, but all require that you prick the tip of your finger with a sterile needle to get a drop of blood. The drop of blood is then placed on a test strip that has been inserted into the meter. Within seconds, the meter gives a reading of your blood glucose level. This test helps you keep track of how well you are balancing your eating, exercise, and medications during the day and over time. This is the most efficient method for helping you to monitor and control your blood glucose levels, as you can adjust your self-management program according to the test results.

Your doctor or other health care team member can advise you on how often to self-test, and what actions to take based on the results. Remember, home glucose monitoring provides daily information and feedback that is useful to you, not just information to give to your doctor. It provides day-to-day feedback on how well you are controlling your blood glucose levels, and the effect of changes in diet, exercise, medications, and illness. Home blood glucose monitoring can help you feel more in control and know what actions to take to prevent symptoms and complications from diabetes.

Urine Testing

When the blood glucose levels are very high, excess glucose is filtered out of the body by the kidneys and passed in the urine. By testing the urine, you can see how much glucose is being lost. Usually this test is done in the morning before eating and the measurement is taken by dipping a test strip into the urine sample. The colour of the strip after testing tells you how much glucose is being lost. But if the blood glucose level is within the target range, or is too low, no glucose is deleted in the urine. Urine testing is useful only to let you know if glucose is being lost in the urine. Blood glucose monitoring is a much more accurate way of knowing how high or how low your blood glucose levels are throughout the day.

Urine testing is useful for many other tests so your doctor may ask you for a urine sample from time to time. The urine may also be tested to check for ketones when the blood glucose levels are high, for example, above 14 mmol/L. If the body is burning excess fat due to a lack of insulin, high levels of both glucose and ketones will be found in the urine. These are danger signs and should be treated immediately.

Ketones can also be measured by using a special strip in a blood glucose monitor that is designed to measure the levels of both blood glucose and blood ketones. Using this type of monitor is more accurate than urine testing. This is a specialized monitor or meter.

WHAT TO DO IF BLOOD GLUCOSE LEVELS ARE TOO LOW OR TOO HIGH

Monitoring your blood glucose levels every day will let you know if your blood glucose is too high, too low, or on target. Blood glucose levels can fluctuate widely. Go back to the section *Maintaining Target Blood Glucose Levels* on page 336 to see what ideal blood glucose levels should be before and after meals for most people with diabetes. Also check Table 19.2 on page 338 to find out the different possible causes, and the signs and symptoms of both hypoglycemia (low blood glucose) and hyperglycemia (high blood glucose).

Hypoglycemia

Hypoglycemia usually occurs in people who are taking insulin or certain types of oral hypoglycemic medications. The low blood glucose can be caused by too much insulin or medication, not enough food, or too much exercise without adjusting food. (see Table 19.2, page 338 for a detailed list of causes).

When the blood glucose falls too low (below 4 mmol/L) you may experience symptoms such as dizziness, shakiness, headaches, etc. (see Table 19.2, page 338 for a detailed list of signs and symptoms). If hypoglycemia is not treated quickly, an emergency situation may occur.

Severity of Hypoglycemia

Mild: when a person feels mild symptoms and can treat themselves.

Moderate: when a person feels moderate to severe symptoms but can still help or treat themselves.

Severe: when a person requires assistance from others and could become unconscious.

How to Treat Hypoglycemia
(Recommended in Canadian Diabetes Association Clinical Practice Guidelines 2008)

Mild To Moderate

When symptoms occur, check your blood glucose if possible. If the blood glucose is below 4 mmol/L, take 15 g of carbohydrate, preferably in the form of glucose tablets but other carbohydrates can be used such as:

- 3 teaspoons or 3 packets of sugar dissolved in water
- ¾ cup of juice or regular pop
- 6 lifesavers
- 1 tablespoon of honey

Wait 15 minutes. Check blood glucose level again. If still below 4 mmol/L, take another 15 g of carbohydrate. Once the hypoglycemia is reversed, eat the usual meal or snack. If the next mealtime is more than one hour away, eat a snack containing 15 g of carbohydrate and a protein such as a peanut butter or cheese sandwich.

Severe Hypoglycemia

If the person is conscious, they should be given 20 g of carbohydrate, preferably as glucose tablets or the equivalent.

Wait 15 minutes if possible. Check blood glucose level. If blood glucose is still below 4 mmol/l, give another 15 g carbohydrate. Continue as for mild to moderate treatment with a carbohydrate and protein snack if the next mealtime is more than one hour away.

Severe Hypoglycemia if Unconscious

If the person is unconscious, immediately call an ambulance at 911 or the local emergency number for your area.

If an individual is at risk for severe hypoglycemia, support persons should be taught how to give an injection of Glucagon (a hormone that releases glucose from the liver and immediately raises the blood glucose level).

Once the person is conscious and able to swallow, follow the treatment for mild to moderate hypoglycemia.

It is important to always carry emergency carbohydrate foods with you, and to know when to get medical help for treating low blood glucose. Therefore, we recommend you call the doctor or nurse for help if:

- you have repeated episodes of low blood glucose (more than three) within a week,

- your blood glucose is repeatedly lower than usual without cause, or

- you need help from another person when your blood glucose is low.

It is also recommended that a person with diabetes wear a medic alert bracelet and/or carry an emergency contact card at all times. The emergency card should also have information about the medication, doctor, and emergency contact person's name and number. This will help people know what to do and whom to contact in case of emergency.

Hyperglycemia

When your blood glucose gets too high (more than 10 mmol/L), this is considered hyperglycemia. This can occur gradually in people with Type 2 diabetes and sometimes does not cause any symptoms. Hyperglycemia can occur rapidly in people with Type 1 diabetes who do not take their insulin, or if their insulin pump malfunctions. If there are symptoms, they can include extreme thirst, frequent urination, fatigue, blurry vision, and so on (see Table 19.2, page 338). Hyperglycemia can be caused by too much food, not enough insulin or oral medication, or lack of exercise, etc. (see Table19.2 on page 338 for more details on the signs and symptoms of hyperglycemia). Fortunately, hyperglycemia can be monitored with daily blood testing. If you begin to notice a pattern in which your blood glucose is rising, you may want to watch carefully how much and what you are eating, increase your exercise, and talk to your doctor or nurse about possible changes in your medication or insulin dose.

When you have diabetes and get another illness (for example, a cold), you should also monitor your blood glucose carefully and follow the recommendations for what to do when you are sick, on pages 352 to 354.

How to Treat Hyperglycemia

Type 1 Diabetes

- Continue to take your insulin dose. You may need to increase your insulin if the hyperglycemia persists

- Eat your regular meals and drink plenty of extra sugar-free fluids

- Check your blood glucose levels every 4 hours. If your blood glucose level is more than 14 mmol/L, check your urine or blood for ketones.

- If ketones are present, you will need extra insulin in order to prevent the serious condition called diabetic ketoacidosis.

- Do not exercise while you have ketones in the blood or urine. This will increase ketone levels.

Type 2 Diabetes

- Continue to take your diabetes medications

- Eat your regular meals and drink plenty of extra sugar-free fluids

- Check your blood glucose levels 4 times a day before meals and at bedtime

- Try to do some extra exercise. Walking is good.

- If you take insulin, check for ketones and follow the treatment for Type 1 diabetes (above).

High blood glucose levels over long periods of time can cause serious diabetes-related complications.

Managing a Healthy Eating Plan

The Canadian Diabetes Association Clinical Practice Guidelines 2008 state that a healthy eating plan is considered to be Nutrition Therapy, which is an important part of the treatment and self-management of diabetes. What you eat can improve and maintain your quality of life and your nutritional and psychological health. Recent research indicates that nutrition therapy can reduce A1c levels by 1.0 % to 2.0 % and, when used with other self-management components of diabetes care, can improve your blood glucose control and help to reduce diabetes-related complications.

Although many people with Type 2 diabetes receive most of their diabetes care from a family doctor, it is recommended that all people with Type 1 or Type 2 diabetes receive nutrition counseling from a registered dietitian. The dietitian can work with you to make good food choices, how to space meals and carbohydrate intake, and how to balance or match food intake with insulin, diabetes medications and activity.

The way you eat makes a big difference in controlling your diabetes. However, for many people with diabetes, going on "diets" or making changes in eating habits can seem overwhelming. Remember, small changes in your eating can make important differences in your blood glucose levels and how you feel. Also, healthy eating can still be tasty, satisfying, and fun.

You do not have to go hungry or deprive yourself of the foods you like best, nor do you have to buy "special" food. An eating plan that is good for diabetes is also a healthier diet for all family members. Rather, you need to be careful only about the quantity and quality of the foods you eat so that each meal is nutritionally balanced. To do this, however, you may need to make changes in some of your eating habits. For example, you may need to eat more of some foods and less of others, eat a greater variety of foods, establish a regular schedule for your meals, and/or eat the same quantity or portions at each meal.

All foods contain nutrients that provide the body with energy. For people with diabetes, there are three types of nutrients that are important to consider when watching the way you eat: carbohydrates, proteins, and fats.

Carbohydrates

Carbohydrate foods cause the blood glucose levels to rise more rapidly than do proteins or fats. For this reason, it is important to be mindful of the total amount and type of carbohydrate foods eaten at each meal. The goal is to choose vegetables, fruits, grains, and pasta. These types of carbohydrates provide good nutrients, energy, and fibre but fewer calories and less fat. Try to limit carbohydrates with simple sugars, such as candy, cakes, cookies, sodas, and ice cream, which not only rapidly raise your blood glucose but also add fat and calories. This doesn't mean you can never have a slice of birthday cake again. Remember, moderation is the key to successful management of blood glucose.

The Glycemic Index
When considering what type of carbohydrates to eat, it is recommended that people with diabetes learn about the glycemic index (GI).

The glycemic index (GI) measures how carbohydrates in food affect blood glucose levels. High GI foods such as white bread, sugar, rice cakes and some cereals, raise the blood glucose quickly. Medium GI foods such as whole wheat bread, brown rice, popcorn and sweet corn, raise the blood glucose more slowly.

Low GI foods such as heavy mixed grain breads, oatmeal, pasta, sweet potatoes and legumes, raise the blood glucose the least of all carbohydrate foods. When you have diabetes, choosing low GI foods more often than high GI foods is recommended. For more information on the glycemic index and for a list of low, medium and high GI foods to

Table 19.3 **Recommended Targets for Glycemic Control**

	A1C* (%)	FPG or preprandial PG (mmol/L)	2-hour postprandial PG (mmol/L
Type 1 and Type 2 diabetes	≤ 7.0	4.0-7.0	5.0-10.0 (5.0-8.0 if AC1 targets not being met)

* Treatment goals and strategies must be tailored to the individual with diabetes, with consideration given to individual risk factors. Glycemic targets for children ≤ 12 years of age and pregnant women differ from these targets. See relevant guidelines for further details. An A1C of 76.0% corresponds to a laboratory value of 0.070.

A1C = glycated hemoglobin; FPB = fasting plasma glucose; PG = plasma glucose

Source: 2008 Clinical Practice Guidelines S30

Table 19.4 **Examples of Standard Alcoholic Drinks**

Drink	Ethanol content (%)	Quantity (mL)
Beer	5	341 (12 oz)
Table wine	12	142 (5 oz)
Spirits	40	43 (1.5 oz)
Fortified wine (e.g. sherry, port)	18	85 (3 oz)

choose from, see Chapter 13, pages 220-221, and Tables 19.3 and 19.4 on page 346. Information is also available from the Canadian Diabetes Association.

Proteins

Proteins are needed to repair muscle tissues, bones, and skin; they also supply energy for the body in the absence of carbohydrates. Generally, proteins are found in animal products like meat, fish, milk, and so on, as well as in vegetables and grain products. As animal proteins tend to be high in fat, try to choose low-fat sources of protein.

Fats

Fats are also used by the body for energy and help absorb certain vitamins. They are necessary for the body but, if consumed in excess, can lead to weight gain and affect the heart and other organs, complicating your diabetes even more. Choose low-fat or nonfat foods often. Reducing your intake of saturated fat sand keeping trans fatty acids to a minimum lowers your risk of developing heart disease. Adding food containing polyunsaturated omega 3 fatty acids (found in fatty fish and plant oils) may provide protection for your heart. You will find more detailed information about nutrition and guidelines for healthy eating in Chapter 13.

* * *

The eating plan for a person with diabetes is similar to that recommended for everyone: one that encourages you to eat a variety of foods. This has many advantages. Besides helping you to maintain an appropriate blood glucose level, it also helps you maintain a healthy weight, as well as reduce your blood pressure and cholesterol.

It is recommended that everyone with diabetes follow the *Eating Well with Canada's Food Guide*. This guide is published by Health Canada to meet the nutritional needs of people of all ages, and contains information of benefit to everyone. Information on *Eating Well with Canada's Food Guide* can be found in Chapter 13: Healthy Eating on pages 217-223.

Table 19.5 found on page 350 of this chapter provides a summary of nutritional considerations for people with diabetes using information from the *Eating Well with Canada's Food Guide*. The table comes from the Canadian Diabetes Association Clinical Practice

Table 19.5 Summary of Nutritional Considerations for People With Diabetes

People with diabetes should follow *Eating Well with Canada's Food Guide*

- Eat at least 1 dark green and 1 orange vegetable each day; have vegetables and fruit more often than juice
- Make at least half of your grain products whole grain, each day
- Drink lower-fat milk or fortified soy beverages
- Have meat alternatives such as beans, lentils and tofu often
- Eat at least 2 servings of fish each week
- Achieve and maintain a healthy body weight by being active
- Enjoy foods with little or no added fat, sugar or salt
- Satisfy thirst with water

Carbohydrates (45–60% of energy)

- Up to 60 g of added fructose (e.g. fructose-sweetened beverages and foods) in place of an equal amount of sucrose is acceptable
- Intake of <10 g/day of sugar alcohols (maltitol, mannitol, sorbitol, factitol, isomalt and xylitol) is acceptable
- The use of acesulfame potassium, aspartame, cyclamates, saccharin and sucralose is acceptable
- Include vegetables, fruit, whole grains and milk
- Within the same food category, consume low-glycemic-index foods in place of high-glycemic-index foods
- Increase dietary fibre to 25-50 g/day from a variety of sources, including soluble and cereal fibres
- Sucrose intake of up to 10% of total daily energy is acceptable

Protein (15-20% of energy)

- There is no evidence to suggest that usual recommended protein intake should be modified

Fat (<35% of energy)

- Restrict saturated fats to <7% of total daily energy intake and restrict trans fat intake to a minimum
- Limit polyunsaturated fat to <10% of energy intake
- Consume monounsaturated fats instead of saturated fats more often
- Include foods rich in polyunsaturated omega-3 fatty acids and plant oils

Vitamin and mineral supplements

- Routine supplementation is not necessary, except for vitamin D in persons aged >50 years and folic acid in women who could become pregnant
- In the case of an identified deficiency, limited dietary intake or special need, supplementation may be recommended

Alcohol

- People using insulin or insulin secretagogues should be aware of the risk of delayed hypoglycemia that can occur up to 24 hours after alcohol consumption
- Limit intake to 1-2 drinks per day (<14 standard drinks per week for men and ≤9 per week for women)

Source: 2008 Clinical Practice Guidelines S43

Guidelines, and provides you with some information on vitamin and mineral supplements and alcohol, as well as information on carbohydrate, protein and fat.

There is a lot to learn about healthy eating. Following are a few simple tips to get you started. These tips talk about starchy foods and fruits, which are carbohydrates, meats and alternatives which are proteins, vegetables which can provide carbohydrates, and protein, fats and milk products.

To keep your blood glucose levels in target range, it is important to balance the food you eat with the insulin or medications that you take, and the amount of activity that you do. Eating breakfast provides a good start to the day. To learn more, you can contact your local Canadian Diabetes Association office, or talk to a certified diabetes educator or dietitian at a Diabetes Education Centre or hospital near you. You may also call Dial-a-Dietitian. Check at the end of this chapter for more information.

Exercise

As with nutrition therapy, regular exercise will benefit you. Include sustained exercise that reaches your target heart rate. This might include swimming, stationary cycling, or dancing, along with brisk walking. Regular physical activity is one of the best things you can do to control diabetes and improve health. Exercise provides all the benefits for the person with diabetes that it does for everyone else. It keeps the joints flexible, strengthens the heart, lungs, and blood vessels to help prevent heart problems; reduces stress; and helps many people deal with sad or unhappy feelings. No one is too old to start some gentle physical activity.

Exercise is an effective way of lowering your blood glucose levels. It also provides the benefit of burning calories (energy), which helps you to lose weight or maintain a healthy weight. Exercise helps with weight control in three ways. First, we burn calories or energy while we are exercising. Second, exercise helps build and maintain muscle. Therefore, a steady supply of energy in the form of glucose needs to be supplied because the muscles are burning calories (using energy) 24 hours a day. This helps manage weight. Third, sustained aerobic exercise, which is exercise that raises your heart rate, makes you breathe harder or perspire and also increases the rate at which the body burns calories. For example, after about 30 minutes, the body will start to burn calories from fat to obtain the energy it needs to function; therefore, you are burning calories through an increase in your metabolism, as well as through exercise. When you stop exercising, your metabolism does not return immediately to normal. It remains slightly elevated for several hours after. Exercise changes the metabolism in the muscles and helps normalize blood glucose levels. Thus, you continue burning calories at an increased rate long after you finish exercising, helping your body use the glucose in the blood as energy. Each week we require a total of 150 minutes of moderate to vigorous-intensity aerobic exercise. This may include walking, bicycling, swimming or dancing, for 30 minutes each day, with no more than 2 consecutive days without exercise. We also benefit from resistance exercises such as lifting weights 3 times a week. The local recreation centre offers orientation programmes for fitness equipment and learning to meet your target heart rate. All ages can safely participate—even if you have not exercised for many years. The social aspect of group sessions provides another benefit. Let's get moving.

If you are just beginning an exercise program, start slowly. Five minutes of gentle physical activity, such as dancing to your favorite songs on the radio each day can make a big difference to your health and physical wellbeing. Before beginning a program of physical activity other than walking, people with diabetes should be assessed for conditions that might restrict certain types of exercise. Discuss your exercise program with your physician, diabetes educator or an exercise specialist.

Walking is the most popular and feasible type of aerobic exercise in most overweight middle-aged and elderly people with diabetes. Moderately brisk walking on level ground is an example of moderate aerobic exercise. For younger people, running would be vigorous aerobic exercise. During all of these activities, make certain that you are meeting your target heart rate. The Clinical Practice Guidelines suggest that several short sessions (lasting at least 10 minutes each) during the course of a day may be as useful as a single longer session.

Exercise is an important part of your self-management program because it helps to lower your blood glucose. Sometimes, particularly in people taking insulin or some oral medications that help them produce more insulin, exercise can lower the blood glucose too much, causing hypoglycemia. Therefore, it is important to find the best time during the day to exercise and to know how to treat hypoglycemia should it occur (see How to Treat Hypoglycemia on pages 341-342 of this chapter). Generally, the best time to exercise is when your blood glucose tends to be the highest, which is usually 1–2 hours after a meal. To reduce the probability of hypoglycemia, eating extra carbohydrates or reducing insulin before vigorous activity may be helpful. Before prolonged activity such as skiing, hiking or playing soccer, you may need to consume extra carbohydrates. In people with Type 1 diabetes, delayed overnight hypoglycemia may occur following vigorous afternoon or evening exercise. Your doctor or diabetes educator can suggest ways to prevent and manage this.

Exercise helps your diabetes by lowering blood glucose levels. It also lowers high blood lipid levels and high blood pressure. Your risk of cardiovascular complications is also reduced by frequent exercise.

For more information on how to develop and maintain an exercise program, see Chapter 6. Also, be sure to read page 159 for some special advice on exercise for people with diabetes.

Stress and Emotions

After learning that you have diabetes, you may be feeling angry, scared, or depressed. These feelings are normal, understandable, and manageable. For people with diabetes, stress and emotions such as anger, fear, frustration, and depression can affect blood glucose levels. For this reason, it is important to learn effective ways to deal with these feelings. Don't try to hide or suppress your emotions; these are a normal part of life and some of the work you will have to deal with in managing your condition. According to recent research released by the Canadian Diabetes Association, depression may be common in persons with diabetes. You may feel as if the adjustment to living with diabetes is overwhelming. Share your feelings. Once you feel as if you have some control in the decision-making, your stress will lessen and the management of your diabetes will seem easier. If you lose interest in doing things that previously gave you pleasure, talk with your physician or diabetes educator. A self-management program gives you the skills to cope and to improve your well being. To help you understand the impact of these feelings on your illness and identify some ways to manage them, read Chapters 4, 5, and 10.

Other Illnesses

Blood glucose levels are affected when we are sick with an infection, a cold or the flu. Blood glucose levels tend to go up with most illnesses, but can also go low if you have a stomach flu or gastritis, are vomiting and cannot eat. Maintaining awareness of your blood glucose level is important when you are sick. Your plan for sick days should include blood glucose testing, knowing what to do and when to seek additional help. Therefore, be sure you have the following on hand to help you manage your sick days:

- A family member or friend who is ready and able to help you when needed. This person should also know what to do to help you and when to call the doctor or when to take you to the emergency room, if needed.

- Have plenty of both sweetened and unsweetened or sugarless liquids on hand.

- Have a thermometer at home and learn how to use it.

- Have acetaminophen or ibuprofen available to treat pain and fever. Have gravol available to treat nausea and vomiting

- Have your blood glucose monitor available and teach your family member or friend how to use it and to interpret the results

- Have your emergency medical information on hand (including doctor's number, list of medications with and/or insulin doses, a list of medications and so on).

Talk with your doctor and/or diabetes educator so you are clear about when they want you to call them.

What to Do When You Are Sick

When you are sick, your self-care management will be different on days when your blood glucose is high compared to days when your blood glucose is low. It will also be different depending on whether you have Type 1 or Type 2 diabetes. Your individual sick day plans should be written out and kept in an easy to find location.

Following are some general guidelines for managing sick days.

Managing Sick Days When Your Blood Glucose Is High

Type 1 Diabetes

- Continue to take your insulin dose. Never omit your insulin—even if you are nauseated and vomiting

- Drink plenty of clear, sugar-free fluids to avoid dehydration

- Eat your regular meals if you are able to, or try frequent snacks

- Check your blood glucose level every 2-3 hours

- If your blood glucose is over 14 mmol/L, check your urine or blood for ketones

- If ketones are present, avoid activity as this will increase ketone production

- If your blood glucose is over 17 mmol/L and you have ketones in your urine or blood, you will need to take extra insulin every 2-3 hours until the blood glucose level comes down below 17 mmol/L and the ketones diminish or disappear. Take the amount of insulin suggested in your sick day plan, or call your doctor for advice

- Acetaminophen or ibuprofen may be taken for pain and fever. Gravol may be taken to relieve nausea or vomiting

- Seek medical help if your condition worsens

- Ask a family member or friend to be with you for support.

- If you do not take your insulin when your blood glucose levels are high, you can very quickly develop the serious condition called diabetic ketoacidosis.

Type 2 Diabetes

- Continue to take your diabetes medications—even when you are sick

- Drink plenty of clear sugar-free fluids, including clear broth

- Eat small, frequent meals or snacks

- Check your blood glucose level at least 4 times a day

- If your blood glucose level is too high, and/or you have a high fever, call your doctor or diabetes educator

- Acetaminophen or ibuprofen may be taken for pain and fever. Gravol may be taken to relieve nausea or vomiting

- Ask a family member or friend to be with you when you are sick; seek medical help if your condition worsens

- If you are taking insulin, check your urine or blood for ketones if your blood glucose level is above 14 mmol/L. If ketones are present, follow the guidelines as for Type 1 diabetes—or seek medical help

Managing Sick Days When Your Blood Glucose Is Low

Type 1 diabetes, or for those with Type 2 diabetes taking insulin

- If you are unable to eat or drink due to flu, gastroenteritis, nausea or vomiting, your blood glucose level may drop.

- Despite low blood glucose levels, it is important to remember that some insulin is always required. Your normal insulin dose may be reduced. Follow the instructions on your sick day plan, or call your doctor or diabetes educator for advice

- Take sips of fluids containing sugar, suck on popsicles or hard candy, or eat small amounts of sweetened Jell-O

- Check your blood glucose level frequently, every 30 minutes to 1 hour

- Keep your blood glucose level above 4 mmol/L

- Gravol may be taken to relieve nausea and vomiting and to allow you to drink frequent sips of sugar-containing fluids

- If blood glucose levels fall below 4 mmol/L, follow the guidelines for treating hypoglycemia found on pages 341-342 of this chapter

- Mini doses of the hormone glucagon (which raises blood glucose levels) can raise and maintain blood glucose levels during illness. Check with your doctor before you become ill - be prepared.

- Keep yourself safe. Ask someone to be with you when you are sick and your blood glucose levels are low

- Resume eating small, frequent meals and snacks containing carbohydrates as soon as possible

Type 2 Diabetes (not on insulin)

- Only certain types of diabetes medications called insulin secretagogues are likely to contribute to very low blood glucose situations. Ask your doctor about the types of diabetes medications you are taking and which you should omit on a day you are nauseated or vomiting

Table 19.6 **Types of Insulin (Approved for Use in Canada)**

Insulin Type/Action (Appearance)	Brand Names (Generic Name in Brackets)	Dosing Schedule
Rapid-Acting Analogue (Clear) • Onset: 10-15 minutes • Peak: 60-90 minutes • Duration: 3-5 hours	Apidra® (insulin glulisine) Humalog® (insulin lispro) NovoRapid® (insulin aspart)	Usually taken right before eating, or to lower high blood glucose
Short-Acting (Clear) • Onset: 30 minutes • Peak: 2-3 hours • Duration: 6.5 hours	Humulin®–R Novolin®ge Toronto	Taken about 30 minutes before eating, or to lower high blood glucose
Intermediate-Acting (Cloudy) • Onset: 1-3 hours • Peak: 5-8 hours • Duration: Up to 18 hours	Humulin®–N Novolin®ge NPH	Often taken at bedtime, or twice twice a day (morning & bedtime)
Long-Acting Analogue (Clear and Colourless) • Onset: 90 minutes • Peak: None • Duration: Up to 24 hours (Lantus 24 hours, Levemir 16-24 hours)	Lantus® (insulin glargine) Levemir® (insulin detemir)	Usually taken once or twice a day
Premixed (Cloudy) A single vial or cartridge contains a fixed ratio of insulin (the numbers refer to the percent of rapid- or fast-acting insulin to the percent of intermediate-acting insulin)	PREMIXED REGULAR INSULIN–NPH • Humulin® (30/70) • Novolin®ge (30/70, 40/60, 50/50) PREMIXED INSULIN ANALOGUES • Humalog® Mix25 and Mix50 • NovoMix 30	Depends on the combination

Adapted from the Canadian Diabetes Association 2008 Clinical Practice Guidelines for the Prevention and Management of Diabetes in Canada.

Table 19.7 **Medications Used for Non-Insulin-Dependent Diabetes**

Name of Medication	How It Works
Biguanides: Metformin (Glucophage)	Decreases glucose production in liver
Sulfonylureas: Tolazamide (Tolinase), tolbutamide (Orinase), glipizide (Glucotrol), glyburide, (DiaBeta, Micronase), chlorpropamide (Diabinese)	Increases insulin secretion
Alpha-glucosidase inhibitors: Acarbose (Precose) *Thiazolidinediones:* Pioglitazone (Actos)	Slows digestion and absorption of carbohydrates Increases use of insulin in muscle cells, decreases insulin resistance
Meglitinides: Repaglinide (Prandin)	Stimulates pancreas to release more insulin right after meals

- Follow the instructions on your individualized sick day plan

- Check your blood glucose levels 4 times a day, if possible

- If your blood glucose level is low, take sips of sugar-containing fluids. If your blood glucose is within target range or higher, switch to sugar-free fluids

- As soon as possible, begin eating small, frequent meals or snacks containing carbohydrates

- Gravol may be used to relieve nausea and vomiting

- Because people with Type 2 diabetes are often taking medications for high blood pressure and high cholesterol levels as well as diabetes medications, it is important to resume taking these as soon as possible

In any illness situation, knowing who and when to call for appropriate medical help is important. Have current blood glucose levels, and the names and doses of all the medications you take, available for medical personnel when you call. Take this information with you if you need to go to the hospital.

Influenza and Pneumococcal Immunizations

The Canadian Diabetes Association recommends:

- an annual influenza vaccine to reduce the risk of potential complications associated with influenza epidemics.

- that you consider a vaccination against pneumococcus.

Insulin Injections

Insulin is a hormone that allows glucose from the blood to pass into the cells of the body to be used for energy and to regenerate body tissue. A person cannot live without insulin. Insulin is used to treat everyone with Type 1 diabetes and for some people with Type 2 diabetes. It is used to replace the insulin that is not produced and/or is inadequately utilized by the body. Insulin is taken by injection. Insulin can be administered by an insulin syringe and needle, an insulin pen or an insulin pump (called continuous subcutaneous insulin infusion [CSII]). When you start on insulin therapy, you will receive both initial and ongoing education that includes:

- how to administer insulin

- how to care for and use insulin

- how to prevent, recognize and treat hypoglycemia

- how to manage sick days

- how to adjust insulin for food intake (e.g. carbohydrate counting)

- how to adjust insulin to control fluctuating blood glucose levels

- how to adjust insulin for vigorous or prolonged exercise

Insulin regimens are tailored to meet your individual needs, and are based on your lifestyle, food intake, age, general health, motivation, awareness of hypoglycemia, and how you self-manage your diabetes. Multiple daily injections or continuous subcutaneous insulin infusions (pumps) are the recommended insulin regimens for all adults with Type 1 diabetes. This intensive treatment can greatly reduce or delay the onset of heart and blood vessel complications. For people with Type 2 diabetes who have high A1c levels, and have difficulty controlling their blood glucose levels with oral medications, the addition of insulin can greatly improve their diabetes control.

Insulin preparations are classified according to the number of hours they work to control blood glucose levels, how long they take to begin to work, and their peak action times. Rapid- and fast-acting insulins are called bolus insulins; intermediate- and long-acting insulins are called basal insulins. Most people take a combination of basal and bolus insulin. There are also premixed insulins where a single cartridge or vial of insulin contains a combination of basal and bolus type insulins. See Table 19.6 on page 355 for an overview of all types of insulin available in Canada.

It is important that you know the type(s) of insulin you are taking, the manufacturer of the insulin, the dose or number of units you require, and how to adjust your dose. Discuss with your doctor or diabetes nurse educator the type of insulin you are taking.

Diabetes Medications/Pills

Because the diagnosis of type 2 diabetes is often delayed, many people already have some heart and blood vessel complications when they are diagnosed. It is possible for some people with Type 2 diabetes to begin treatment with lifestyle changes such as healthy eating, increased exercise and loss of weight. Usually, though, if blood glucose targets are not achieved within 2-3 months of making lifestyle changes, then antihyperglycemic (diabetes) medications should be started.

There are many different types of diabetes medications that control the blood glucose levels in different ways. Your doctor will adjust and might combine different antihyperglycemic (diabetes) medications in order to help you attain a target A1c level of 7 % or less within 6 to 12 months of your being diagnosed. A combination of healthy eating, increased activity or exercise, the loss of just 5 % of your pre-diagnosis body weight, and taking diabetes medications, can greatly improve your blood glucose control. This will also reduce your risk of developing serious diabetes complications.

Because many people diagnosed with Type 2 diabetes also have high blood pressure, high cholesterol levels and, possibly, some damage to the cardiovascular system, they may also be required to take medications for these conditions as well. Taking all your prescribed medications at the correct times is an important part of your self-management program. Keep a record of all the medications you take, including the dosages and times of day they should be taken. Some medications should be taken just before eating, or with a meal, to reduce the chance of stomach upsets.

Diabetes medicines are categorized according to how they work in the body. Some slow the absorption of glucose from the gut (stomach and intestines), some stimulate your pancreas to produce more insulin, some reduce the amount of glucose produced by the liver, while some sensitize your cells and make them less resistant to the insulin you make. There are also new Incretin agents that work in the intestines, and antiobesity agents. Talk with your doctor about the type of medication(s) he/she has prescribed for you and why. See Table 19.7 on page 356 for a list of antihyperglycemic medications for use in Type 2 diabetes.

Complementary and Alternative Medicines

Many people with diabetes may use complementary and alternative medicines (CAM) such as herbs and dietary supplements in the belief that they will help lower their blood glucose levels. Currently, there is not enough science-based evidence available to show that they are safe and effective. Recent research, reported by the CDA, indicated that popular products containing chromium, magnesium, and vanadium were ineffective for glycemic control. There may be side effects and interactions with other medications. Discuss these products with your doctor before using them.

Timing and Balance

We have talked about healthy eating, exercise, emotions, illnesses, insulin and medications, now let's look at timing and balance. All of these factors are related and interact in helping to maintain the blood glucose level. For example, increased exercise may lower blood glucose, and this may allow you to increase the amount you eat or reduce (under the guidance of your doctor) the dosage of your diabetes medications or insulin. Knowing your blood glucose levels is important for understanding how well you are balancing healthy eating, exercise, illnesses, insulin and/or medications. Blood glucose monitoring forms an important part of your successful self-management program.

You will find that working with your doctor, diabetes educator and dietitian to achieve this balance and to maintain blood glucose targets may help to prevent or to delay some of the serious complications of diabetes. Resources at the end of this chapter will help you find the best plan for you and keep you positive.

The ABC's of Diabetes Management

We have learned that the risks for diabetes and heart disease are partners. It is our job to control blood glucose levels and to also meet blood pressure targets and LDL (low density) cholesterol targets. Each visit with our doctor or diabetes educator is an opportunity to help us reach the following targets:

- A. A1c (A measure of the average blood glucose levels over the past 3 months): 7 %, or less

- B. Blood pressure: 130 / 80 mm Hg, or less

- C. Cholesterol: 2.0 mmol/ (LDL-C), or less

(These targets are recommended in the *Canadian Journal of Cardiology*, 2006: 22 (11) and in the Canadian Diabetes Association publication *Diabetes Dialogue*, 2009: 56 (1) that can be found on the web site www.diabetes.ca.)

PREVENTING THE COMPLICATIONS OF DIABETES

Unfortunately, poor diabetes control can lead to other complications. These complications include damage to the cardiovascular system such as heart disease, heart attacks or strokes; nerve damage (neuropathy, which causes burning, tingling or numbness in the hands and feet); kidney damage and chronic kidney disease; eye damage and eye disease (retinopathy);

foot problems which could lead to foot ulcers, infections and even amputation; erectile dysfunction in men with diabetes; bladder infections, and gum disease. Because diabetes can silently progress and damage other organs of the body, it is important to practise the following measures to prevent or delay these more serious complications:

- Maintain your blood glucose levels between 4.0-7.0 mmol/L before meals and between 5.0 - 10.0 mmol/L two hours after a meal, or as recommended by your doctor

- Do home blood glucose testing regularly and keep a written record.

- Do not smoke or, if you smoke, take steps to quit.

- Take all prescribed insulin and/or medications, including medications to control high blood pressure, lower cholesterol levels, and to prevent heart disease, stroke and kidney disease (such as low-dose aspirin, statins and ACE inhibitors).

- Make sure your blood pressure is in good control, 130/ 80 (see the ABC's of Diabetes Management on page 360 of this chapter). Control of your blood pressure is as important as control of your blood glucose levels if you have diabetes. Have your blood pressure checked at every diabetes-related doctors visit, and at least once a year.

- Make sure your cholesterol levels are in good control. For LDL (low density) or bad cholesterol, the recommended target is 2.0 mmol/L (see the ABC's of Diabetes Management on page 360 of this chapter). Your blood should be tested for cholesterol levels every 1-3 years, or more frequently if you are taking medications to lower cholesterol.

- Practice proper foot care at home (see the section on Foot Problems/ Foot Care on page 367 of this chapter). Have an annual testing of nerve sensation in your feet.

- Have regular check-ups with your doctor. At every visit, remind the doctor and nurse that you have diabetes. This is the time to request the following tests and procedures to be ordered and done:

  - The doctor or nurse checks your blood pressure at every visit and at least once a year

  - The doctor examines your feet at every visit and tests the nerve sensation in your feet once a year

  - You take along your home glucose testing results for the doctor to see and compare with your A1c results

Table 19.8 **Recommended Regular Screening Tests**

	Recommended Screening
Blood Glucose	Self-monitoring of blood glucose daily according to the schedule recommended. A1c measured every 3-6 months depending on your blood glucose control
Blood Pressure	At every diabetes-related doctors visit, and at least once a year
Cholesterol	Blood test every 1-3 years. More frequently if you are on medications to lower cholesterol levels
Heart Disease	A resting electrocardiogram at age 40 years followed by repeat testing and/ or an exercise stress test every 2 years for those at risk
Nerve Damage	Yearly testing of sensation in feet
Foot Problems	Yearly foot exam or more frequently for people at high risk for foot problems
Eye Disease	An eye exam through dilated pupils every 1-2 years by an eye care professional. More frequently if eye disease is present
Kidney Disease	Blood and urine tests to check for protein in the urine once a year, or every 6 months if you have chronic kidney disease
Erectile Dysfunction	When a man is diagnosed with diabetes and, if problems are evident
Depression/ Anxiety	People with diabetes should be checked periodically for signs of depression, and at any point when symptoms arise (see page 351 of this chapter under Stress and Emotions)

- Check that the doctor has ordered the following blood and urine tests for you:

  – An A1c level. Should be done every 3 months if your blood glucose levels are in poor control, Can be done every 6 months if your blood glucose levels are in good control

  – A blood cholesterol level. Should be done every 1-3 years but more frequently if you are taking medications to lower your cholesterol levels. (For A1c, blood pressure and cholesterol level targets, see the ABCs of Diabetes Management on page 360 of this chapter)

  – Blood and urine tests to check your kidney function. Should be done once a year or every 6 months if you have chronic kidney disease

  – A referral to an eye care specialist for examination of your eyes (including the retina at the back of the eye). Every 1-2 years or more frequently if you have eye complications

  – Annual influenza vaccination

  – A pneumococcal (pneumonia) vaccination. This can be repeated once if you are over 65 years of age

- Protect your skin. Don't get sunburned, and keep your skin clean.

- Clean and floss your teeth daily. Have regular checkups with the dentist.

- Set personal goals to control your diabetes, and review/revise them regularly.

- Attend a diabetes education program to learn more about your condition.

Before reading about the complications of diabetes in more detail, it might be useful to review the recommended regular screening tests used to identify early problems in adults with diabetes

Cardiovascular Disease/Heart Disease

People with diabetes have a greater chance of getting cardiovascular disease such as heart disease, heart attacks and stroke. In fact, heart disease is the number one cause of death for people with diabetes. Heart disease occurs because the walls of the blood vessels tend to harden and become blocked when blood glucose levels are elevated over many years. This leads to poor circulation and obstruction to the blood vessels of the heart or other parts of the body, which can result in heart disease, heart attacks, and stroke. The risk of cardiovascular disease can be lessened by not smoking, controlling your blood pressure, following a healthy diet, exercising regularly, achieving a healthy weight, controlling your blood glucose levels and by taking medications as prescribed by your doctor, such as low-dose aspirin, statins, ACE inhibitors or ARBs, which provide further protection for your heart and blood vessels. For example, recent research suggests that people with diabetes have less risk of having a heart attack if they take a statin medication, even if their cholesterol levels are already low. Be sure to discuss with your doctor if taking low dose aspirin, statins, ACE inhibitors, or ARBs are right for you.

The Canadian Diabetes Association recommends that all people with diabetes have a resting electrocardiogram if they are:

- 40 years or older

- Have lived with diabetes for 15 years or more

- Have high blood pressure

- Have protein in their urine indicating kidney damage

- Have any signs of peripheral vascular disease

The electrocardiogram (ECG) measures the electrical activity of the heart. This test may be repeated every two years for people considered at high risk for cardiovascular disease, or as your physician determines.

Kidney Disease

Kidney damage followed by chronic kidney disease is one of the more common and serious complications of diabetes. The kidneys are responsible for filtering the blood, and are continuously filtering excess glucose from the body when the blood glucose levels are high. This excess glucose can block and quickly damage the tiny blood vessels of the kidneys, leading to loss of kidney function and eventually to chronic kidney disease (CKD).

Often there are no signs or symptoms until kidney damage is severe. It is important to perform regular screening tests to identify kidney damage and to start treatment early to delay or prevent loss of kidney function.

See the recommended schedule for kidney screening tests on page 362 of this chapter. Achieving the best possible blood glucose and blood pressure control through self-management of diabetes can help to prevent the onset and delay the progression of CKD. Urine tests determine how well the kidneys are functioning. The same medications that can protect against heart disease can also be used to protect against kidney disease. The Canadian Diabetes Association recommends that adults with diabetes who show persistent protein in their urine receive ACE inhibitors or ARBs to delay the progression of CKD— even if their blood pressure is within normal limits.

Eye Disease/Vision Problems

Blurred vision is very common with high blood glucose levels but can also occur with low blood glucose. The blurring goes away, however, when the blood glucose is brought under control. Of more concern is a condition called diabetic retinopathy, in which the small blood vessels of the eye become blocked and break, causing bleeding and damage to the retina (the light-sensitive membrane located at the back of the eye). This damage can cause vision problems and sometimes blindness. Diabetes eye disease or retinopathy is the main cause of new cases of legal blindness in people of working age. As with kidney disease, often there are no symptoms until serious damage to the eye has occurred. The condition can often be controlled if it is detected and treated early.

Like cardiovascular disease and kidney disease, diabetic eye disease is caused by high blood glucose levels over a period of time that block and damage the tiny blood vessels in the eye. Also, as with cardiovascular disease and kidney disease, achieving good control of your blood glucose levels can reduce the risk of developing serious vision problems. It is recommended that everyone with diabetes have a regular eye examination (see the recommended schedule for eye screening tests on page 362). When you go for this exam, be sure to tell the doctor that you have diabetes and that you especially want him or her to check for diabetic retinopathy. This examination of the retina is different from the test to check your vision to see if you need glasses or corrective lenses. If you are found to have diabetic retinopathy, more frequent eye examinations will be necessary.

Erectile Dysfunction (ED)

ED affects approximately 34-45 % of men with diabetes. It is caused by damage to the blood vessels and may also be one of the earliest signs of cardiovascular disease. This is not the time to be shy if you are a man with diabetes. Your doctor is a good resource on methods of coping with this condition. Diabetes does not mean an end to sexual activity.

Nerve Damage

Nerve damage, or neuropathy, is very common in people with diabetes. Forty to 50 per cent of people with diabetes will develop nerve damage or neuropathy within 10 years of being diagnosed with diabetes. The symptoms range from burning pain and numbness in the feet, legs, or hands to dizziness upon standing. A person with neuropathy may also have sexual problems such as impotence or vaginal dryness. Everything that is controlled by the nerves can be affected one way or another by diabetes. Their doctor should screen all people with diabetes for neuropathy at least once a year. To prevent the onset or to delay the progression of neuropathy, optimal control of blood glucose levels is recommended. Pain due to nerve damage can be difficult to treat, but medications prescribed by your doctor may help. Discuss any symptoms with your doctor.

Infection

Infections of the skin, bladder, kidneys, vagina or gums occur because the immune system is not as effective at killing the bacteria or viruses that enter the body when blood glucose levels are high. Also, if your blood glucose is high, there is likely to be more glucose in your urine, which stimulates the growth of microorganisms that can cause infections of the bladder and kidneys. If your diabetes is poorly controlled, your body's capacity to defend itself against infection is diminished. For this reason, it is important to control your blood glucose levels and to treat any injury or infection immediately. It is also important to take good care of your skin, keeping it clean and dry and using a moisturizer to keep it from drying out. This is especially necessary when taking care of your feet.

Foot Problems/Foot Care

People with diabetes have several reasons for being concerned about their feet. A decrease in blood circulation to the legs and feet can result in infection in the legs and feet. This is

For Proper Foot Care, Remember to . . .

- **Check your feet every day.** You or someone else should look between the toes and on the tops and bottoms of the feet for cuts, cracks, sores (e.g., corns, calluses, or blisters), ingrown toenails, extreme dryness, bruises, redness, swelling, or pus.

- **Wash your feet every day.** Use mild soap and warm (not hot) water. Be sure to test the water's temperature with your elbow first. DO NOT SOAK your feet.

- **Gently dry your feet well between the toes.**

- **Cut your toenails straight across.** Do not cut the back corners of the nail. If you can't safely trim your toenails, ask a family member to do it or get professional help. Also, do not clean under your toenails or remove skin with sharp objects.

- **Rub a mild lotion on your feet before bed if the skin is dry (except between the toes).**

- **Wear comfortable shoes and socks (never go barefoot except when bathing or in bed).** Your shoes should support, protect, and cover your feet. If your feet sweat, use powder. Check inside your shoes before putting them on, and break in new shoes gradually. Also, avoid socks with tight, elastic tops.

- **Have your doctor or other clinician check your feet.** When you go to the doctor, take off your shoes and socks so that your feet can be easily examined.

- **Always get early treatment for foot problems.** A minor irritation can lead to a major problem if not properly cared for early.

why little cuts and sores do not heal well and become infected. Next, since the feet are a long way from the heart, sometimes they do not get all the blood they need. This is especially true if there is some narrowing of the blood vessels. The narrowing of the blood vessels can be due to blood vessel damage caused by high blood glucose levels when our diabetes is not well controlled. When the feet do not get enough blood, they do not get sufficient oxygen. Oxygen is needed to prevent tissue damage and to help the healing process.

When people also have nerve damage (neuropathy) from diabetes, they often have numbness in the feet. This can cause the feet to be less sensitive to heat, cold, and pain. Thus, when any injury occurs, you may not be able to feel it until the damage is quite severe.

Fact or Myth?

Fact or Myth? Diabetes is caused by eating too much sugar.
Answer: Myth. Eating too much sugar does not cause diabetes. However, too much sugar may contribute to obesity. Obesity causes insulin resistance (making it more difficult for your own insulin to work) and this is a leading cause of diabetes.

Fact or Myth? If I don't have to take insulin, my diabetes really isn't that bad.
Answer: Myth. Taking insulin is just one way to help manage diabetes, just like exercising, eating well, and taking medications by mouth. Some people think that if they don't take insulin, their diabetes is not really that bad. Regardless of whether someone takes insulin or not, there is still a risk for developing complications from diabetes. This risk is directly linked to how well your blood glucose is controlled.

Fact or Myth? People with diabetes have about the same risk as anyone else for heart disease.
Answer: Myth. Heart disease and stroke are the biggest killers of people with diabetes. The good news is that there are many things you can do to help reduce this increased risk.

Fact or Myth? It is important to monitor my blood glucose so that my health provider will know how I am doing.
Answer: Myth. In fact, glucose monitoring is a day-to-day self-management tool for YOU. Your provider gets a much better idea of how you are doing from your A1c. Your daily measures help you understand the effect of diet, exercise, stress, medications, and illness as well as how well you are doing in controlling your diabetes. Of course, you should share with your provider any information you get from your monitoring that you do not understand or that concerns you.

Learning about choosing proper footwear and caring for your feet, along with preventing injury and recognizing signs and symptoms (such as cuts, infections and ingrown toenails) that warrant a visit to the doctor, will help to keep your feet in good health. You will benefit from a thorough foot exam at least once a year, which includes testing of sensation in the feet, by a health care professional. Some community health clinics offer this service, as do foot specialists (podiatrist).

Obesity

Even a very moderate weight loss of 5 to 10 % of initial body weight can result in improved blood glucose levels, blood pressure and cholesterol levels according to the Canadian Diabetes Association. Losing weight is a slow process—1 to 2 kg/month is the optimal target. Lifestyle changes including healthy eating and increasing activity levels helps to achieve a healthy weight and improves your sense of well being. Once you feel more in control of your weight, self-management becomes easier, and you are on your way to becoming the best of self-managers. Find the resources in your community to help you reach your goal. An estimated 80 to 90 % of people with Type 2 diabetes are overweight or obese, which increases the risk of developing cardiovascular disease, or other diabetes-related complications.

Preventing Diabetes

This chapter has been concerned with individuals who already have diabetes. Can diabetes be prevented?

Ongoing research indicates that there are no proven ways to prevent or delay the onset of Type 1 diabetes at this time. But it may be possible to prevent or delay the onset of Type 2 diabetes. This would involve regular screening of those considered at risk for developing Type 2 diabetes. Screening tests include a simple fasting blood glucose test every 3 years for individuals over 40 years of age, and for others who may be at risk.

Risk factors for diabetes include; being overweight, having a large waist circumference, having high blood pressure, high cholesterol levels, being inactive and having a strong family history of diabetes. Lifestyle changes including being more active, eating healthy foods, losing weight and, possibly, taking certain medications prescribed by your doctor, could reduce your risk of developing Type 2 diabetes.

Diabetes is a complex disease that can result in serious complications if the blood glucose levels are not well controlled. The Canadian Diabetes Association Clinical Practice Guidelines 2008 provide guidance and recommendations on how to manage diabetes successfully and how to prevent or delay many of the complications discussed here.

YOUR ROLE IS IMPORTANT

Please note that most of the problems mentioned above can be treated and prevented, but you have an important role in doing so. First, maintain your blood glucose level within your target range. This will help prevent or reduce complications; if problems occur, good blood glucose control can prevent them from becoming worse. Second, be aware of your body and symptoms. With early detection and reporting of problems such as an infection or eye problem, it will be easier to treat.

As with all chronic conditions, diabetes is a disease that can be greatly controlled through good self-management. The path is not always easy, but successfully following it can be beneficial to your overall health.

To become a good diabetes self-manager, there is much more to learn than what is discussed in this chapter. Be sure to talk to your doctor or diabetes educator about your questions, problems, and/or concerns. Try to find other information and resources in your community to help you become the best of self-managers. Some resources are listed at the end of this chapter to help you start.

Community Resources

Canadian Diabetes Association
National Office
15 Toronto Street, Suite 800
Toronto, Ont. M5C 2E3
Toll Free: 1-800-BANTING (226-8464)
http://www.diabetes.ca
E-mail: info@diabetes.ca

The Nutrition Section of The Canadian Dietitians Association:
www.dietitians.ca

Both of these web sites contain information important to all people with diabetes. Financial Coverage Charts for diabetes supplies and medication outline the vast differences in what provincial and territorial drug plans cover. Knowing which medications you need to pay for will help you with your financial planning. The website has translation capabilities for many different languages, reflecting Canada's diversity. Medications currently prescribed in Canada are outlined in detail. For the most up-to-date information, visit the local Diabetes Education Centre or a Diabetes Educator at your regional or district office.

BC & Yukon
Toll Free: 1-800-665-6526

Alberta & NWT
Toll Free: 1-800-563-0032

Saskatchewan
Toll Free: 1-800-996-4446

Manitoba
Toll Free: 1-800-BANTING

New Brunswick
Toll Free: 1-800-884-4232

Nova Scotia
Toll Free: 1-800-326-7712

Community Resources

Ontario
Toll Free: 1-800-BANTING

Prince Edward Island
Telephone: 902-894-3005

Newfoundland
Telephone: 709-754-0953

Joslin Diabetes Foundation, Inc.
One Joslin Place
Boston, MA 02215
http://www.joslin.harvard.edu/

This world-famous facility has separate divisions for research, education, and youth. Their efforts involve all facets of diabetes management and research.

DIAL-A-DIETITIAN
www.dialadietitian.org

British Columbia: 1-800-667-3438, or 604-732-9191

Ontario: 1-877-510-5102

Other Provinces use Dietitians of Canada: www.dietitians.ca

Suggested Further Reading

Canadian Diabetes Association. *Beyond the Basics: Meal Planning for Healthy Eating, Diabetes Prevention and Management,* 2007. A series of binder inserts that can be ordered on line at www.diabetes.ca/literature.

Canadian Diabetes Association. *The Glycemic Index.* 2007. Handout and binder insert. Email: www.diabetes.ca.

Copeland, Glenn. *Healthy Feet: The Foot Doctor's Complete Guide for Men and Women.* Toronto: Key Porter, 2004.

Diabetes Dialogue. This is the quarterly journal published by the Canadian Diabetes Association. 1-year subscription with CDA membership is $29.95, or $27.95 for subscription only. Contact CDA at 416-363-3373. or email to: dialogue@diabetes.ca

HEALTH CANADA. EATING WELL WITH CANADAS FOOD GUIDE. www.healthcanada.gc.ca/foodguide. Tel. 1-866-225-0709.

Rosenthal, M. Sara. *The Canadian Type 2 Diabetes Sourcebook, 2nd ed.* Mississauga, Ont.: John Wiley & Sons, Ltd., 2004.

Walker, Rosemary, and Jill Rodgers. *Living with Diabetes: A Practical Guide to Managing Your Health.* New York, Toronto: Dorling Kindersley Limited, 2006.

PLANNING FOR THE FUTURE: Fears and Reality

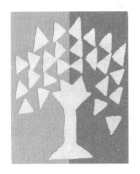

20

PEOPLE WITH CHRONIC ILLNESSES OFTEN WORRY ABOUT WHAT WILL HAPPEN TO THEM IF THEIR DISEASE BECOMES REALLY DISABLING. They fear that at some time in the future they may have problems managing their lives and their illness. One way people can deal with fears of the future is to take control and plan for it. They may never need to put their plans into effect, but there is reassurance in knowing that they will still be in control if the events they fear come to pass. Here are the most common concerns and some suggestions that may be useful.

WHAT IF I CAN'T TAKE CARE OF MYSELF ANYMORE?

Becoming helpless and dependent is one of the most common fears among people with a potentially disabling health problem. This fear usually has physical as well as financial, social, and emotional components.

Physical Concerns of Day-to-Day Living

As your health condition changes over time, you may need to consider changing your living situation. These changes may involve hiring someone to help you in your home or moving to a living situation where help is provided. The decision about which alternative is best will be related to your needs and how best these can be met.

The first thing you will need to do is carefully *evaluate what you can do for yourself* and what activities of daily living (ADLs) will require some kind of help. ADLs are the everyday things like getting out of bed, bathing, dressing, preparing and eating your meals, cleaning house, shopping, paying bills, and so on. Most people can do all of these, even though they may have to do them slowly, with some modification, or with some help from gadgets.

Some people, though, may eventually find one or more of these no longer possible without help from somebody else. For example, you may still be able to fix meals, but your mobility may be impaired to the degree that shopping is no longer possible. Or, if you have problems with fainting or sudden bouts of unconsciousness, you might need to have somebody around at all times. Using the problem-solving steps discussed in Chapter 2, analyze and make a list of what the potential problems might be. Once you have this list, problem-solve the problems one at a time, first making a list of every possible solution you can think of.

Example:

Can't go shopping
- Get daughter to shop for me
- Find a volunteer shopping service
- Shop at a store that delivers
- Ask neighbor to shop for me
- Use the Internet
- Get home-delivered meals

Can't be by myself
- Hire an around-the-clock attendant
- Move in with a relative
- Get a "Life-Line" emergency response system
- Move to an assisted living facility
- Move to a retirement community

When you have listed your problems, and the possible solutions to the problems, select the solution that seems the most workable, acceptable, and least expensive for your needs (step 3 of problem solving).

The selection will depend upon your finances, the family or other resources you can call on, and how well any of the potential solutions will in fact solve your problem. Sometimes, one solution will be the answer for several problems. For instance, if you can't shop and can't be alone, and household chores are reaching the point of a need for help, you might consider that a retirement home will solve all of these problems. It offers meals, regular house cleaning, and transportation for errands and medical appointments.

Even if you are not of "retirement" age, some facilities may accept younger people, depending on their criteria for admission. Some facilities for the "retired" take people as young as 50, or younger if one member of a couple is the minimum age. If you are a young person, the local centre for persons with disabilities or independent living organization may be able to direct you to an out-of-home facility appropriate for you.

Your appraisal of your situation and needs may be aided by sitting down with a trusted friend, relative or, social worker and discussing your abilities and limitations. Sometimes another person can spot things we ourselves overlook or would like to ignore. A good self-manager often utilizes other resources, which is step 6 in the problem-solving steps in Chapter 2.

Make changes in your life slowly, one step at a time. You don't need to change your whole life around to solve one problem. Remember, too, that you can always change your mind. Don't burn your bridges behind you. If you think that moving out of your own place to another living arrangement (relatives, care home, etc.) is the thing to do, don't give up your present home until you are settled in your new home and are sure you want to stay there.

If you think you need help with some activities, hiring help at home is less drastic than moving out and may be enough for quite a while. If you can't be alone, and you live with a family member who is away from home during the day, maybe going to an adult or senior day care centre will be enough to keep you safe and comfortable while your family is away. In fact, adult day care centres are ideal places to find new friends and activities geared to your abilities.

A social worker at your local senior centre, centre for people with disabilities, or hospital social services department can be very helpful in providing information about resources in your community and also in giving you ideas about how to deal with your care needs. There are several kinds of professionals who can be of great help. As previously mentioned, *social workers* are good for helping you decide how to solve financial and living arrangement problems and locating appropriate community resources. Some social workers are also trained in counselling the disabled and/or the elderly in relation to emotional and relationship problems that may be associated with your health problem.

A licensed occupational therapist can assess your daily living needs and suggest assistive devices or rearrangements in your environment to make life easier.

A lawyer specializing in family law, specifically elder issues, should be on your list for helping you set your financial affairs in order to preserve your assets, to prepare a legal will, and to help with enduring power of attorney and/or representation agreements for financial, health and personal care. If finances are a concern, ask your local senior centre for the names of lawyers or notaries who offer low-cost services to seniors. Your local Bar Association can also refer you to lawyers specializing in this area. Even if you are not a "senior," your legal needs are similar to those of an older person.

Finding In-Home Help

If you find that you cannot manage alone, the first option is usually to hire somebody to help. Most people just need a person called a *home aide* or some similar title. These are people who provide no medically related services needing special licensing, but do help with bathing, dressing, meal preparation, and household chores.

Throughout Canada, many of these services are available through the local hospital social work department or health authority. The services are delivered through a mix of not-for-profit agencies and private agencies. You may hire someone privately, through any of the agencies listed under Home Support Services in the yellow pages telephone book. By using an agency, all of the insurance, bonding, and employee benefits are assumed by the agency. Of course, this is included in the fee you are charged. If you qualify for subsidized home support services, you will be assessed and will pay on a sliding scale for the service. Whether you hire through an agency or qualify for a subsidy, remember that you do not pay the worker directly. You will be sent an invoice and you pay the agency.

The fees are usually about double what you would expect to pay for someone you hire directly. One advantage, if you can afford the agency, is that the agency assumes responsibility for the skill and integrity of the attendant, and can replace an ill or no-show attendant right away.

Registered nurses (RNs) hired this way are very expensive, but it is rare that home care for a chronically ill person requires a registered nurse. Licensed practical nurses (LPNs) cost somewhat less, but are still expensive and are usually not needed unless there are nursing services required (such as dressing changes, injections, ventilator management, etc.). Certified Care Attendants have some basic training, are much less expensive, and can provide satisfactory care for all but the most critically ill person at home.

Most of these agencies supply home aides as well as licensed staff. Unless you are bedridden, or require some procedure that must be done by someone with a certain category of license, a home aide most likely will be the most appropriate choice for your needs.

There are registries that supply pre-screened lists of attendants or caregivers, from which you select the one you wish to hire. The agency will charge a "placement fee," usually equal to one month's pay of the person hired. The agency will assume no liability for the skill or honesty of these people, and it will be necessary to check references and to interview carefully, just as you would for someone from any other source. This type of resource can be found in the yellow pages under the same listing as "home nursing agencies" or "registries." Some agencies provide both their own staff and registries of staff for you to select from.

Other resources that may provide help at home include senior centres and centres serving the disabled population. They often have listings of people who have called them to say they want work as a home attendant, or who have put a notice up on a bulletin board there. These job seekers are not screened, and need to be interviewed carefully and to have references checked before they start on the job.

Many experienced home care attendants use the local newspaper's classified "employment wanted" section to find new jobs. Home attendant jobs tend to be temporary, since one's patient usually progresses to a need for more or sometimes less care than the attendant can provide, so the attendant must then look for a new job. Again, one can find a competent helper through the newspaper, but the advice to interview carefully is valid here, too.

Probably the best source of help is word of mouth, from somebody who has employed a person or knows of somebody who has worked for someone he or she knows. Putting the word out through your family and social network may result in a jewel.

A home-share may also benefit you, if you have space and feel comfortable offering a home to someone who may help out with household and garden chores. Check with a voluntary agency, or a local church or religious organization. Be very clear on what you require, and ask your family or a close friend to help you make a safe choice.

You may qualify for the Disability Tax Credit Certificate (Form T2201 E), issued by the Canada Revenue Agency. The criteria for this credit are very specific, and it is best to discuss this with your doctor. If you are a Canadian Armed Forces Veteran, you may be eligible for services, which will allow you to remain in your home. Contact the Veterans Affairs Canada office closest to you, and enquire about the VIP program and other services for veterans.

Finding Out-of-Home Care

Retirement Communities

The person who needs very little personal care, but recognizes the need to live in a more protected setting, with security, emergency response services, and so on, and who is older (usually 50-plus) may wish to consider a retirement community. These may consist of self-owned apartment units, or rental units. They may be developed by a for-profit company, or sponsored by a service organization. These are options requiring a lot of thought, and your decision should not be left until you are in a panic or recently bereaved. Questions to ask include: are pets allowed, are there rules about overnight visitors, what are the additional costs should I require the next level of care, is housecleaning included in the monthly fee, are television cable service and telephone service included? Some subsidized units are available through provincial ministries of health.

There are almost always waiting lists for retirement communities, especially subsidized units. If you think such a place might be right for you, you should get on the waiting list right away. You can always change your mind or decline if you are not ready when a space is offered. To locate seniors housing, call your local seniors centre or advocacy group, or contact the provincial ministry responsible for housing.

Residential Care Homes

Throughout Canada, there are different levels of care available, and a lot of change is underway. A new category is Assisted Living, which is similar to an apartment building with individual units. A central dining area is available, but you must be able to make your way to the dining room. Activities are offered in common rooms, and some level of supervision is offered through minimal staff levels. Take the time to learn about the different levels of care offered. For those who require supervision with medications, or assistance getting out of bed or getting into the bath, some facilities will offer this care for an additional fee. You may also hire a caregiver to provide this assistance to you, while you live in Assisted Living. It is important when considering residential care to evaluate the type of residents already living there to make sure you will fit in. For example, some residents may have a level of mental confusion. If you are mentally clear, you would not find much companionship there. Because corporately-operated care homes are new to Canada, and some do not have a long history of service, visit a variety of facilities, ask a lot of questions, and listen carefully to what your circle of friends say about each facility. Each facility is required to maintain a certain standard of nutrition in the meals served, but make sure the menu is one you like. If you need a salt-free or diabetic diet, for instance, be sure these are available at each meal. Monthly fees vary widely for assisted living, depending on the level of luxury and services offered. The lowest fees are consistent with Federal pension amounts and the range goes up to about $5,000 monthly. The more luxurious the furnishings, neighbourhood, and services, the greater the cost. Compare costs, review your budget, and take your time making a decision.

Extended Care Facilities

This is a category of care that has undergone a lot of change in Canada. Typically, if you require some nursing care, or are severely restricted in mobility, or have some level of mental confusion, this is the type of facility you will need. These facilities differ from rehabilitation centres, where you may stay after you have had a hip replacement or a serious traumatic accident. Some hospitals have units for recovering from trauma or a stroke. Here, education is key. Approach your local hospital and find out what level of care you might expect, before you need it. We have all heard "nursing home" horror stories, and seen media reports detailing the misfortunes of those who have been mistreated. However, the level of care required when we are looking at nursing home care means no other facility will meet this need. This level of care is provided for people who are no longer able to be in a non-medical care situation. This means there may be medications to be administered, either by injection or intravenously, or monitored by professional nursing staff. An extended care facility is necessary if you are physically limited, needing to have help getting in and out of bed, eating, bathing, or dealing with bladder and/or bowel control. Care of feeding tubes, respirators, and other medical equipment can be monitored here. If you have become acutely ill, and are in a regional hospital, consult the hospital discharge planner or social worker to help you locate a space for when you are discharged, if you are unable to continue to live on your own. In most provinces and territories, the Ministry of Health monitors all levels of care facilities. If you are not satisfied with the level of care you are receiving, contact your local elected representative or a seniors advocacy group.

WILL I HAVE ENOUGH MONEY TO PAY FOR MY CARE?

Next to the basic fear of physical dependency, the greatest fear most people experience is the fear of not having enough money to pay for their needs. Being sick often requires expensive care and treatment. If you are too ill or disabled to work, the loss of income, and especially the loss of your extended health benefits, may present an overwhelming financial problem. You can, however, avoid some of the risks by planning ahead and knowing your resources.

The Federal pension amount and the Provincial Pension Supplement will pay for most of the cost of institutional care. Some retirees have extended health benefits. If you are eligible for Veterans Benefits, your facility fees will be paid.

Some insurance policies are available to pay for sickness or disability. If you plan to buy such insurance for yourself, carefully read the sections on limitations and exclusions. Be sure the policy covers nursing-home care at a daily rate level that is realistic for your community. Check that it will cover treatments or care for "pre-existing conditions." Some policies have a waiting period for such pre-existing conditions, usually three to six months. Others won't cover you at all for any condition that was diagnosed before the start date of the policy.

If you are too sick to work, you may be entitled to Sickness Benefits from Employment Insurance, or, if your sickness worsens, you may be eligible for a Disability Pension from the provincial or the Federal Government. If you have dependent children, the provincial government will provide a modest monthly amount for you and your family. Eligibility for programs differs widely from province to province. An elder care lawyer may also be able to help.

The social services department in the hospital where you have obtained treatment can advise you about your own situation and the probability of your being eligible for these programs. The local agency serving the disabled usually has advisors who can refer you to programs and resources for which you may be eligible. Senior centers often have counselors knowledgeable about the ins and outs of health care insurance.

One last thought: If you own a home, you may be able to get a "reverse mortgage." This is where the bank pays you a monthly amount based on the value of your home. The nice thing is that, no matter how long you live, they can never throw you out of your home.

I NEED HELP, BUT DON'T WANT HELP— NOW WHAT?

Let's talk about the emotional aspects of becoming dependent. Every human being emerges from childhood reaching for and cherishing every possible sign of independence—the driver's licence, the first job, the first checking account, the first time we go out and don't have to tell anybody where we are going or when we will be back, and so on. In these and many other ways, we demonstrate to ourselves as well as to others that we are "grown up"—in charge of our lives and able to take care of ourselves without any help from parents.

If a time comes when we must face the realization that we need help, that we can no longer manage completely on our own, it may seem like a return to childhood and having to let somebody else be in charge of our lives. This can be very painful and embarrassing.

Some people in this situation become extremely depressed and can no longer find any joy in life. Others fight off the recognition of their need for help, thus placing themselves in possible danger and making life difficult and frustrating for those who would like to be helpful. Still others give up completely and expect others to take total responsibility for their lives, demanding attention and services from their children or other family members. If you are having one or more of these reactions, you can help yourself to feel better and develop a more positive response.

The concept "*. . . change the things I can change, and accept the things I cannot change, and have the wisdom to know the difference*" is really fundamental to being able to stay in charge of our lives. You must be able to correctly evaluate your situation. You must identify those activities requiring the help of somebody else (going shopping and cleaning house, for instance) and those activities you can still do on your own (getting dressed, paying bills, writing letters).

This means making decisions, and as long as you keep the decision-making prerogative, you are in charge. It is important to make a decision and take action while you are still able to do so, before circumstances intervene and the decision gets made for you. That means being realistic and honest with yourself.

Some people find that talking with a sympathetic listener, either a professional counselor or a sensible close friend or family member, is very comforting and helpful. An objective listener often helps by pointing out alternatives and options you may have overlooked or were not aware of. She or he can provide information, or another point of view or interpretation of a situation that you would not have come upon yourself. This is part of the self-management process.

Be very careful, however, in evaluating advice from somebody who has something to sell you. There are many people whose solution to your problem just happens to be whatever it is they are selling—health or burial insurance policies, annuities, special and expensive furniture, "sunshine cruises," special magazines, or health foods with magical curative properties.

In talking with family members or friends who offer to be helpful, be as open and reasonable as you can be and, at the same time, try to make them understand that you will reserve for yourself the right to decide how much and what kind of help you will accept. They will probably be more cooperative and understanding if you can say, "Yes, I do need some help with . . . , but I still want to do . . . myself." More tips on asking for help can be found in Chapter 10, "Communicating."

Insist on being consulted. Lay the ground rules with your helpers early on. Ask to be presented with choices so that you can decide what is best for you as you see it. If you try to objectively weigh the suggestions made to you, and don't dismiss every option out of hand, people will consider you able to make reasonable decisions and will continue to provide you the opportunity to do so.

Be appreciative. Recognize the good will and the efforts of those who want to help. Even though you may be embarrassed, you will maintain your dignity by accepting with grace the help that is offered, if you need it. If you are truly convinced that you are being offered help you don't need, you can decline it with tact and appreciation. For example, you can say, "I appreciate your offer to have Thanksgiving at your house, but I'd like to continue having it here. I could really use some help, though—maybe with the clean-up after dinner."

If you are at length unable to come to terms with your increasing need to be dependent on others for help in managing your living situation, you should consult a professional counsellor. This should be someone who has experience with the emotional and social issues of people with disabling health problems.

Your local agency providing services to the disabled should be able to refer you to the right kind of counsellor. The local or national organization dedicated to serving people with your specific health condition (Canadian Lung Association, Heart and Stroke Foundation, Canadian Diabetes Society, etc.) can also refer you to support groups and classes to help you in dealing with your condition. You should be able to locate the agency you need through the telephone book yellow pages under the listing "social service organizations." Also, don't forget the Internet.

Akin to the fear and embarrassment of becoming physically dependent is the fear of being abandoned by family members who would be expected to provide needed help. Tales of being "dumped" in a nursing home by children who never come to visit haunt many, who worry that this may happen to them.

We need to be sure that we do reach out to family and friends and ask for the help we need when we recognize that we can't go on alone. It sometimes happens that in expectation of rejection, people fail to ask for help. Some people try to hide their need in fear that their need will cause loved ones to withdraw. Families often complain, "If we'd only known . . . ," when it is revealed that a loved one had needs for help that were unmet.

If you really cannot turn to close family or friends because they are unable or unwilling to become involved in your care, there are agencies dedicated to providing for such situations. Through your local social services department's "adult protective services" program or Family Services Association, you should be able to locate a "case manager" who will be able to organize the resources in your community to provide the help you need. The social services department in your local hospital can also put you in touch with the right agency.

GRIEVING:
A NORMAL REACTION TO BAD NEWS

When we experience any kind of a loss—small ones (such as losing one's car keys) or big ones (such as losing a life partner or facing a disabling or terminal illness)—we go through an emotional process of grieving and coming to terms with the loss.

A person with a chronic, disabling health problem experiences a variety of losses. These include loss of confidence, loss of self-esteem, loss of independence, loss of the lifestyle we knew and cherished, and, perhaps the most painful of all, loss of a positive self-image if our condition has an effect on appearance (such as rheumatoid arthritis or the residual paralysis from a stroke).

Elizabeth Kübler-Ross, who has written extensively about this process, describes the stages of grief:

- **Shock,** when one feels both a mental and a physical reaction to the initial recognition of the loss.

- **Denial,** when the person tells himself, "No, it can't be true," and proceeds to act for a time as if it were not true.

- **Anger,** the "why me?" feelings and searching for someone or something to blame (if the doctor had diagnosed it early enough, I'd have been cured; or the job caused me too much stress; etc.).

- **Bargaining,** when we say to ourselves, to someone else, or to God, "I'll never smoke again," or "I'll follow my treatment regimen absolutely to the letter," or "I'll go to church every Sunday," "if only I can get over this."

- **Depression,** when the real awareness sets in; we confront the truth about the situation and experience deep feelings of sadness and hopelessness.

- **Acceptance,** when we eventually recognize that we must deal with what has happened and make up our minds to do what we have to do.

We do not pass through these stages in a linear, out-of-one-into-the-next fashion. We are more apt to have several, or even many, flip-flops back and forth between them. Don't be discouraged if you find yourself angry or depressed again, when you thought you had reached acceptance.

I'M AFRAID OF DEATH

Fear of death is something most of us begin to experience only when something happens to bring us face to face with the possibility of our own death. Losing someone close, having an accident that might have been fatal, or learning we have a health condition that may shorten our lives usually causes us to consider the inevitability of our own eventual passing. Many people, even then, try to avoid facing the future because they are afraid to think about it.

Our attitudes about death are shaped by our own central attitudes about life. This is the product of our culture, our family's influences, perhaps our religion, and certainly our life experiences.

If you are ready to think about your own future—about the near or distant prospect that your life will most certainly end at some time—then the ideas that follow will be useful to you. If you are not ready to think about it just yet, put this aside and come back to it later.

As with depression, the most useful way to come to terms with your eventual death is to take positive steps to prepare for it. This means to get your house in order by attending to all the necessary small and large details. If you continue to avoid dealing with these details, you will create problems for yourself and for those involved with your situation in a significant way.

There are several components to getting your house in order:

- **Decide, and then convey to others your wishes** about how and where you want to be during your last days and hours. Do you want to be in a hospital or at home? When do you want procedures to prolong your life stopped? At what point do you want to let nature take its course when it is determined that death is inevitable? Who should be with you—only the few people who are nearest and dearest, or all the people you care about and want to see one last time?

- **Make a will.** Even if your estate is a small one, you may have definite preferences about who should have what. If you have a large estate, the tax implications of a proper will may be very significant.

- **Make arrangements,** or at least plans, for your funeral. Your grieving family will be very relieved not to have to decide what you would want and how much to spend. There are prepaid "future need" funeral plans available, and you can purchase burial space in the location and of the type you prefer.

- **Make an enduring power of attorney for health care,** and also a representation agreement or mandate that will allow someone to manage your financial affairs. (See Chapter 12.) You should also discuss your wishes with your physician, even if he or she doesn't seem very interested. (Your physician may also have trouble facing the prospect of losing you.)

Be sure that some kind of document or notation is included in your medical records that indicates your wishes in case you can't communicate them when the time comes.

Be sure that the persons you want to handle things after your death are *aware of all that they need to know* about your wishes, your plans and arrangements, and the location of necessary documents. You will need to talk to them, or at least prepare a detailed letter of instructions and give it to someone who can be counted on to deliver it to the proper person when needed. This should be a person close enough to you to know when that time is at hand. You may not want your spouse to have to take on these responsibilities, for example, but your spouse may be the best person to keep your letter and know when to give it to your designated agent.

You can purchase at any well-stocked stationery store a pre-organized kit, in which you place a copy of your will, your enduring power of attorney, important papers, and information about your financial and personal affairs. There are forms that you fill out about bank and charge accounts, insurance policies, the location of important documents, your safe deposit box and where the key is kept, and so on. This is a handy, concise way of getting everything together that anyone might need to know about.

- **Finish "business" with the world around you.** Mend your relationships. Pay your debts, both financial and personal. Say what needs to be said to those who need to hear it. Do what needs to be done. Forgive yourself. Forgive others.

- **Talk about your feelings about your death.** Most family and close friends are reluctant to initiate such a conversation, but will appreciate it if you bring it up. You may find that there is much to say to and to hear from your loved ones. If you find that they are unwilling to listen to you talk about your death and the feelings that you are experiencing, find someone who will be comfortable and empathetic in listening to you. Your family and friends may be able to listen to you later on. Remember, those who love you will also go through the stages of grieving when they have to think about the prospect of losing you.

A large component in fear of death is the fear of the unknown. "What will it be like?" "Will it be painful?" "What will happen to me (after I die)?"

Most people who die of a disease are ready to die when the time comes. Painkillers and the disease process itself weaken body and mind, and the awareness of self diminishes without the realization that this is happening. Most people just "slip away," with the transition between the state of living and that of no longer living hardly identifiable. Reports from people who have been brought back to life after being in a state of clinical death indicate they experienced a sense of peacefulness and clarity and were not frightened.

A dying person may sometimes feel very lonely and abandoned. Regrettably, many people cannot deal with their own emotions when they are around a person they know to be dying and so deliberately avoid his or her company, or they may engage in superficial chitchat, broken by long, awkward silences. This is often puzzling and hurtful to those who are dying, who need companionship and solace from those they counted on.

You can sometimes help by telling your family and friends what you want and need from them—attention, entertainment, comfort, practical help, and so on. Again, when a person has something positive to do, they are more able to cope with their emotions. If you can engage your family and loved ones in specific activities, they can feel needed and can relate to you around the activity. This will give you something to talk about, to occupy time, or it will at least provide a definition of the situation for them and for you.

If you choose to die at home, a hospice can be very helpful. These organizations provide both physical and emotional care to people who are dying, as well as for their families. A hospice can arrange for setting up your home to meet your needs and take care of the details of your care both before and at the time of death. This can be a great help to loved ones and is one of the greatest gifts you can give them. To find a hospice near you, ask the hospital social worker, your doctor, or community service information and referral.

Hospice care, as with everything else discussed in this chapter, can be arranged before the time it's needed. Planning ahead can be a comfort to both you and your loved ones.

Suggested Further Reading

Kuhl, David. *Facing Death, Embracing Life: Understanding What Dying People Want.* Toronto: Doubleday Canada, 2006.

Kuhl, David. *What Dying People Want: Practical Wisdom for the End of Life.* Toronto: Doubleday Canada, 2002.

Simpson, Sheila. *Saying Goodbye with Love: How to Take Care of the Details of Death.* Surrey, B.C.: Sea Breeze Press, 1996.

Other Resources

Canadian Palliative Care Association
www.cpca.net

Health Canada
www.hc-sc.gc.ca/homecare/english/link.html
includes links to many research sites providing clear and unbiased information

Veterans Affairs Canada
1 866 522 2122

200+ HELPFUL HINTS

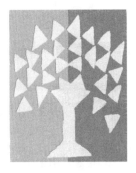

21

THERE ARE MANY WAYS TO ORGANIZE YOUR LIFE TO MAKE THINGS EASIER. Necessity, they say, is the mother of invention. If so, then creativity must be the father. Fortunately for us, creative people before us have invented "shortcuts" to make things a little easier for us. Here are a few. These suggestions are offered to jog your imagination and problem-solving abilities. Not everything works for everyone. Use what is helpful.

WAKING UP

Try some stretching and strengthening exercises while you are still in bed.

Get a clock radio and set it to awaken you with music rather than an alarm. Some can wake you with a prerecorded tape of your choice. Record the tape with your own "pep talk."

Make half of your bed while you are are still in it. Pull the top sheet and blanket up on one side and smooth them out. Exit from the unmade side, which is then easy to finish.

A quilted comforter and matching pillow cases or pillow shams can replace a bedspread. They are easy to pull up, and carefully smoothing the sheets and blankets underneath is unnecessary, since the thick quilting hides any irregularities in the surface.

Do some of your dressing sitting on the edge of your bed before you get up. Leave the clothes within reach of your bed the night before.

Consider an electric mattress pad for your bed. Turn it on just before you do your exercises to help loosen morning stiffness.

Keep a cane or chair next to your bed to help pull yourself out of bed in the morning.

BATHING AND HYGIENE

If standing in a shower or sitting down in a tub are too demanding, get a bath stool. It is waterproof and goes right in the tub. You can sit while you bathe.

Shower heads or bath faucets can be replaced with a unit that incorporates hand-held sprayers.

A "sponge bath" can be taken in place of a tub bath and can be a lot less taxing.

If you are weak, don't take a bath or shower unless someone else is at home with you.

A long, absorbent, cotton terry robe will eliminate the effort of drying with a towel.

An oxygen tube can be kept out of the way while bathing by passing it over the shower curtain rod.

Soap on a rope enables you to use soap with one hand, and keeps it from falling.

A liquid soap dispenser may be easier to use than a bar of soap.

If excess humidity bothers you, leave the bathroom door open while you bathe.

Replace difficult twist tops on shampoo or lotions with pump tops.

A shower caddy keeps bathing supplies within easy reach.

Use nonskid safety strips or a rubber bath mat in the tub or shower.

Consider having grab bars installed in your tub or shower to minimize the risk of falling.

Install touch-free or automatic faucets and flushers that eliminate the need for turning knobs or levers while washing or using the toilet.

Get a long-handled sponge or brush.

Suctioned soap holders make it possible to soap up without grasping the soap or needing to use two hands.

Suctioned brushes are useful for cleaning dentures with one hand.

Electric toothbrushes and "water pic" appliances make brushing easier.

Get a dental-floss holder if flossing is difficult with two hands.

It is possible to open a toothpaste tube with one hand by holding the tube in the palm of the hand and using the thumb and index finger to open the cap. Use the heel of the hand to squeeze out the toothpaste.

Look for special long- and/or curved-handled toothbrushes.

Toothbrush handles can be made easier to grasp by wrapping a small sponge or foam hair curler around them.

Ask family members to fold the end of the toilet paper into a "V" to make it easier to grasp.

Have a grab bar or safety frame installed next to the toilet. A free-standing towel rack next to the toilet can also help you when getting off the toilet.

"Le Funelle" or "Sani-Fem" makes it possible for women to urinate standing up.

Women who are troubled by occasional accidents of losing urine find that small panty liners or sanitary pads with adhesive backs help avoid potentially embarrassing situations.

Women who find tampons difficult to remove might try winding the tampon string around a pencil and gently pulling with both hands. Some brands have looped strings, making removal with either fingers or a pencil easier.

Women who use pads for feminine hygiene can keep the genital area clean by using a squeeze bottle of water kept by the toilet. These bottles can be found with a variety of spray nozzles.

GROOMING

A small sponge or a foam hair roller around the handle of a razor or an eyeliner pencil can make them easier to grasp.

Long-handled brushes and combs make it easier to reach hair.

Shaving or applying makeup is easier if you have a low mirror so that you can sit down while doing either.

Talk to a hair stylist about a "drip-dry" style. Special haircuts and/or permanents can eliminate rollers and/or hairdryers and still be very stylish.

If you have respiratory problems, switch to non-aerosol toiletries. You can get liquid or gel hair dressings and roll-on or solid deodorants.

Many toiletries can be purchased that are unscented or hypoallergenic.

DRESSING

Use the dresser drawers that are easiest to reach.

Lower the rod in your closet or get a closet organizer to bring clothes within easier reach.

It is safer and easier to pull underpants and trousers up when lying flat in bed, if balance or mobility is a problem. Graduate to a chair.

Shop for clothes with dressing in mind. Look for easy-to-reach fasteners, front openings, and elastic waistbands loose enough to be pulled over the hips.

Look for clothes with Velcro or elastic instead of buttons.

Replace the buttons on your garments with Velcro. Move the buttons to the top part of the opening for decoration.

Bras can be fastened in front and then turned around and pulled into place, or buy front-opening bras.

When putting on pantyhose or a girdle, roll them down from top to bottom, then step in and pull onto your hips and unroll.

Dusting powder on the thighs makes pulling on pantyhose or girdles easier.

Avoid tight belts, bras, or girdles that restrict chest and abdominal expansion.

Avoid tight neck bands. Ties should be loose, or replaced with a bolo or loosely tied scarf or kerchief.

Suspenders (braces) may be more comfortable than a belt.

Put rings or loops on zipper pulls, or get a special "zipper puller."

Many who are bothered by extreme temperatures may find cotton underclothing more comfortable than synthetic.

Use a bent coathanger, reacher, or "dressing stick" to help with pulling up pants or retrieving clothes that are out of reach.

Most women find that wearing slacks and socks is much easier than struggling into panty hose.

Avoid socks or stockings with elastic bands or garters, which may bind the leg and restrict circulation.

Use a "sock donner" to put on socks and stockings.

Get a long-handled shoehorn.

Slip-on shoes are easy and require no bending over to tie.

Convert your lace-up shoes to slip-ons with elastic shoelaces.

When shopping for clothes, take a tape measure with you that is already marked with your measurements. By measuring the garments, you may not have to try on so many before you buy.

To avoid exposure to cold, dress in layers when outdoors. Thermal underwear is great for winter.

Choose women's pants or skirts with pockets, and carry money, driver's license, and so on in the pockets instead of carrying a large, heavy purse. A photographer's vest is good for this.

GETTING AROUND

Lead with your stronger leg when going up stairs. Lead with your weaker leg when going down.

Remove all throw rugs—they can cause falls.

Doorways inside your home can be made wider by removing the doors, making them easier to get through with a wheelchair, walker, or other equipment.

Consider installing stair rails on both sides of the stairway to increase safety.

A small ramp can replace a couple of stairs at the entrance to your home or elsewhere.

Carry a folding cane seat with you when you go out. It gives you both something to lean on and something to sit on when necessary.

Look for a walker that has a large basket in front and a small bench seat to sit on when you get tired.

Consider installing a mechanical lift chair on your stairs.

Place a chair or table near the top of stairs for you to lean or sit on when you reach the top.

To lift and carry:

1.   Lift or carry while exhaling through pursed lips.

2.   Rest and inhale through the nose; continue this pattern of intermittent work and rest until you get the job done.

DOING HOUSEHOLD CHORES

Get a small utility cart—some fold, and most have at least two shelves. As you move about doing your chores, use the cart to carry your supplies or things that need to be put away. If you live in a two-storey house, keep a cart on each level.

Pick-up tongs can retrieve things from hard-to-reach places. The tongs can be purchased from most medical supply houses or rented from the Canadian Red Cross Society.

A magnet tied to a string can help pick up thumbtacks, hairpins, and so forth. It will stick to your cart, refrigerator, or washing machine for quick availability.

Plan your chores so that you go in a circle, rather than back and forth.

Keep a set of cleaning supplies in each area where they are to be used to avoid carrying them around.

Long-handled sponges are good for hard-to-reach areas.

To clean your bathtub, sit on a low stool next to the tub and use a long-handled sponge, or clean it at the end of your bath. Then rinse both you and it.

Consider a battery-powered "scrubber" for bathtub, sink, and so on.

Get a long-handled dustbin and a small broom for dry spills. Small brooms can be found in toy stores.

Foam floor mats can be placed where you may need to stand often, such as at the sink, ironing board, or telephone. They can reduce foot and ankle pain and low back pain.

Use an adjustable-height ironing board so that you can sit down while ironing. Attach a "cord minder" to keep the cord out of your way.

Small items such as socks or underwear can be washed in laundry bags to avoid having to search in the washer or dryer.

If lifting heavy detergent boxes is difficult, have someone pour some into a small container, or put a large container on the floor and use a scoop.

For some, a front-loading washer is easier to use than a top-loader.

Use gravity to get clothes out of the dryer or front-loading washer. Put a basket under the door and scoop the clothes into it with a reacher or stick.

Try old-fashioned push-on clothespins rather than pinch clothespins.

Fitted bed sheets are difficult to put on the bed; slit one corner and fasten with a tie.

Use a large, wide spatula or oven shovel to tuck in sheets.

Use a vacuum cleaner with disposable bags, and remove the bag with extreme care, if you have respiratory problems.

A small, battery-powered hand vacuum is easy to use for spot clean-ups and can be kept on your cart.

Those with breathing problems should avoid sweeping and dusting. If you feel you must do it, wrap the working end of the broom or mop with a damp cloth.

A damp cloth is also good for dusting. If you don't want to use anything damp on wood surfaces, get a roll of crinkly paper towels and a bottle of lemon oil. Tear the towels in sections and fold in quarters, put 4 or 5 coin-sized dots of oil on each towel and roll up tight. Store in a zip-lock bag or a jar. Use and discard.

If you must do a dusty job, wear a mask.

Have good ventilation and an adequate supply of fresh air at all times.

People with respiratory problems should observe the "no aerosol" rule for cleaning products.

Avoid harmful substances that can vaporize, such as mothballs, solvents, and kerosene.

Put lockable casters on furniture you wish to move to clean around.

COOKING

Microwave and convection ovens save time and energy.

Replace the twist-ties on bread or other foods with clothespins.

Avoid lifting heavy pots of food along with the water they were cooked in. Place food in a basket to lower into the water for cooking, or get a spaghetti cooker provided with a perforated insert. You can lift the basket out to drain food. Someone else can drain the pot later, or you can ladle the water out.

Ask family members not to close jars too tightly. A jar opener can be mounted under a countertop, or you can get a rubber disk to help you open jars.

Try to replace any heavy cast-iron or ceramic utensils with lightweight pots, bowls, and dishes.

Don't try to get everything done at once. Almost all jobs can be divided into small tasks. For instance, clean the top shelf of the refrigerator today and the bottom shelf tomorrow.

Plan your meals when you are neither hungry nor tired. Light, well-balanced meals are too important to leave to impulse.

A number of small meals is better than large ones, especially for a person with limited lung capacity, to allow more room for lungs than for the stomach.

Use convenience food when desired, but remember that many packaged foods have high salt and sugar contents. Read the labels.

Keep plenty of water in the refrigerator. You can get containers to sit on your shelf that have spigots near the bottom so that you won't have to lift the container to fill your drinking glass.

For many recipes, it's just as easy to cook double or triple quantities as small ones. Freeze the excess in meal-sized containers and enjoy some cook-free meals when you feel like a day off. In a microwave, they can be easily thawed and heated without drying out.

A slow-cooker or crockpot can make many meals easier to prepare, as can a pressure cooker.

Always use an exhaust fan when cooking, especially if you have respiratory problems.

A small, portable fan can help you overcome shortness of breath from exertion or cool you off in a warm kitchen or laundry room. Some are battery-powered and can clip onto a shelf or counter.

Use your cart when tidying up after a meal. For example, gather all the items that need to go into the refrigerator, and then sit down with the cart and put them away all at once.

Put your most-used pots and pans back on the stove and leave them there. Instead of putting dishes and silverware away, reset the table for the next meal.

Try a cutting board with spikes sticking up that will hold meat firmly in place while you cut it. If necessary, you will be able to carve meat with one hand.

Select appliances with levers or pushbuttons that are easy to operate.

Store canned goods so that the same items are lined up behind one another. Storing them upside-down allows you to see the labels more easily.

Get attractive cooking pots that double as serving pieces.

Disposable foil pie tins, loaf pans, and so on save clean-up effort.

Line pans with aluminum foil for easier clean-up.

Get pans with nonstick surfaces for quicker clean-up.

Stabilize mixing bowls by placing them on a wet washcloth or by placing them in an open drawer at work height.

Put flour and sugar in conveniently located containers so that you won't have to lift the heavy bags.

Oven mitts allow you to lift hot pans with both hands.

Use a bent coathanger or a dowel with a hook on the end to pull out hot oven racks.

Attach a spray hose at the kitchen sink, and fill pots with water while they sit on the countertop or stove.

When friends pop in for a visit, ask them to peel and cut up vegetables for you. You can blanch and freeze them for use later

A pizza wheel can cut more than pizza easily!

A small food processor can make short work of grating, chopping, or slicing.

One- or two-wheeled stools or chairs in the kitchen will make work easier—at counter height or low enough to allow you to get into lower cabinets with minimal bending.

EATING

If you have difficulty using a knife, try a "rocker knife" or pizza cutter, which requires the use of only one hand.

Use a scoop dish with a nonskid bottom to avoid shoving food off of the plate.

Boating supply stores are a good source for stable, nonskid dishes.

For easier grip, build up utensil handles with pieces of foam and tape.

ENTERTAINING

Buffets are easy. Let guests serve themselves.

Party supply stores have very attractive and festive disposable plates, utensils, and serving pieces.

Plan a potluck rather than doing it all yourself.

Dessert potlucks are especially popular.

Buy two tickets for an event and ask a friend.

REMEMBERING MEDICATIONS

A pillbox with a separate compartment for each day of the week is useful. A pillbox like this can be made out of an egg carton or purchased at your pharmacy.

Take-out food places often have 1-oz plastic containers for salad dressing and ketchup that can be labelled and used for each pill-taking occasion during the day.

Some electronic pillboxes can be programmed to "beep" you when it's time to take your medication.

Combine your medication-taking with a normal, daily habit, such as brushing your teeth or watching the news. Put your pills next to the things you use for that activity (making sure your medications are out of the reach of children).

Whenever you get a prescription filled, figure out how long it will last and mark the time to reorder on a calendar. This may prevent you from running out in the middle of the night or on a weekend or holiday.

Shopping

Find grocery stores and pharmacies that deliver, or buy on the Internet.

If you are shopping with an oxygen carrier, find a shopping cart on your way in and put the oxygen in it while you shop.

When you are grocery shopping, have all the perishables packed in a separate bag. When you get home, put them away and leave the rest for later.

Some supermarket chains are now offering motorized, riding shopping carts.

Community service clubs and churches will sometimes offer shopping services for people with disabilities. Volunteers will shop for you.

Mail-order catalogues offer just about everything you would want and are fun to look through, too. You need only be able to plan ahead a little.

If you have a home computer with a modem, you can do a lot of shopping by computer.

Order stamps through the mail or on the Internet.

GOING OUT

Get assertive about exposure to other people's tobacco smoke. You have a right to breathe smoke-free air. Ask smokers near you to stop.

Wash your hands well when you get home. Colds and other diseases are often spread by touch.

Find out where you can get a daily air-quality report for your area, and use it when making your plans for the day.

Before going out, prepare for your homecoming. Lay out your comfortable clothes and slippers, leave a drink in a handy thermos, set out whatever utensils you will need for your evening meal, and even turn down your bed. Homecoming can then be a real relief.

If you don't already have one, ask your doctor about getting a handicapped parking permit. Even if you don't drive, a friend can use this when you go places together.

If you will have to sit in the car for a long period of time, make up a kit of helpful things such as a pad and pencil, paperback book, tissues, and so on. A coffee can with a snap-on plastic lid can be an emergency urinal.

If you must fill the gas tank, get upwind so that you don't inhale the fumes.

If you worry about being away from a phone in an emergency situation, consider a mobile phone.

When shopping for a new car, look for easy-to-open doors and easy-to-adjust seats.

Attach a loop to the inside handle of your car door to make it easier to pull closed.

Wide-angle rear-view mirrors allow for increased visibility without straining your neck.

A back support device (such as Sacro Ease) can make a car seat more comfortable.

GARDENING

A riding mower, preferably with a self-starter, can be a real morale booster.

Find lightweight, easy-to-handle tools. Many tools now come in lighter, durable plastic.

Use a folding stool or one with wheels. There are wheeled stools made especially for gardening, with a tool storage area under the seat.

Many tools can be purchased with a long handle, or you can have a short handle replaced with a long one.

Replace flower beds with containers on legs and balcony gardens.

ENJOYING RECREATION AND LEISURE

If you like to play cards, try a card holder.

Get to know your neighbours. Think of a signal, such as a pulled-down shade at night, to let them know you are OK.

Start a buddy phone system. Regular calls to and from friends are good for you, and these contacts will be able to aid in case of an emergency.

Somewhere near you, there is someone who needs your friendship and help, too. Look for these opportunities.

You can play board games long distance by mail, over the phone, or by computer.

Home computers and Web TV are getting more and more reasonable to own. Many games, including card and board games we all grew up with, are now available for home computers. You can have your own "Wheel of Fortune" game, with music and colour graphics, right at home.

Your computer can also introduce you to other people by e-mail.

Learn to use your computer or take art classes in an adult education program in your community. Your mind needs exercise, too, and you can meet interesting people in class.

Many adult education classes are offered through television or correspondence.

If you find your previous hobbies too demanding, try scaling them down for the time being. Start a container garden or try bonsai or orchids rather than a full-sized garden, for example.

If you like to paint, consider watercolours, watercolour pencils, or coloured pencils. They are lightweight, are odourless, and dry quickly.

An embroidery frame and stand will allow you to do needlework without having to use your hands to stabilize the piece you are working on.

Self-threading needles are available at yardage stores and through catalogs. Ask a grandchild to give you two dozen threaded needles for your birthday.

TRAVELLING

Ask your doctor about your tolerance to altitude before you travel. Be aware of the altitudes of your destination, as well as altitudes while travelling to your destination.

You can arrange in advance with airlines for a wheelchair, oxygen tank, special boarding and seating, or special meals. Be sure to call at least 24 hours in advance of your flight.

Travel light. Get suitcases with wheels, or get a rolling luggage rack.

Ask your local disability access community group if there is a travel agent in your area who specializes in travel arrangements for people with physical limitations.

Instead of a purse, use a vest with lots of pockets.

Make sure you do ankle and leg exercises on long trips to avoid dangerous blood clots.

GETTING SLEEP

Go to bed in stages so that you arrive there relaxed, not worn out. Put on your night clothes and then relax by reading or watching TV for a little while.

Have everything you need handy near your bed, such as a telephone and light. Have emergency numbers attached to the phone, or use a phone with an auto-dial feature. A clock radio with earphones, a glass of water, and a urinal are also nice to have handy.

A night-light will help to prevent falls or disorientation in the dark.

Keep a flashlight (torch) near the bed for emergencies.

Bedtime is often a good time to do some gentle, muscle relaxation exercises.

KEEPING WARM

Heating pads come in a variety of shapes and sizes, to fit just about any part of your body.

Soak stiff, sore hands or feet in warm water.

Thermoelastic gloves are good for warming. They are available in some pharmacies. Thermoelastic products are also available for knees and elbows.

Electric blankets and electric mattress pads are lightweight and warm.

Sleeping inside a sleeping bag placed under a blanket will help to keep you warm.

Consider long underwear. They come in many colours and styles. Silk is great!

Pre-heat your bathroom before your bath or shower in the morning with a small space heater or heat lamp.

A large shawl is great for the occasional shivers, and much easier to put on and take off than a sweater.

Avoid really frigid temperatures if you have respiratory problems. Cold air can cause bronchospasms.

If you have a great suggestion to add to this chapter, please let us know, and we will add it in our next edition. Write to: self-management@stanford.edu.

INDEX